Frontiers in Anti-Cancer Drug Discovery

Volume 4

Editor

Atta-ur-Rahman, *FRS*

Honorary Life Fellow
Kings College
University of Cambridge
UK

Co-Editor

M. Iqbal Choudhary

H.E.J. Research Institute of Chemistry
International Center for Chemical and Biological Sciences
University of Karachi
Pakistan

CONTENTS

PREFACE

Development of safe and effective anti-cancer drugs is one the most active areas of scientific research today and it is likely to remain so for years to come. Cancers cause more deaths than any other single disease, both in the developed and developing world. Prognosis in many forms of cancers is often glimpsed, despite major development in surgery and radiotherapy. Development of cancer chemotherapy remains an important challenge. The major bottleneck in the development of safe and effective anti-cancer drugs is the complex nature of the disease, involving still far from perfect understanding of the disease process at the molecular level, heterogeneity, and environmental factors. Emergence of resistance against existing drugs is yet another challenge to be faced.

Research and development in the area of anti-cancer therapies are overwhelming. For researchers working in this field, it is often difficult to keep track of and benefit from the key developments. The eBook series, *"***Frontiers in Anti-Cancer Drug Discovery***"*, is intended to represent the most notable developments in the field in the form of cutting edge reviews written by the leading experts.

Volume 4 of the eBook series, *"***Frontiers in Anti-Cancer Drug Discovery***"*, is a compilation of six well written and well referenced chapters contributed by some of the most prominent researchers in the field of cancer chemotherapy. Munoz and Coveñas skillfully review the role of peptide substance P (SP), and the NK-1 receptor in cancer progression, especially migration of tumor cells, angiogenesis and antiapoptotic effects. Based on this, they have discussed the relevance of NK-1 receptor antagonists in blocking the function of SP, thus serving as "Intelligent Bullets" against cancer.

Bouattour and Wassermann have contributed a review on the understanding of the hepatocellular carcinoma (HCC) at the molecular level, and identification of targets for drug development against this "orphan disease". Angiogenesis plays an important role in the progression of HCC due to the well-vascularized nature of the tumor. They review the results of pre-clinical and clinical studies on some novel agents against HCC targeting angiogenesis.

Metal complexes play an important role in cancer chemotherapy. The best known example is cisplatin. However, platinum based drugs are known for severe adverse effects, lack of tolerability and emerging resistance. Oliveira Silva reviews the anticancer and antitumor activities of ruthenium based drugs against cancer. Several of these complexes have entered into clinical trials and have shown great promise.

Fujii *et al.* have contributed a comprehensive review on the development of chemotherapy or endocrine therapy against breast cancer. The overall theme is the effectiveness of molecularly-targeted therapy. These therapies exert their effects anticancer/anti-tumor effects by targeting human epidermal growth factor receptor (HER), mammalian target of rapamycin (mTOR) and vascular endothelial growth factor (VEGF).

Wu *et al.* review the role of intracellular signaling transduction pathways (Purinergic signaling) in cancer and associated inflammation and immune response. Recent advances in the development of purinergic modulators as cancer therapies have also been comprehensively discussed.

Last but not the least, the role of HER2 (Human epidermal growth factor receptor 2) in breast cancer is extensively reviewed by O'Donovan *et al.* HER2 is over-expressed in breast cancer, particularly in aggressive types. In the last decade, the HER2 has been a popular target for the development of breast cancer therapies. Some of these drugs, along with their mechanisms of action, limitations and effectiveness in various stages of breast and other cancers are discussed in this article.

This volume of the eBook series represents the results of a considerable amount of work by many eminent contributors. We wish to thank them all for their excellent contributions and their commitment to complete the writing assignments in time. We would also like to thank the excellent team of the Bentham Science Publishers, especially Ms. Fariya Zulfiqar. The team is led by Mr. Mahmood Alam, Director Bentham Science Publishers, who deserves all appreciation.

Prof. Atta-ur-Rahman, *FRS*
Honorary Life Fellow
Kings College
University of Cambridge
UK

Prof. M. Iqbal Choudhary
H.E.J. Research Institute of Chemistry
International Center for Chemical and Biological Sciences
University of Karachi
Pakistan

LIST OF CONTRIBUTORS

Alexandra Canonici
National Institute for Cellular Biotechnology, Dublin City University, Ireland

Brigid C. Browne
The Kinghorn Cancer Centre, Garvan Institute of Medical Research, Sydney, Australia

Denis M. Collins
National Institute for Cellular Biotechnology, Dublin City University, Ireland

Denise de Oliveira Silva
Department of Fundamental Chemistry, Institute of Chemistry, University of São Paulo, Av. Prof. Lineu Prestes, 748, 05508-000, São Paulo, SP, Brazil

Elliot B. Tapper
Division of Gastroenterology, Department of Medicine, Beth Israel Deaconess Medical Center, Harvard Medical School, Boston, MA, USA

Hiroki Takahashi
Department of Surgery, Kurume University, Kurume, Japan

Johanna Wassermann
Department of Medical Oncology, La Pitié Salpêtrière University Hospital, Assistance Publique-Hôpitaux de Paris, France

John Crown
National Institute for Cellular Biotechnology, Dublin City University, Ireland; St. Vincent's University Hospital, Dublin, Ireland

Karen Howe
National Institute for Cellular Biotechnology, Dublin City University, Ireland

Keisuke Miwa
Multidisciplinary Cancer Treatment Center, Kurume University, Kurume, Japan

Kotaro Yuge
Multidisciplinary Cancer Treatment Center, Kurume University, Kurume, Japan

Lili Feng
Division of Gastroenterology, Department of Medicine, Beth Israel Deaconess Medical Center, Harvard Medical School, Boston, MA, USA; Department of Hematology, Provincial Hospital Affiliated to Shandong University, Jinan, P.R. China

Mai Mishima
Department of Surgery, Kurume University, Kurume, Japan

Maki Tanaka
Kurume General Hospital, Kurume, Japan

Marina Gehring
Division of Gastroenterology, Department of Medicine, Beth Israel Deaconess Medical Center, Harvard Medical School, Boston, MA, USA

Martina S.J. McDermott
Department of Drug Discovery and Biomedical Sciences, South Carolina College of Pharmacy, University of South Carolina, Columbia

Masaru Fukahori
Multidisciplinary Cancer Treatment Center, Kurume University, Kurume, Japan

Masayoshi Kage
Center for Innovative Cancer Therapy, Kurume University, Kurume, Japan; Department of Pathology, Kurume University, Kurume, Japan

Miguel Muñoz
Research Laboratory on Neuropeptides (IBIS), Virgen del Rocío University Hospital, Sevilla, Spain

Miki Takenaka
Department of Surgery, Kurume University, Kurume, Japan

Mohamed Bouattour
Department of Hepatology, Beaujon University Hospital, Assistance Publique-Hôpitaux de Paris, France

Mototsugu Matsunaga
Multidisciplinary Cancer Treatment Center, Kurume University, Kurume, Japan

Neil A. O'Brien
Department of Medicine, Division of Hematology/Oncology, Geffen School of Medicine at UCLA, Los Angeles, CA, USA

Nobutaka Iwakuma
Department of Surgery, Kurume University, Kurume, Japan

Norma O'Donovan
National Institute for Cellular Biotechnology, Dublin City University, Ireland

Rafael Coveñas
Laboratory of Neuroanatomy of the Peptidergic Systems (Lab. 14), Institute of Neurosciences of Castilla y León (INCYL), University of Salamanca, Salamanca, Spain

Ryuji Takahashi
Department of Surgery, Kurume University, Kurume, Japan

Shino Nakagawa
National Hospital Organization Kyushu Medical Cancer, Breast Care Center, Clinical Research Institute, Fukuoka, Japan

Simon C. Robson
Division of Gastroenterology, Department of Medicine, Beth Israel Deaconess Medical Center, Harvard Medical School, Boston, MA, USA

Teruhiko Fujii
Multidisciplinary Cancer Treatment Center, Kurume University, Kurume, Japan; Center for Innovative Cancer Therapy, Kurume University, Kurume, Japan

Tomoyuki Ushijima
Multidisciplinary Cancer Treatment Center, Kurume University, Kurume, Japan

Uhi Toh
Department of Surgery, Kurume University, Kurume, Japan

Xiaofeng Sun
Division of Gastroenterology, Department of Medicine, Beth Israel Deaconess Medical Center, Harvard Medical School, Boston, MA, USA

Yan Wu
Division of Gastroenterology, Department of Medicine, Beth Israel Deaconess Medical Center, Harvard Medical School, Boston, MA, USA

Yoshito Akagi
Department of Surgery, Kurume University, Kurume, Japan

CHAPTER 1

Substance P, the NK-1 Receptor and NK-1 Receptor Antagonists in Cancer Treatment

Miguel Muñoz[*,1] and Rafael Coveñas[2]

[1]Research Laboratory on Neuropeptides (IBIS), Virgen del Rocío University Hospital, Sevilla, Spain; [2]Laboratory of Neuroanatomy of the Peptidergic Systems (Lab. 14), Institute of Neurosciences of Castilla y León (INCYL), University of Salamanca, Salamanca, Spain

Abstract: Despite the great efforts made in research into cancer, in the last two decades therapeutic progress has unfortunately been very limited. It is crucial to seek new avenues of enquiry able to provide solutions to this scientific challenge. Currently, the term "Magic Bullet", coined by Paul Ehrlich, should be revisited and applied to new, more selective and effective cancer treatments. The peptide substance P (SP) exerts an important role in cancer progression. After the binding of SP to the tachykinin neurokinin-1 receptor (NK-1 receptor), the peptide exerts a mitogenic action on tumour and endothelial cells (inducing angiogenesis). It also regulates the migration of tumour cells and exerts an antiapoptotic effect on them. However, when NK-1 receptor antagonists bind to NK-1 receptors, these antagonists block the functions regulated by SP. These antagonists inhibit tumour cell proliferation (tumour cells die by apoptosis), angiogenesis, and tumour cell migration. These antagonists are broad-spectrum antitumour drugs. It is known that the administration of NK-1 receptor antagonists in combination with cytostatics exerts a synergic effect and decreases the side effects induced by cytostatics to a considerable extent. Many authors have suggested that these antagonists should be called "Intelligent Bullets", because cancer cells overexpress the NK-1 receptor and hence NK-1 receptor antagonists could act as specific anticancer drugs. The aim of the present study is to update knowledge of the involvement of the SP/NK-1 receptor system in cancer progression. We also suggest the use of NK-1 receptor antagonists as an anticancer therapy.

Keywords: Antitumour, aprepitant, cancer, metastasis, mitogenesis, neoangiogenesis, NK-1 receptor antagonists, substance P, tachykinin NK-1 receptor.

***Corresponding Author Miguel Muñoz:** Research Laboratory on Neuropeptides (IBIS), Virgen del Rocío University Hospital, Pediatric Intensive Care Unit, Av. Manuel Siurot s/n, 41013 – Sevilla, Spain; Tel: 34-955012965; Fax: 34-955012921; E-mail: mmunoz@cica.es

Atta-ur-Rahman / M. Iqbal Choudhary (Eds.)

INTRODUCTION

Although the therapeutic arsenal for cancer treatment has been expanding steadily, at present it is necessary to search for new drugs able to solve the many currently existing therapeutic challenges underlying this disease. Research into cancer has advanced considerably in the recent decades, but in general the prospects for the patients are not very promising. Recently, an analysis of the contribution of chemotherapy in adult malignancies with respect to 5-year survival has reported that in 22 adult malignancies treated between 1990 and 2004, cytotoxic chemotherapy afforded an only minor contribution to the survival of cancer patients [1]. Moreover, it is known that the administration of cytostatic drugs elicits severe side effects (*e.g.*, leukopenia, anaemia) and such drugs have a very low safety profile, because they are not specific against cancer cells. Thus, research should focus on drugs showing a specific action against tumour cells. In this sense, anticancer drugs will be fully effective when the drug used is directed against a specific target located in cancer cells. If this can be achieved, the side effects exerted by this type of anticancer drug will be considerably decreased. It is therefore crucial to explore other avenues of enquiry to improve this global problem in cancer.

In this sense, the involvement of peptides in cancer progression has gained increasing interest because these substances influence tumour proliferation [2-7]. In cancer research, new ways for translational research are emerging. For example, many data indicate that the substance P (SP)/tachykinin neurokinin-1 receptor (NK-1 receptor) system is involved in cancer progression [2-6, 8-11]. SP is a universal mitogen in tumour cells and inhibits apoptosis in these cells. It is known that the peptide elicits endothelial cell proliferation, promoting angiogenesis, and that it is involved in the migration of tumour cells for invasion and metastasis [2-4, 8, 10-12]. Thus, in the future, a novel strategy in cancer treatment must be exploited by using NK-1 receptor antagonists. Our study focuses on cancer progression and, in particular, on the involvement of the SP/NK-1 receptor system in cancer. We also suggest the clinical use of NK-1 receptor antagonists to block such progression.

SP/NK-1 RECEPTOR SYSTEM

SP belongs to the tachykinin family of peptides. SP is derived from the preprotachykinin A gene and the expression of this gene is increased in breast cancer when compared with normal mammary cells [3]. Three tachykinin receptors have been reported: NK-1 (the natural ligand of SP), NK-2 and NK-3. Through the NK-1 receptor, SP is involved in pain, neurogenic inflammation, anxiety, emesis, movement control, stress, depression, mitogenesis, angiogenesis, gastric motility, pruritus, salivation, micturition, neuronal survival and degeneration. SP is also involved in the regulation of respiratory mechanisms, in the control of the cardiovascular system, in cell motility (*e.g.*, monocytes, eosinophils, natural killer cells), and in the control of the cellular shape, including blebbing [11, 13-24]. SP is also implicated in human immunodeficiency virus replication [25, 26]. SP has a widespread distribution in both the central and peripheral nervous systems acting as a neurotransmitter and/or neuromodulator, but it is also present in cells not belonging to the nervous system (*e.g.*, immune cells, liver, lung). The expression of SP has also been demonstrated in numerous cancer cell lines [2, 8, 27, 28]. In fact, SP has been observed in both the cytoplasm and the nucleus of tumour cells [2, 28]. SP has also been observed in the tumour mass and in the peri-tumoural tissue [29, 30] and the undecapeptide exerts a mitogenic action on endothelial cells, stimulating vessel growth and promoting migration and invasion of MKN45 gastric carcinoma cells *in vitro* [4, 29]. SP is also located in the body fluids such as blood, cerebrospinal fluid, breast milk, *i.e.*, SP is ubiquitous throughout human body. Thus, SP can regulate cell function by autocrine, paracrine, endocrine, and/or neuroendocrine mechanisms [2].

The NK-1 receptor has a widespread distribution throughout the body (*e.g.*, central and peripheral nervous systems, heart, lung, gut, pancreas, liver, and placenta) [25, 31]. This receptor is coupled to a G-protein and acts as an allosteric molecule, where agonists and antagonists stabilize different conformations. It has been reported that human tumour cells (*e.g.*, glioma, melanoma, neuroblastoma, pancreas carcinoma, retinoblastoma, larynx carcinoma, gastric and colon adenocarcinoma, lung cancer, leukaemia) express isoforms of the NK-1 receptor [2, 30, 32, 33]. The full-length and the truncated forms of the NK-1 receptor have been described in humans. In the truncated subtype, the C terminus of the full-length subtype is missing. The full-length form mediates the slow growth of tumour cells, whereas the truncated subtype mediates malignancy in tumour cells and increases the growth of cancer cells, stimulating the synthesis of cytokines [5, 9]. These latter substances activate the transcription factor called NF-κB, which in turn upregulates the truncated subtype but slightly increase the full-length subtype [34, 35]. NK-1 receptors have been identified in human primary tumours and neoplastic cells, in human cancer cell lines and in intra- and peri-tumoural blood vessels (*e.g.*, smooth muscle cells, endothelial cells) of most of tumours investigated [13, 29, 30]. NK-1 receptors have been located in the cytoplasm of tumour cells [27, 28, 32, 33, 36, 37]. When SP is bound to the NK-1 receptor, this complex is internalized into the cell through endosomes, after which SP is degraded, whereas the NK-1 receptor is recycled to the cell surface [see 13]. NK-1 receptors have also been located in the plasma membrane and in the nuclei of tumour cells [2, 32]. The keratinocytes of the thorny and granular strata of the supratumoural epidermis (melanoma) show an evident nuclear immunoreactivity for the NK-1 receptor [32]. Cancer cells overexpress NK-1 receptors [2, 30, 38, 39] and this is extremely important because with the application of immunohistochemical techniques the observation of NK-1 receptors should facilitate, first, the location of tumours for diagnostic purposes and, second, the therapeutic action by administering NK-1 receptor antagonists.

HOW IS THE SP/NK-1 RECEPTOR SYSTEM INVOLVED IN CANCER PROGRESSION?

As reported above, many data support the idea that the SP/NK-1 receptor system is involved in cancer progression. Many *in vivo* and *in vitro* studies have demonstrated this involvement [2-6, 8-11]. Thus, SP is expressed in cancer cells; the NK-1 receptor is overexpressed in tumour cells; the NK-1 receptor is involved in the viability of cancer cells, and SP is involved in the proliferation and migration of tumour cells and also stimulates neoangiogenesis.

SP and the NK-1 Receptor are Expressed in Cancer Cells

SP has been observed in normal and tumour cells (Fig. **1B**), as well as in peri-tumoural tissue [30]. SP is expressed at high level in breast cancer cells in comparison to non tumourigenic cells, which showed low levels of SP [3]. In tumour cells, the immunoreactivity for SP was observed in the cytoplasm and in the nucleus [27, 28, 30, 37]. In fact, in these cells SP is more strongly expressed in the nuclei than in the cytoplasm (Fig. **1B**). The functional significance of the presence of SP in the nucleus of tumour cells requires further investigation. The presence of SP in tumour cells indicates that the peptide could be secreted by primary tumours. This is extremely important. Moreover, SP can be released from nerve terminals and/or may be released into the blood stream [see 2 for review]. It is known that the peptide is rapidly degraded in blood [40], but it is also known that SP could form a complex with fibronectin and this molecule protects the undecapeptide from the action of peptidases, increasing its half-life [41].

It has been reported that the NK-1 receptor is expressed/overexpressed in tumour cells (*e.g.*, glioblastoma, breast cancer, retinoblastoma, melanoma, acute lymphoblastic leukaemia, lung cancer, larynx, pancreatic, gastric and colon carcinomas) (Fig. **1A**); that human tumour samples showing advanced tumour stages express more NK-1 receptors; that astrocytoma and glioblastoma tumours containing the most malignant phenotypes show a higher rate of NK-1 receptor expression; that the level of *TAC1R* cDNA is higher in human lymphoblastic leukaemic cell lines than in normal cells; that astrocytoma and glioma primary tumours show more NK-1 receptors than astrocytoma and glioma cell lines in culture; that cancer cells have more NK-1 receptors than normal cells, and that astrocytomas express a lower number of NK-1 receptors than glioblastomas [2, 10, 13, 33, 42, 43]. In addition, the expression of the NK-1 receptor has been reported to be increased in lung cancer cell lines in comparison with a normal cell line [30], and increased levels of mRNA receptor expression have been observed in malignant tissues, but not in benign ones [3, 43]. In fact, the level of mRNA NK-1 receptor expression is lower in normal cells than in tumour cells and it is also known that melanoma cells overexpress NK-1 receptors in comparison with the expression found in non-cancer cells [39, 43]. All these data suggest that the expression of the NK-1 receptor is fairly well correlated with the degree of malignancy and that this receptor is a specific target for the treatment of tumours using NK-1 receptor antagonists, because cancer cells overexpress NK-1

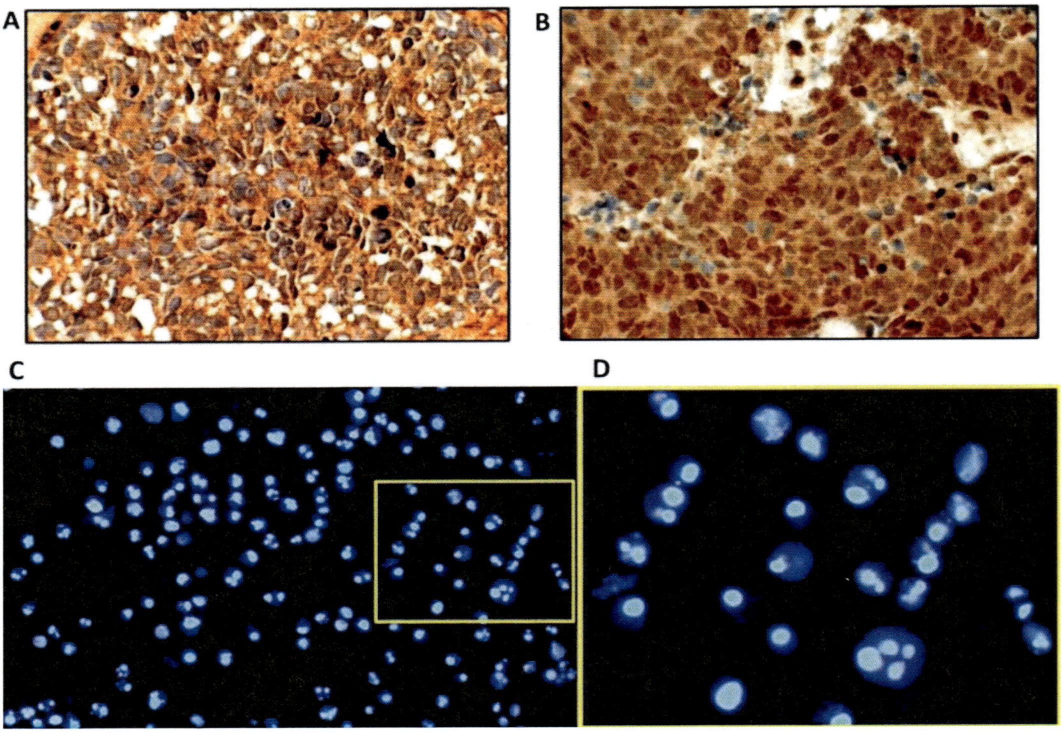

Fig. (1). Presence of NK-1 receptors (**A**) and SP (**B**) in small-cell lung carcinoma (40x). The immunoreactivity for the NK-1 receptors was predominantly found in the cytoplasm of tumour cells, whereas the immunoreactivity for SP was mainly located in the nucleus. In both cases, the sections were counterstained with hematoxylin. The immunocytochemical protocols for the demonstration of NK-1 receptors and SP and the immunocytochemical controls (omission of the first antibodies, preabsorption of the primary antibodies with the corresponding synthetic peptides) demonstrating the specificity of the immunoreactivity observed here, have been previously reported [28, 30, 32]. Sections were incubated overnight at 4° C with 1/1,000 diluted anti-NK-1 receptor antibody (Sigma-Aldrich, Madrid, Spain) or 1/3,000 diluted anti-SP antibody (Sigma-Aldrich, Madrid, Spain). Culture breast carcinoma cells treated with the NK-1 receptor antagonist aprepitant (**C**). Note apoptotic figures: nuclear fragmentation and chromatin condensation are observed (40x). A high power magnification of the region delimited by a rectangle in **C** is also shown (**D**).

receptors. By contrast, cytostatic drugs elicit severe side effects since they are not specific against cancer cells. Cytostatics induce cell death by necrosis. It has been also reported that the immunosuppressive cyclic undecapeptide cyclosporin A, *via* the NK-1 receptor, exerts a broad-spectrum antitumour action (cells die by apoptosis) against many human cancer cell lines (*e.g.*, glioma, neuroblastoma, retinoblastoma, larynx carcinoma, pancreas carcinoma, gastric carcinoma, colon carcinoma and melanoma) [39, 44]. However, in clinical practice this interesting therapeutic action of cyclosporin A is not possible because the high dosage necessary to exert an antitumour action is associated to a dangerous side effect: a renal failure.

The NK-1 Receptor is Involved in Cancer Cell Viability

It has been reported that following the use of a knockdown gene-silencing method the number of non-transfected cells increases significantly in comparison with the number of transfected cells, and hence apoptotic cells are more numerous in transfected cells [30, 32, 39, 43]. This means that the NK-1 receptor is involved in cancer cell viability. It seems that the overexpression of NK-1 receptors by tumour cells renders them highly dependent upon the mitotic signal induced by SP. This potent signal counteracts the death signal pathways activated in cancer cells by their own suppressor gene losses, oncogene activation, genetic damage, *etc*. Thus, by increasing the phenotypic expression of NK-1 receptors tumour cells could neutralize the pathways leading to cell death, since the different death signals are overridden by the SP-mediated mitotic stimulus. Thus, after the blockade of NK-1 receptors by NK-1 receptor antagonists, the cell dies because the balance inside the cell is favourable to apoptotic/death signals [see 45, 46] (Fig. **2**).

SP is Involved in the Proliferation, the Antiapoptotic Effect and the Migration of Tumour Cells and Stimulates Neoangiogenesis

SP exerts, *via* the NK-1 receptor, a mitogenic action in both normal and tumour cells (*e.g.*, glioma, neuroblastoma, retinoblastoma, melanoma, larynx, pancreatic, gastric, colon carcinoma, small-cell lung cancer and non-small-cell lung cancer, acute lymphoblastic leukaemia B and T cells, osteosarcoma, hepatoblastoma) [2, 13, 30, 38, 43, 45, 47] (Table **1**). The undecapeptide could be secreted from tumour cells (autocrine action); SP could exert a mitogenic action in endothelial cells (paracrine action, promoting neoangiogenesis); the peptide could be secreted from nerve terminal; SP, *via* the bloodstream, reaches the whole body (in this process the limbic system is involved), and/or through an endocrine action the

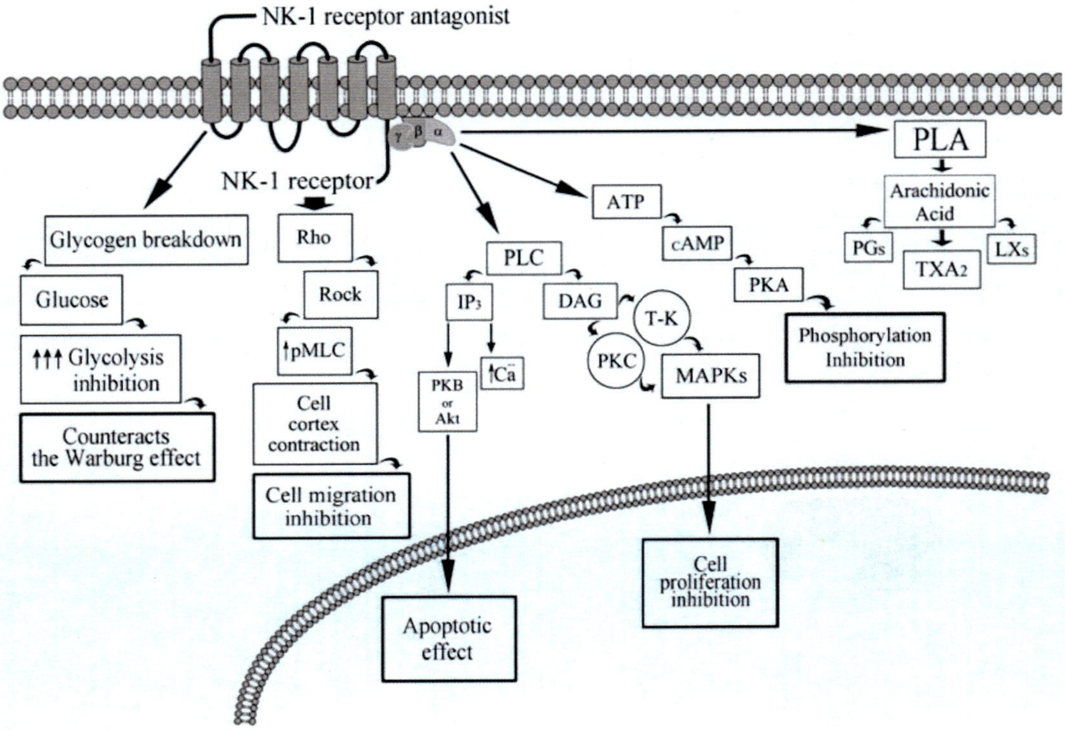

Fig. (2). After binding to the NK-1 receptor, SP induces cell proliferation, an antiapoptotic effect and cell migration. The downstream signaling pathways involved in these mechanisms are indicated. By contrast, after binding to the NK-1 receptor, NK-1 receptor antagonists exert an apoptotic effect and block these pathways, inhibiting both the proliferation and the migration of cancer cells. In addition, NK-1 receptor antagonists could counteract the Warburg effect. ATP: adenosine triphosphate; cAMP: cyclic adenosine monophosphate; DAG: diacylglycerol; IP_3: inositol triphosphate; LXs: leukotrienes; MAPKs: mitogen-activated protein kinase; PGs: prostacyclin; PKA: protein kinase A; PKB or Akt: protein kinase B; PKC: protein kinase C; PLA: phospholipase A; PLC: phospholipase C; pMLC: myosin regulatory light chain phosphorylation; TK: tyrosine-kinase; TXA_2: thromboxane A_2.

peptide is released into the blood vessels from the tumour mass [see 2 for review]. In cancer cells, SP increases DNA synthesis and activates members of the MAPK (mitogen-activated protein kinase) family (*e.g.*, ERK1/2 (extracellular signal-regulated kinases 1 and 2), p38MAPK) [10] (Fig. **2**). ERK1/2 protects the cell from apoptosis and also induces cell proliferation [6]. Moreover, in cancer cells, SP increases the phosphorylation and activity of Akt or protein kinase B (Fig. **2**); the activation of this protein kinase suppresses apoptosis [48, 49].

Table 1. Tumour Cells, Cytotoxicity, Mitogenic Effect and NK-1 Receptor Isoforms

Tumour	Cell Line	L-732,138		L-733,060		Aprepitant		SP	*NK-1 Receptor* Isoforms kDa
		IC_{50} *μM*	IC_{100} *μM*	IC_{50} *μM*	IC_{100} *μM*	IC_{50} *μM*	IC_{100} *μM*	*nM*	
Glioma	GAMG	48.1	100	21.3	43	33.1	66.2	50	54, 38, 33
Neuroblastoma	SKN-BE(2)	41	80.5	11.6	21	24.6	48.8	100	54
	IMR-32	45.7	99			19.6	45.1	5	75, 54, 33
	KELLY	53.2	103.4			27.7	49.5	10	54, 33
Retinoblastoma	Y-79	56.8	132	12.2	25	30.4	59	100	75, 58, 33
	WERI-Rb-1	60.5	119	17.4	35	23	53.1	100	75, 58, 33
Melanoma	MEL-HO	76.3	140.6	27.5	54	29.6	56.5	500	75, 58, 33
	COLO 858	44.6	97.6	8.7	17.5	24.3	52.1	10	75, 58, 33
	COLO 679	64.2	124.7	33.8	67	32.1	58.6	10	75, 58, 33
Pancreatic Carcinoma	PA-TU-8902			18.1	38.4	31.2	63	100	75, 58, 46, 33
	CAPAN-1			20	39.7	27.4	52	100	75, 58, 46, 33
Larynx Carcinoma	HEp-2	38	77.3	21.3	42	22.7	46.5	50	75, 58, 46, 34
Gastric Carcinoma	23132-87			14.3	29.6	24.2	52.5	10	75, 58, 46, 34
Colon Cancer	SW-403			14.5	25.8	30.5	60.5	50	75, 58, 46, 34
Small Cell lung cancer	H-69	51.9	109	18.7	39.2	21.8	45.2	5-100	75, 58, 46, 34
Non-small Cell Lung Cancer	COR-L23	87	102.3	22	41.5	30	60	5-100	75, 58, 46, 34
T Acute Lymphoblastic Leukaemia	BE-13	63.9	124	15.4	40	19.5	50	5-50	58, 33
B Acute Lymphoblastic Leukaemia	SD-1	49.7	103.5	18.4	50	29.4	59.2	5-50	75, 58, 33
Osteosarcoma	MG-63	58.6	100	14.5	30	28.6	80	5-500	46
Hepatoblastoma	HUH6, HepT1, HepG2	110		25		28.5, 31.1, 33.18		10-100	58,50

In addition, the activation of the NK-1 receptor by SP generates second messengers that trigger several effector mechanisms involved in the regulation of cellular function as well as in cellular excitability [see 2, 13 for review] (Fig. **2**).

In human astrocytoma cells, the activation of NK-1 receptors by SP produces the following actions: the mobilization of intracellular calcium, increases in intracellular Ca^{2+} concentrations, the release of IL (interleukin)-8 and IL-6, the synthesis of inositol phosphates, the release of taurine, the activation of phospholipase D, the release of glutamate, the regulation of glutamate and K^+ transport, and the stimulation of glycogen breakdown [see 13 for review]. The release of interleukins, taurine and glutamate by tumour cells is very important, since these substances induce inflammatory processes; the level of SP increases and hence cancer cell proliferation also increases. It is also known that chronic inflammation increases the risk of cancer, because an increase in mitogenesis and mutagenesis occurs during inflammatory processes [50-53]. SP induces oedema and it is known that the SP/NK-1 receptor system is upregulated in inflammatory processes [14, 54-57]. The data suggest that this system is altered in inflammatory processes and that this alteration could facilitate cancer progression.

Another important point is that SP stimulates glycogen breakdown in cancer cells in a concentration-dependent manner. However, this effect is blocked upon using NK-1 receptor antagonists [58] (Fig. **2**). Tumour cells mainly produce energy by means of a high rate of glycolysis followed by lactic acid fermentation; this mechanism is called the Warburg effect [59]. It is known that the glycolytic rates of growing cancer cells are higher than those of their normal tissues of origin. In cancer cells, SP induces glycogen breakdown, after which the glucose obtained is used by cancer cells to increase their metabolism [58], but NK-1 receptor antagonists block this breakdown [58], and in this way these antagonists can counteract the Warbur effect because without glucose glycolysis is not possible.

Moreover, *via* the NK-1 receptor SP is involved in cancer cell migration: *i.e.*, in metastasis [2-4, 8, 13, 25, 45]. It is known that the migration of cancer cells is regulated by SP, dopamine and noradrenalin and hence after the administration of NK-1 receptor, D_2 receptor, or adrenoceptor antagonists, this migration is inhibited [45, 60] (Fig. **2**). It is also known that SP induces the migration of pancreatic tumour cells [12]; and that the peptide promotes changes in cellular shape (*e.g.*, blebbing) [11, 24]. Membrane blebbing is very important in cell movement and spreading, as well as in cancer cell infiltration [11, 24].

SP is also involved in neoangiogenesis, because the peptide promotes the mitogenesis of endothelial cells [15], but this action is not carried out by NK-2/NK-3 receptor agonists [42, 45]. In neoangiogenesis, it is known that an increased expression of NK-1 receptors occurs; that SP increases tumoural blood flow; and that SP and these receptors are located in intra- and peri-tumoural blood vessels [15, 42, 45].

NK-1 RECEPTOR ANTAGONISTS

Many studies have focused on the development of highly selective antagonists for the NK-1 receptor with a view to shedding light on the physiological/ pathophysiological actions in which the SP is involved. These antagonists are known to exert antiemetic and antidepressive effects [2, 13, 19, 20, 61-65]. NK-1 receptor antagonists have also been used in inflammatory diseases (*e.g.*, arthritis, cystitis, inflammatory bowel disease, urinary incontinence) [2, 23, 57]. Two types of these antagonists have been reported: peptide or non-peptide NK-1 receptor antagonists.

Peptide Antagonists

Numerous peptide antagonists (also called SP analogue antagonists, synthetic analogues of SP or broad-spectrum peptide antagonists) derived from SP have been developed. However, for many reasons the use of these antagonists is limited in clinical practice: their inability to cross the blood-brain barrier, mast cell-degranulation activity, neurotoxic effects, partial residual agonist activity, metabolic instability, poor potency, and poor ability to discriminate between tachykinin receptors [13].

The main chemical characteristic of peptide NK-1 receptor antagonists is that in the sequence of SP an L-aminoacid is replaced by a D-amino acid. Some of these NK-1 antagonist peptides are: Spantide I ([D-Arg^1, D-$Trp^{7,9}$, Leu^{11}] SP) (this exerts a neurotoxic effect and facilitates the release of histamine from mast cells); Spantide II (H-D-Lys(Nicotinoyl)-Pro-[3-(3-pyridyl)-Ala]-pro-D-Phe83,4-Cl_2-Asn-D-Trp-Phe-D-Trp-Leu-Nle-NH_2); [Arg^6, D-$Trp^{7,9}$, $MePhe^8$] SP (6-11); [D-Pro^2- $Trp^{7,9}$] SP; [D-Arg^1, D-Phe^5, D-$Trp^{7,9}$, Leu^{11}] SP; NY-3460 (D-MePhe-D-

Trp-Phe-D-Trp-Leu(CH_2NH)Leu-NH); NY-3238 (p-HOPA-DTrp-Phe-DTrp-Leu-Leu-NH_2); [D-Arg^1, D-Pro^2, D-Trp ^{7,9}, Leu^{11}] SP; [D-Pro^4, D-Trp ^{7,9,10}, Phe^{11}] SP (4-11); and [D-Arg^1, D-$Trp^{5,7,9}$, Leu^{11}] SP.

Non-Peptide Antagonists

Benzylamino piperidines (GR-203,040, CP-99,994, CP-122,721…), benzylamino and benzylether quinuclidine (L-709,210, CP-96,345…), steroids (WIN-51,708…), benzylether piperidines (L-733,060, L-741,671, L-742,694…), tryptophan-based (L-732,138, L-737,488…), and perhydroisoindolones (RPR-100,893, RP-67,580, RP-73,467…) are non-peptide NK-1 receptor antagonists (Fig. **3**).

L-733,060, which shows a high affinity for the NK-1 receptor, is a 3, 5-bistrifluoromethyl benzylether piperidine (Fig. **4**) developed from CP-99,994 [13].

L-733,060 exerts anti-inflammatory, and antitumour effects [2, 13, 33, 36, 66] (Table **1**). L-732,138 (N-acetyl-L-tryptophan 3, 5-bis (trifluoromethyl) benzyl ester) is more potent in human NK-1 receptors than in rat NK-1 receptors, and more potent in human NK-1 receptors than in human NK-2/NK-3 receptors.

Other non-peptide NK-1 receptor antagonists are MEN-11,467, MEN-11,149, CJ-11,974 (Ezlopitant), CJ-12,458, CJ-12,764, L-703,606, L-754,030 (MK-869, aprepitant, Emend), L-758,298 (fosaprepitant, an aprepitant salt for intravenous use), L-759,274, SR-1,400,333, GW-679,769 (casopitant), GW-823,296 (orvepitant), GR-205,171 (vofopitant), maropitant and GW-597,599 (vestipitant) (Figs. **3-5**).

Aprepitant (Fig. **4**) shows a high affinity for the NK-1 receptor and it is more selective for the human NK-1 receptor (IC_{50} = 0.1 nM) than for the human NK-2 (IC_{50} = 4,500 nM) and NK-3 receptors (IC_{50} = 300 nM). Aprepitant exerts antiemetic, antidepressive and antitumour effects [13, 32, 43, 61, 63-65, 67-69] (Table **1**). At present, aprepitant and fosaprepitant (this is converted to aprepitant by the action of ubiquitous phosphatases) [70] (Fig. **4**) are the only agents commercially available for the prevention of CINV (chemotherapy-induced

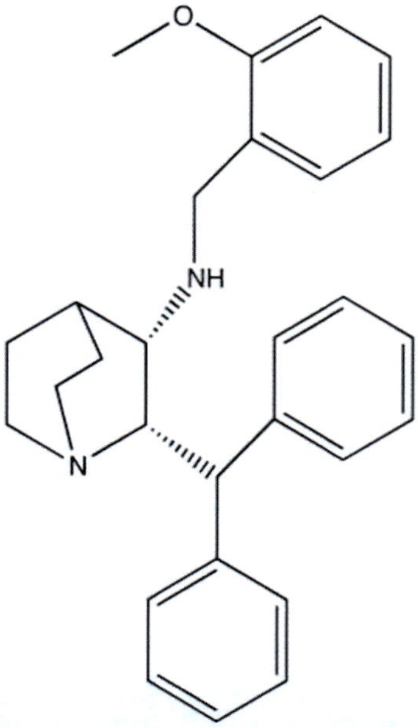

CP-96,345

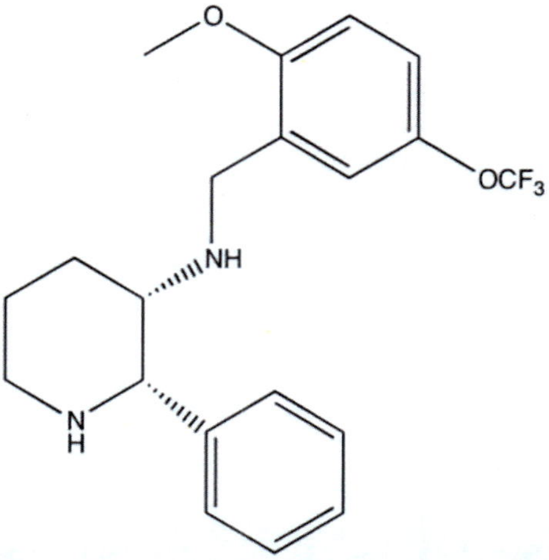

CP-122,721

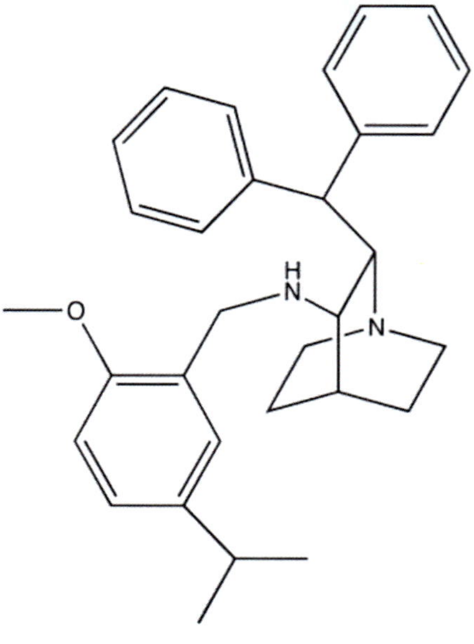

Ezlopitant
(CJ-11,974)

Fig. (3). Chemical structures of CP-96,345, CP-122,721 and ezlopitant (CJ-11,974).

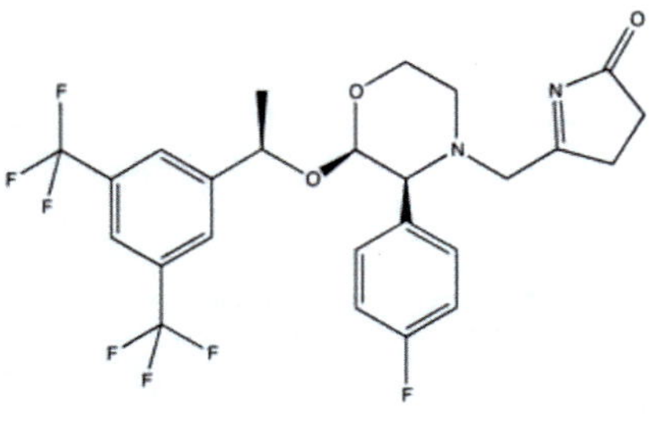

Aprepitant
(MK869 or L-754,030)

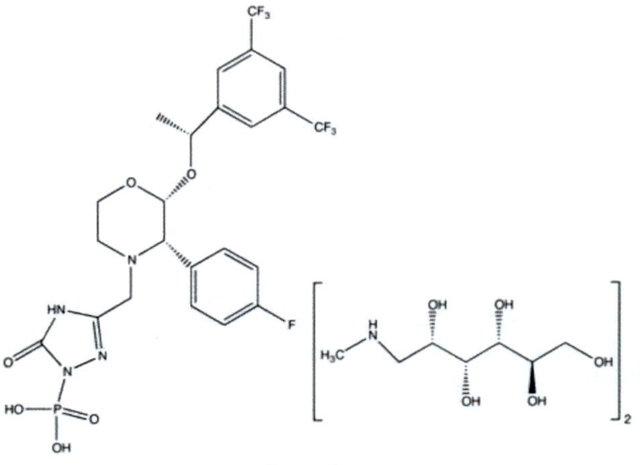

Fosaprepitant

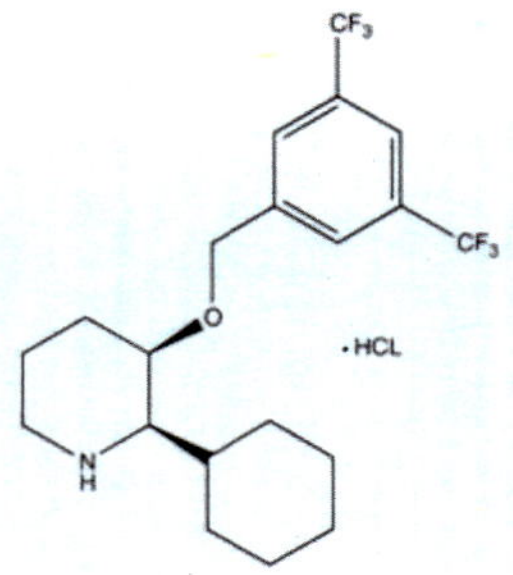

L-733,060

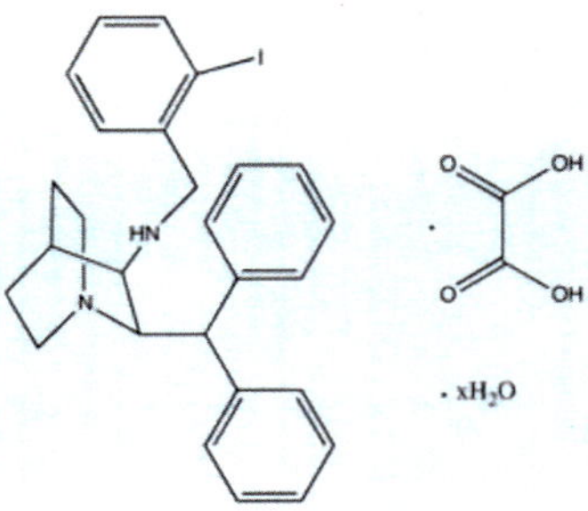

L-703,606

Fig. (4). Chemical structures of aprepitant (MK 869 or L-754,030), fosaprepitant (L-758,298), L-733,060 and L-703,606.

nausea and vomiting) and PONV (post-operative nausea and vomiting). It has been reported that a single intravenously dose of fosaprepitant (150 mg) was as safe and effective as the 3-day oral aprepitant regimen [61, 62]. Aprepitant is mainly metabolized in the liver by cytochrome P450, family 3, subfamily A (CYP3A4) [71]. It is an inhibitor and a substrate of the CYP3A4 metabolic pathway, which in humans is involved in the metabolism of a broad range of drugs. This pathway affects both dosage over time and drug-drug interactions; this is important from a clinical point of view [see 72 for review]. Aprepitant is a mild inducer of CYP2C9 and when used for more than 7 days it may act as an inducer of CYP3A4. Its half-life ranges from 9 to 13 h and it binds to plasma proteins [61, 63]. Moreover, aprepitant has been developed as a nanoparticle formulation to enhance exposure and to minimize food effects [64]. In humans, the nanoparticle formulation increased 3-4 times the bioavailability of aprepitant [64].

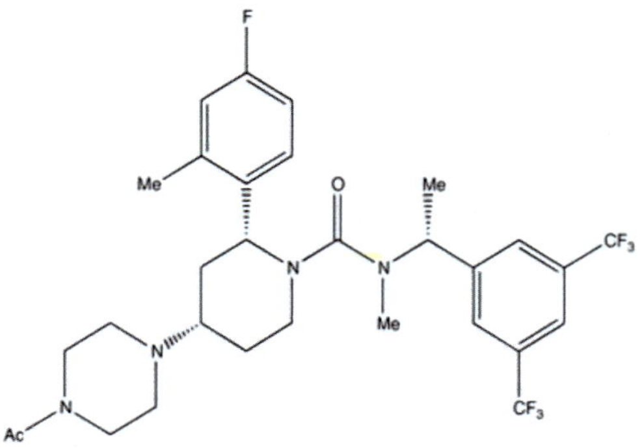

Casopitant (Rezonic)
(GW-679,769)

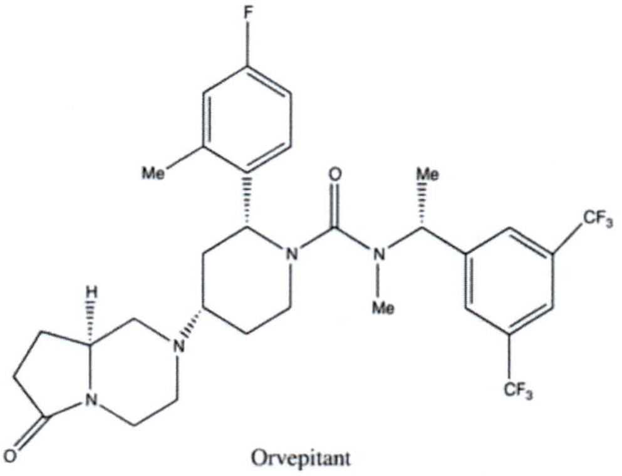

Orvepitant
(GW-823,296)

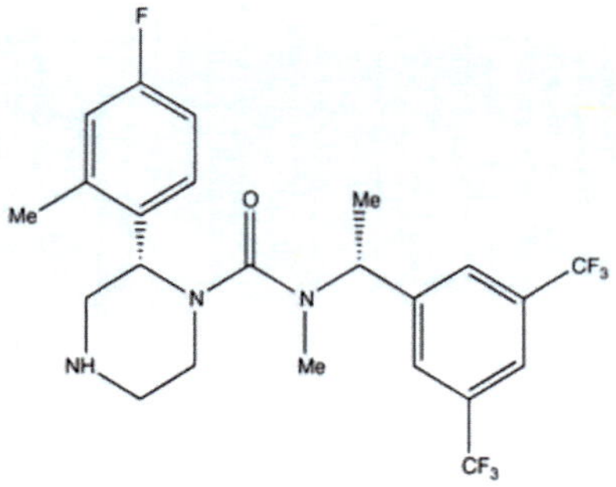

Vestipitant
(GW-597,599)

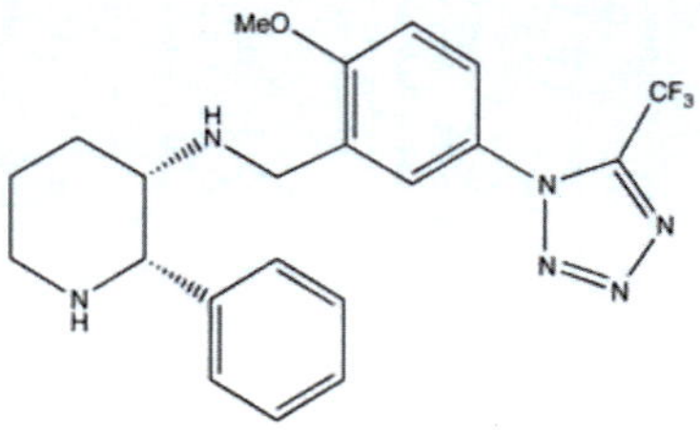

Vofopitant
(GR-205,171)

Fig. (5). Chemical structures of casopitant (GW-679,769), orvepitant (GW-823,296), vestipitant (GW-597,599) and vofopitant (GR-205,171).

NK-1 receptor antagonists are a growing family of compounds. The molecules belonging to this family are structurally unrelated compounds. However, the antitumour action of non-peptide NK-1 receptor antagonists is linked to stereochemical features and not to the chemical composition. All have one aspect in common, namely their affinity for the NK-1 receptor. This is a seven-transmembrane receptor. It is known that SP and non-peptide NK-1 receptor antagonists bind to different regions of the NK-1 receptor: the peptide binds to the extracellular loops of the receptor, whereas the antagonists bind more deeply between the III, IV, V and VI transmembrane segments (Fig. **6**). Thus, very little overlap occurs between SP and non-peptide NK-1 receptor antagonists because NK-1 receptor antagonists act as allosteric molecules, where agonists and antagonists stabilize different conformations [see 45 for review].

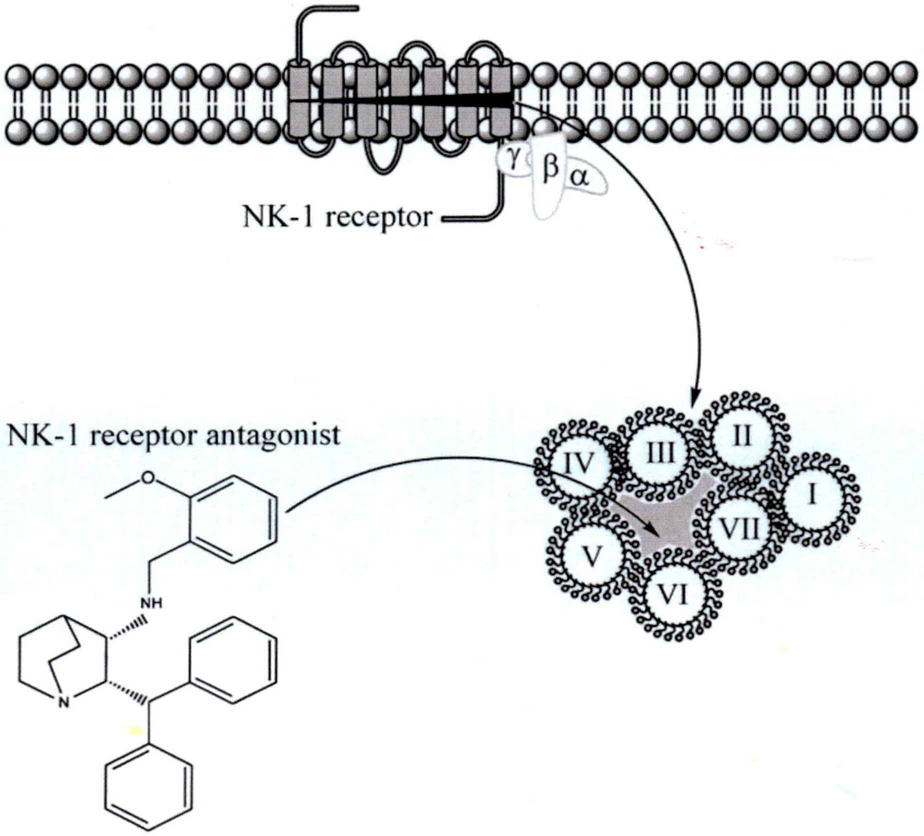

Fig. (6). NK-1 receptor antagonists bind more deeply, between the transmembrane segments, whereas SP binds to the extracellular loops of the NK-1 receptor.

COULD AN ANTIEMETIC ACT AS AN ANTITUMOUR DRUG?

In *in vitro* studies it has been demonstrated that NK-1 receptor antagonists exert an antitumour action (cancer cells die by apoptosis) against different human tumour cell lines (*e.g.*, osteosarcoma, retinoblastoma, melanoma, lung, glioma, neuroblastoma, hepatoblastoma) [2, 7, 13, 25, 30, 32, 36, 38, 47, 72-75] (Table **1**). NK-1 receptor antagonists block the mitogenic action exerted by SP on tumour cells and also inhibit cancer cell growth in a dose-dependent manner. Thus, NK-1 receptor antagonists induce apoptosis in tumour cells and this strategy could represent a new approach to cancer treatment [2, 13, 25, 30, 32, 36, 38, 47, 72] (Fig. **1C**, **D**). It has been reported that NK-1 receptor antagonists inhibit cell proliferation and DNA synthesis and that they decrease the basal phosphorylation of Akt [6, 45, 76] (Fig. **2**). In the near future, it will be very important to investigate the cellular signaling pathways downstream from the NK-1 receptor, after the binding of NK-1 receptor antagonist/SP, in particular regarding the involvement of both compounds in glucose metabolism because this process is crucial for tumour cells [58].

Many studies have also been carried out *in vivo* [7, 38, 47, 73-75, 77, 78]. Thus, in athymic nude mice NK-1 receptor antagonists elicit tumour regression by means of antiproliferative and antiangiogenic mechanisms [74, 75, 78]. In addition, when nude mice transplanted with human glioma U373 MG xenografts were treated with NK-1 receptor antagonists (MEN 11,467 or MEN 11,149), the antagonists inhibited the tumour growth. It has also been demonstrated that subcutaneous or intravenous administrations of NK-1 receptor antagonists are effective in preventing tumour growth [7, 73] and that these antagonists diminish tumour volume [38, 47]. In nude mice, the treatment of MG-63 human osteosarcoma xenografts with fosaprepitant (peri-tumoural subcutaneous injection) showed a significant reduction in tumour volume [47]. The animals received fosaprepitant the days 0 (when tumours became visible), 7, 14, 21 and 28. At these days, tumour volume in the control group (treated with phosphate-buffered saline) was higher than in the treated group. Moreover, in a similar *in vivo* model (hepatoblastoma xenograft nude mice) it has been reported that the treatment with 80 mg/kg/day of aprepitant for 24 days resulted in a significant reduction of tumour growth, as evidenced by reduced tumour volume and weight, lowered tumour-specific alpha-fetoprotein serum levels, and decreased number of Ki-67 positive cells [38]. Recently, in mice another *in vivo* study has reported that the administration of the NK-1 receptor antagonist Emend IV decreased both tumour volume and cancer cell proliferation [79]. All these experiments demonstrate that, *in vivo*, NK-1 receptor antagonists exert an antitumour action. However, in a murine model of melanoma it has been reported that SP prevents tumour growth and that this action is mediated by T and natural killer cells [77]. The findings reported in this *in vivo* study are not in agreement with those mentioned above, although it should be noted that in this latter study [77] SP was administered prior to the development of the tumour. It has been suggested that SP could exert a beneficial action in the early stages of DNA damage [see 79]. However, no experiment has been carried out to study the action of SP in well established tumours [see 79]. Thus, new experiments should be developed to clarify the issue.

NK-1 receptor antagonists not only exert an antitumour effect, but also inhibit the migration of cancer cells [4, 11, 12, 45, 60] (Fig. **2**) by blocking SP-mediated changes in cellular shape, including blebbing. This is extremely important because these mechanisms are directly involved in cell spreading and cancer cell invasion [24, 45]. These findings open up new clinical perspectives for tackling tumour cell invasion and metastasis. In fact, it has been reported that in patients with breast cancer the risk of recurrence or metastasis decreases when surgery is associated with paravertebral anaesthesia [80], which blocks the migration, invasion and metastasis of tumour cells induced by SP [see 81]. The results suggest that the SP/NK-1 receptor system plays an important role in this process. This hypothesis is quite interesting because the use of paravertebral anaesthesia prior to surgical interventions for cancer could reduce the number of recurrences and metastases, and hence pretreatment with NK-1 receptor antagonists prior to surgery could have synergic effects [see 81].

In brain metastasis, the blood brain barrier (BBB) is a handicap for the treatment with chemotherapy because the drugs do not cross this barrier. SP promotes BBB breaching by breast tumour cells *via* changes in endothelial cell tight junctions. SP, which is secreted from breast cancer cells, induces the migration of these cells across the BBB, leading to the secretion of TNF-α and Ang-2 and promoting BBB impairment and the colonization of the central nervous system by tumour cells [82]. In another study the authors suggested that the extravasation of tumour cells into the brain to form brain metastases was a SP-mediated process [8].

It is known that NK-1 receptor antagonists block the mitogenesis of endothelial cells and decrease angiogenesis [13, 45, 74] and that SP stimulates vessel growth by inducing mitogenesis in endothelial cells [15]. It has also been reported in *in vivo* experiments that aprepitant inhibits angiogenesis [38].

The data reported above indicate that NK-1 receptor antagonists exert an antitumour activity, an antimigratory action on tumour cells and inhibit neoangiogenesis and suggest that these compounds could be considered as possible pharmacological tools in the treatment of cancer. Moreover, the data suggest that the NK-1 receptor is a therapeutic target in cancer (Figs. **1C**, **D** and **2**). Currently, there are more than 300 NK-1 receptor antagonists [29] and this means that there are more than 300 potential drugs against the treatment of cancer. Then two questions should be answered: Which is the most appropriate NK-1 receptor antagonist to be tested in human clinical trials regarding its antitumour action? And are NK-1 receptor antagonists safe?

Despite the large number of non-peptide NK-1 receptor antagonists reported, aprepitant and its intravenously administered prodrug fosaprepitant are currently the only NK-1 receptor antagonists approved for clinical practice [see 72 for review]. It is known that fosaprepitant is rapidly converted to aprepitant [70, 72]. Both are administered for the prevention of CINV and PONV; aprepitant, orally, and fosaprepitant intravenously. This means that aprepitant is a good candidate for testing its antitumour activity in future human trials, because the drug is currently used in clinical practice for the treatment of emesis and hence the required safety studies for this drug have already been carried out [see 29]. In fact, NK-1 receptors have been found at high concentrations in the vomiting centre of the brain [25, 83]. Moreover, it is known that aprepitant exerts *in vitro* an antitumour action against many different human tumour cells [67] (Fig. **1 C**, **D** and Table **1**) and that, *in vivo*, fosaprepitant and aprepitant diminish tumour volume [38, 47]. In sum, aprepitant is an excellent candidate for human clinical trials in order to test its antitumour action, its antimigratory activity on tumour cells and its antiangiogenic action. Moreover, in brain metastasis, the treatment with aprepitant could have beneficial therapeutic effects in primary and metastatic brain tumours, since the drug diffuses well through the BBB. In fact, it seems that NK-1 receptor antagonists like aprepitant may prevent breaching of the BBB by cancer cells (that secretes SP) and their brain colonization.

In general, NK-1 receptor antagonists do not induce serious side effects (headaches, hiccupping, drowsiness, vertigo) [16, 45, 65, 68, 72, 84]. Many clinical trials have focused on the antiemetic action of aprepitant in cancer patients treated with chemotherapy. However, it should be noted that the efficacy and safety of aprepitant have not been studied in other diseases (*e.g.*, cancer) in which the SP/NK-1 receptor system plays an important role. Currently, it is known that aprepitant is well tolerated and elicits minimum side effects [see for 72 review]. The majority of the adverse events are mild or moderate and are consistent with the side effects brought about by chemotherapy [72]. In addition, the safety of aprepitant against human fibroblasts has been demonstrated: the IC_{50} for tumour cells is lower than the IC_{50} for fibroblasts and the IC_{50} for non-tumour cells is 90 μM whereas the IC_{100} for tumour cells is 60 μM [67]. It has also been shown that the administration of aprepitant (300 mg/day) is well tolerated and no difference in the frequency of adverse events was observed in comparison to placebo [20, 72]. Thus, in order for NK-1 receptor antagonists to exert an effective antitumour action, it has been suggested that higher doses of aprepitant than those used in CINV should be used and that the number of days on which aprepitant is currently administered should be increased [72]. These issues should be investigated in-depth in order to demonstrate if an antiemetic could be used as an antitumour drug. It has also been reported that aprepitant does not alter the metabolism of ondansetron, granisetron, palonosetron, hydrodolasetron, vinorelbine, thiotepa, dinaciclib or digoxin, but oral doses of dexamethasone or methylprednisolone should be reduced when administered with aprepitant (aprepitant increases the plasma level of corticosteroids) [61, 85-87]. Regarding the interaction between ifosfamide and aprepitant, a case-control study reported no correlation between ifosfamide-induced neurotoxicity and coadministration with aprepitant, but in another study it was concluded that aprepitant should be used with caution, since it induced the accumulation of toxic metabolites [69]. Moreover, aprepitant increases the plasma levels of some chemotherapeutic agents (*e.g.*, docetaxel, paclitaxel, irinotecan, midazolam) [71]. In adolescents with malignancies, aprepitant was generally well-tolerate and thus it seems that the adult dose regimen is adequate [17, 88]. However, further studies in adolescents should be carried out, because to date the number of the adolescents patients studied has been too small [72]. Carcinogenicity studies have been carried out for aprepitant and the carcinogenetic effects of this drug have been related to hepatic CYP metabolism [2, 71]. It has been reported that the administration of aprepitant (125-2,000 mg/kg/day) to male rats/mice increases thyroid follicular cell adenomas and carcinomas; thyroid parafollicular cell carcinoma; skin fibrosarcomas; and hepatocellular adenomas and/or carcinomas, whereas administration of the drug (125-2,000 mg/kg/day) to female rats induces an increase in hepatocellular adenomas and carcinomas and thyroid follicular adenomas. It is known that thyroid and liver tumours are a result of hepatic CYP enzyme induction in rodents, and this is consistent with the results observed in rodents with other compounds that induce hepatic CYP enzymes. However, judging by the concentration of aprepitant that exerts an antitumour effect in *in vitro* experiments, the doses of the drug that could be used in clinical practice would be very low (40-50 mg/kg/day for cancer treatment) in comparison with the doses used in carcinogenicity studies (125-2,000 mg/kg/day for carcinogenesis) [see 2 for review]. Regarding other NK-1 receptor antagonists (*e.g.*, casopitant, vofopitant, ezlopitant), in general these are well tolerated, but further safety data are required [72].

It should be noted that a few patents regarding the use of NK-1 receptor antagonists as antitumour drugs have been reported, as well as other patents using antibodies against SP or against tachykinin receptors or using proteins able to bind to SP have been developed [see 29 for review]. A patent, based on many published experimental data, has been reported concerning the use of non-peptide NK-1 receptor antagonists as antitumour drugs by inducing tumour cell death through apoptosis [29]. These antagonists showed antitumour action against primary neuroblastoma cells, astrocytoma cells, Burkitt's lymphoma cells, invasive malignant melanomas, metastatic melanoma cells, glioma cells, breast cancer cells, rhabdomyosarcoma cells, small-cell lung cancer cells, osteosarcoma cells, acute lymphoblastic leukaemia B and T cells, Hodgkin's lymphoma cells and Ewing's sarcoma cells [29]. Other patent on the anticancer effects exerted by neurokinin receptor antagonists has been reported. This invention is related to the inhibition of the growth of cancer cells (the growth inhibition capacity of the NK-1 receptor antagonist SR-140,333 was tested in MEL and K562 erythroleukaemia cell lines) [29]. Another patent focused on libraries of thiophene and pyrrole-based heterocyclic compounds has been reported. These substances bind to tachykinin receptors, are non-peptide, and they show an antitumour effect against small-cell lung cancer cells [29]. Yet another patent reports the use of an antibody, or a specific fragment thereof, against NK-1, NK-2 and/or NK-3 cell receptors to produce a drug for the therapeutic treatment of human cancer *via* direct administration to a mammalian species, including humans [29]. The antibody induces apoptosis in tumour cells [29]. In another patent a monoclonal antibody against SP was used. The antibody induced apoptosis in cancer cells and it was obtained for the treatment of mammalian cancer cells expressing an ErbB receptor family member and/or the NK-1 receptor [29]. Finally, another patent has been filed in which the hematopoietic growth factor-inducible NK-1 (HGFIN) was used; this compound is a protein that can bind to SP [29]. This strategy could be beneficial in the treatment of cancer [29] and by this way, SP would be unavailable for mediating mitogenesis in cancer cells.

SYNERGIC EFFECT OF NK-1 RECEPTOR ANTAGONISTS WITH CHEMOTHERAPY

It has been reported that, *in vitro*, microtubule destabilizing agents (MDA) and NK-1 receptor antagonists have a synergic effect [45, 89]. The combination of both compounds could be useful in the treatment of cancer, since this combination is synergistic for the growth inhibition of cancer cells overexpressing the NK-1 receptor, but not for normal cells. MDA, such as vinblastine, trigger apoptotic signaling through c-jun N-terminal kinases, and the modulation of MAPK pathway elements can enhance or inhibit MDA-induced apoptosis. In addition, it has been reported that L-733,060 reduces antiapoptotic NK-1 receptor signaling and hence enhances vinblastine-induced cell death [see 45]. Thus, the results found suggest that the coadministration of NK-1 receptor antagonists and MDA could be useful in chemotherapy [45, 89].

An *in vitro* study has recently demonstrated the synergism of NK-1 receptor antagonists and common cytostatics in malignant human cells [47]. In this study, MG-63 human osteosarcoma cells were cultured with the NK-1 receptor antagonists L-733,060 and with cytostatic drugs (adriamycin, mitomycin, ifosfamide or cisplatin). For example, in the case of adriamycin, a low cell inhibition was observed for the cytostatic drug alone, but this inhibition was higher when was administered together with the NK-1 receptor antagonist. However, this synergism was not found in non-malignant immortal HEK 293 cells. A low cell inhibition for the L-733,060 was observed in HEK 293 cells, whereas a robust cell inhibition exerted by the cytostatic drugs was observed. In contrast to what it was observed in the malignant MG-63 cell line, when combined with L-733,060, cytostatic drugs in HEK 293 induced similar (for adriamycin and mitomycin) or less (for cisplatin and ifosfamide) cell inhibition compared to the cytostatic applied alone [47]. It should be noted that compared to malignant cells, the growth inhibition of the benign cell line HEK 293, induced by L-733,060, was only minimal. Whether this selectivity is exclusively due to the fact that one cell is malignant and the other benign, is currently unknown. However, such a specific selectivity between malignant and benign cells has been previously hypothesized regarding the overexpression of the NK-1 receptors in several malignant cells compared to benign cells [67]. Moreover, it has also been demonstrated that the pretreatment of HEK 293 cells with L-733,060 prior to exposure to cytostatic drugs partially protected these cells from the inhibition mediated by these drugs [47].

NK-1 RECEPTOR ANTAGONISTS DECREASE THE SIDE EFFECTS OF RADIOTHERAPY AND CHEMOTHERAPY

The antineoplastic agent cyclophosphamide and X-ray radiation may elicit neurogenic inflammation, which is mediated by NK-1 receptors. Antineoplastic drugs facilitate the extravasation of plasma proteins, which is reduced by NK-1 receptor antagonists [see 45]. Radiation therapy and cytostatics mediate neurogenic inflammation, which is induced by the release of SP from nerve terminals. *Via* NK-1 receptors, SP increases the permeability of blood vessels and causes the extravasation of plasma proteins. Thus, the blockade of NK-1 receptors with NK-1 receptor antagonists could inhibit the triggering of the inflammatory cascade as well as the lysis of neutrophils, which is mediated by inflammatory mediators. This is extremely important, since X-ray radiation and cytostatics induce a breakdown of the mucosal barrier and an inflammation of the mucosa, providing a gateway for germs and eliciting systemic infection, which is exacerbated by neutropenia. However, NK-1 receptor antagonists improve the neurogenic inflammation induced by radiation or by inflammatory mediators. It has also been reported that the cytostatic placlitaxel, *via* SP, exerts adverse effects in the lung, and that cisplatin impairs renal function, but in both cases an improvement in pulmonary and kidney functions was observed after the administration of NK-1 receptor antagonists [90-92].

In sum, the combination of radiation therapy and/or chemotherapy and NK-1 receptor antagonists has a double effect: a decrease in the side effects induced by the radiation therapy and chemotherapy and the induction of a synergistic antitumour action [45, 89].

OTHER THERAPEUTIC ACTIONS OF NK-1 RECEPTOR ANTAGONISTS

SP and the NK-1 receptor are involved in many human pathologies [see 25 for review]. Thus, NK-1 receptor antagonists exert a broad-spectrum of therapeutic actions since after binding to the NK-1 receptor; NK-1 receptor antagonists block the SP function.

Antiemetic

A high density of NK-1 receptors has been observed in the vomiting centres of the central nervous system and when these are activated the vomiting reflex occurs. In this sense, it is known that CP-99,994, an NK-1 receptor antagonist, prevents emesis generated by many emetic stimuli (copper sulphate, cyclophosphamide, motion, cisplatin, nicotine, radiation…). This means that SP plays an important role in the emetic reflex pathway [see 25 for review]. It has also been demonstrated that the NK-1 receptor antagonist CJ-11,974 controls the acute emesis (< 24 h post-chemotherapy) induced by cisplatin. Regarding the control of acute emesis and nausea, the efficacy of CJ-11,974, when combined with dexamethasone and with a 5-hydroxytryptamine-3 receptor antagonist, was better than placebo [18]. It has also been reported that NK-1 receptor antagonists (*e.g.*, CP-99,994) abolish not only acute emesis, but also delayed (> 24 h post-chemotherapy) emesis after cisplatin administration [93]. It has been described that 80% of patients who received chemotherapy suffered an important side effect, CINV, but also that aprepitant blocked the NK-1 receptor and exerted an antiemetic action, preventing acute and delayed CINV and PONV. Aprepitant is the first NK-1 receptor antagonist to be approved by the FDA (US Food and Drug Administration) for its antiemetic effect in CINV and PONV. Fosaprepitant has been also marketed. This is a prodrug (fosaprepitant dimeglumine) of aprepitant and it is administered intravenously to patients receiving chemotherapy. The piperidine analogue vofopitant and the carbamoxyl-piperazine/carbamolypiperidine analogues vestipitant, casopitant and orvepitant are also important compounds. Casopitant has been studied in clinical trials addressing CINV and PONV. However, despite its positive effects in controlling CINV, the use of this NK-1 receptor antagonist has been discontinued because further safety studies have been demanded. Moreover, ezlopitant, and rolapitant have been tested in CINV.

Antidepressant Effect

It is known that the level of SP increases in depression; that the administration of antidepressant drugs induces a decrease in the level of SP in certain regions of the central nervous system, and that almost complete NK-1 receptor occupancy is necessary for NK-1 receptor antagonists to exert an antidepressant action [20, 94]. It has been reported that L-733,060, aprepitant and other NK-1 receptor antagonists (oral administration, preclinical assay) exert an antidepressant action [19] and that the administration of aprepitant (300 mg/day) (placebo-controlled trial) to patients suffering from moderate-to-severe major depression also exerts an antidepressant effect [20]. However, another study showed the absence of antidepressant effect for aprepitant (160 mg) [95]. Both studies reported contradictory results and it seems that the different doses used are the responsible for the contradictory findings. Thus, further studies on the antidepressant effect of aprepitant should be carried out in order to check the clinical efficacy of this NK-1 receptor antagonist.

Anti-Inflammatory Effect

Up to date, cancer prevention is only possible through an early clinical diagnostic when the tumour mass is still small and metastasis does not occur. However, the use of NK-1 receptor antagonists could prevent cancer. It is known that there is a high possibility of cancer development when chronic inflammation occurs; that the SP/NK-1 receptor system plays a crucial role in chronic inflammatory diseases (*e.g.*, viral hepatitis, ulcerative colitis, chronic pancreatitis...); and that the risk of developing pancreatic cancer is high in patients suffering from chronic pancreatitis [96]. *Via* the NK-1 receptor, SP induces inflammation and elicits cell proliferation. Thus, chronic inflammation could facilitate the development of cancer through the SP/NK-1 receptor system because this system is upregulated in inflammatory processes [see 25]. Thus, overexpression of the NK-1 receptor could be involved in chronic pancreatitis-associated cancer. By contrast, NK-1 receptor antagonists exert an anti-inflammatory and an antimitotic effect and hence the treatment with these antagonists could prevent the appearance/progression of cancer. This means that a new strategy in the prevention of cancer could be possible: a prophylaxis therapy using NK-1 receptor antagonists.

SUBSTANCE P, EMOTIONAL STRESS AND CANCER

Very frequently cancer and depression occur in the same person and, in fact, the development of cancer is more likely in patients suffering from severe or chronic depression. Moreover, in cancer patients the prevalence of depression increases with the severity of the disease. Many data support the idea that depression predicts cancer progression and mortality and that psychosocial support increases the survival time of patients with cancer by reducing anxiety and depression. Therefore, there must be a bi-directional relationship between depression and cancer, and new strategies are now emerging for adequate therapeutic intervention [see 97]. In this sense, it has been reported that mammary tumourigenesis is related to exposure to several forms of stressors together with factors associated to life-style. The latter is quite important because breast cancer mortality is increasing throughout the world and the development of curative therapies for this disease is currently not very promising. A crucial factor regarding tumour progression is the interaction among the following three factors: psychosocial support, personality and stress, as well as the result of this interaction on an individual's ability to cope with stress [98, 99]. In sum, all these data support the notion that psychological factors play an important role in cancer progression [98].

In several regions of the central nervous system the expression of NK-1 receptors and that of the genes encoding the synthesis of tachykinins are modified after the administration of psychotropic drugs [100-102]. Thus, in the central nervous system (*e.g.*, substantia nigra, amygdala, and striatum) chronically administered antidepressant drugs decrease the concentration of SP in these regions. This means that by decreasing the level of SP in several central nervous regions antidepressant drugs could exert a beneficial effect in the treatment of affective disorders through this mechanism [103].

Owing to the involvement of SP in depression, the NK-1 receptor antagonists L-733,060 and aprepitant have been used as antidepressive agents [19, 20], and it has been reported that both NK-1 receptor antagonists have antitumour activity against human glioma, retinoblastoma, melanoma, larynx, pancreatic, gastric and colon carcinomas, T and B cells of acute lymphoblastic leukaemia, osteosarcoma and hepatoblastoma cell lines [2, 13, 30, 32, 38, 47]. Moreover, in the treatment of depression it has been reported that aprepitant is as efficient as the antidepressant drug paroxetine [see 2, 72].

Both SP and NK-1 receptors are widely distributed in the limbic system (amygdala, hypothalamus...). Moreover, SP plays an important role in the integration of emotional responses to stress, and this suggests that an alteration in the SP/NK-1 receptor system could be responsible for the pathogenesis of depression [20]. In fact, an increase in the level of SP has been reported in this disease [20]. The data also suggest that in depression the SP/NK-1 receptor system could be activated and hence the disease could facilitate the proliferation of cancer cells. Thus, with the administration of NK-1 receptor antagonists both depression and tumour cell proliferation could be treated. In addition, the data show that emotional behaviour (*e.g.*, depression, anxiety) [104, 105], cancer progression and metastases [60] might be related through alterations in the SP/NK-1 receptor system. Thus, an interrelationship between cancer progression and cerebral mechanisms could take place through this system. SP binds to the NK-1 receptors located in the limbic system and to those located in tumour cells. In the first case, this induces anxiety and depression and in the second case it promotes cancer progression; *i.e.*, tumour cell proliferation, neoangiogenesis and metastasis. However, these actions are blocked by NK-1 receptor antagonists; these compounds exert antitumour and antidepressant actions.

CONCLUDING REMARKS

Many *in vitro* and *in vivo* studies have demonstrated that NK-1 receptor antagonists exert an antitumour action against numerous human cancer cell lines and that this action is dose-dependent. These antagonists inhibit the growth of cancer cells by inducing apoptosis and the same NK-1 receptor antagonist (*e.g.*, aprepitant) exerts its antitumour action against different human cancer cell lines. NK-1 receptor antagonists suppress cell proliferation and DNA synthesis *via* the MAPK pathway, and they also suppress the formation of a β-arrestin-containing complex, leading to the nuclear translocation of ERK1/2, inhibiting cell proliferation, and promoting apoptosis. In addition, NK-1 receptor antagonists decrease the basal phosphorylation of Akt and cause the proteolysis of poly (ADP-ribose) polymerase and the cleavage of caspase-3. It should be mentioned that after genetic (applying the small interfering RNA gene-silencing methodology) and pharmacological (using NK-1 receptor antagonists) treatments, cancer cells die by apoptosis. It has also been demonstrated that SP, *via* the NK-1 receptor, promotes mitogenesis in many human cancer cell lines. This means that a common mechanism for cancer cell proliferation through the SP/NK-1 receptor system occurs; that NK-1 receptor antagonists inhibit cancer progression by inducing apoptosis in many human cancer cell lines overexpressing the NK-1 receptor, and that such antagonists are excellent candidates for broad-spectrum antineoplastic drugs.

Tumour cell migration, which is regulated by substances synthesized in the nervous, immune and neuroendocrine systems, is necessary for invasion mechanisms and metastasis. The latter could be explained because G protein-coupled receptors could regulate the migratory activity of cancer cells after the binding of their respective ligands (*e.g.*, SP) to these receptors. In this way, these ligands could promote the migration of cancer cells, and hence the administration of NK-1 receptor antagonists could prevent such migration. In fact, it has been demonstrated that these antagonists fully suppress the metastasis of tumour cells, this effect being mediated by SP; that SP promotes modifications in the cellular shape (*e.g.*, blebbing); and that these modifications are blocked by NK-1 receptor antagonists. It is known that membrane blebbing is crucial for cell movement and spreading, as well as for tumour cell invasion and metastasis.

Tumour development is associated with angiogenesis. During angiogenesis, both an increase in the expression of NK-1 receptors and an increase in tissue innervation have been reported. In addition, it is known that NK-1 receptor agonists mimic angiogenesis, which is inhibited by NK-1 receptor antagonists; that SP promotes vessel growth by increasing the proliferation of the endothelial cells, but that this angiogenic effect is blocked by NK-1 receptor antagonists, and that both SP and NK-1 receptors are located in the intra- and peri-tumoural blood vessels. The data suggest that NK-1 receptor antagonists exert an antiangiogenic action.

In sum, many data suggest that the SP/NK-1 receptor system regulates the growth of cancer cells, angiogenesis and metastasis, because this system is upregulated in tumour cells and in peri-tumoural tissues. The data also show that NK-1 receptor antagonists act through three mechanisms: 1) an antiproliferative action: they inhibit the tumour cell growth by inducing apoptosis in cancer cells; 2) an antiangiogenic effect: they inhibit angiogenesis in the tumour mass; and 3) an antimetastatic action: they block the migration of tumour cells, and in the brain they may prevent breaching of the BBB by cancer cells (which secrete SP) and their colonization of the brain. That is, the NK-1 receptor is a therapeutic target in cancer. In addition, in the near future the combination of NK-1 receptor antagonists and cytostatics should be studied, and the antitumour action of the drug aprepitant should be tested in human clinical trials because the use of NK-1 receptor antagonists in oncology therapy is very promising.

ACKNOWLEDGEMENTS

The authors wish to thank Mr. Nicholas Skinner (University of Salamanca) for supervising the English text and Mr. Javier Muñoz (University of Sevilla) and Mr. Manuel Sánchez for technical assistance.

CONFLICT OF INTEREST

USPTO Application no. 20090012086 “Use of non-peptidic NK-1 receptor antagonists for the production of apoptosis in tumor cells” (Miguel Muñoz).

REFERENCES

[1] Morgan G, Ward R, Barton M. The contribution of cytotoxic chemotherapy to 5- year survival in adult malignancies. Clin Oncol 2004; 16: 549-60.

[2] Muñoz M, Coveñas R. Involvement of substance P and the NK-1 receptor in cancer progression. Peptides 2013; 48: 1-9.

[3] Singh D, Joshi DD, Hameed M, Qian J, Gascón P, Maloof PB, *et al.* Increased expression of preprotachykinin-I and neurokinin receptors in human breast cancer cells: implications for bone marrow metastasis. Proc Natl Acad Sci USA 2000; 97: 388-93.

[4] Feng F, Yang J, Tong L, Yuan S, Tian Y, Hong L, *et al.* Substance P- immunoreactive nerve fibers are related to gastric cancer differentiation status and could promote proliferation and migration of gastric cancer cells. Cell Biol Int 2011; 35: 623-9.

[5] Patel HJ, Ramkissoon SH, Patel PS, Rameshwar P. Transformation of breast cells by truncated neurokinin-1 receptor is secondary to activation by preprotachykinin-A peptides. Proc Natl Acad Sci USA 2005; 102: 17436-41.

[6] DeFea KA, Vaughn ZD, O'Bryan EM, Nishijima D, Dery O, Bunnett NW. The proliferative and antiapoptotic effects of substance P are facilitated by formation of a beta-arrestin-dependent scaffolding complex. Proc Natl Acad Sci USA 2000; 97: 11086-91.

[7] Palma C, Bigioni M, Irrissuto C, Nardelli F, Maggi CA, Manzini S. Anti-tumour activity of tachykinin NK1 receptor antagonists on human glioma U373 MG xenograft. Br J Cancer 2000; 82: 480-7.

[8] Lewis KM, Harford-Wright E, Vink R, Nimmo AJ, Ghabriel MN. Walker 256 tumour cells increase substance P immunoreactivity locally and modify the properties of the blood-brain barrier during extravasation and brain invasion. Clin Exp Metastasis 2013; 30: 1-12.

[9] Ramkissoon SH, Patel PS, Taborga M, Rameshwar P. Nuclear factor-κB is central to the expression of truncated neurokinin-1 receptor in breast cancer: implication for breast cancer cell quiescence within bone marrow stroma. Cancer Res 2007; 67: 1653-9.

[10] Luo W, Sharif TR, Sharif M. Substance P-induced mitogenesis in human astrocytoma cells correlates with activation of the mitogen-activated protein kinase signaling pathway. Cancer Res 1996; 56: 4983-91.

[11] Meshki J, Douglas SD, Lai JP, Schwartz L, Kilpatrick LE, Tuluc F. Neurokinin 1 receptor mediates membrane blebbing in HEK293 cells through a Rho/Rho- associated coiled-coil kinase-dependent mechanism. J Biol Chem 2009; 284: 9280- 9.

[12] Li X, Ma G, Ma Q, Li W, Liu J, Han L, *et al.* Neurotransmitter substance P mediates pancreatic cancer perineural invasion *via* NK-1R in cancer cells. Mol Cancer Res 2013; 11: 294-302.

[13] Muñoz M, Rosso M, Coveñas R. A new frontier in the treatment of cancer: NK-1 receptor antagonists. Curr Med Chem 2010; 17: 504-16.

[14] O'Connor TM, O'Connell J, O'Brien DI, Goode T, Bredin CP, Shanahan, F. The role of substance P in inflammatory disease. J Cell Physiol 2004; 201: 167-80.

[15] Ziche M, Morbidelli L, Pacini M, Gepetti P, Alessandri G, Maggi CA. Substance P stimulates neovascularization *in vivo* and proliferation of cultured endothelial cells. Microvasc Res 1990; 40: 264-78.

[16] Ständer S, Siepmann D, Herrgott I, Sunderkötter C, Luger TA. Targeting the neurokinin receptor 1 with aprepitant: a novel antipruritic strategy. PLoS One 2010; 5: e10968.

[17] Jin Y, Wu X, Guan Y, Gu D, Shen Y, Xu Z, *et al.* Efficacy and safety of aprepitant in the prevention of chemotherapy-induced nausea and vomiting: a pooled analysis. Support Care Cancer 2012; 20: 1815-22.

[18] Hesketh PJ, Gralla RJ, Webb RT, Ueno W, DelPrete S, Bachinsky ME, *et al.* Randomized Phase II study of the neurokinin 1 receptor antagonist CJ-11,974 in the control of cisplatin-induced emesis. J Clin Oncol 1999; 17: 338-43.

[19] Varty GB, Cohen-Williams ME, Hunter JC. The antidepressant-like effects of neurokinin NK1 receptor antagonists in a gerbil tail suspension test. Behav Pharmacol 2003; 14: 87-95.

[20] Kramer MS, Cutler N, Feighner J, Shrivastava R, Carman J, Sramek JJ, *et al.* Distinct mechanism for antidepressant activity by blockade of central substance P receptors. Science 1998; 281: 1640-5.

[21] King KA, Hu C, Rodríguez MM, Romaguera R, Jiang X, Piedimonte G. Exaggerated neurogenic inflammation and substance P receptor upregulation in RSV-infected eanling rats. Am J Respir Cell Mol Biol 2001; 24: 101-7.

[22] Yu J, Cadet JL, Angulo JA. Neurokinin-1 (NK-1) receptor antagonists abrogate methamphetamine-induced striatal dopaminergic neurotoxicity in the murine brain. J Neurochem 2002; 83: 613-22.

[23] Green SA, Alon A, Ianus J, McNaughton KS, Tozzi CA, Reiss TF. Efficacy and safety of a neurokinin-1 receptor antagonist in postmenopausal women with overactive bladder with urge urinary incontinence. J Urol 2006; 176: 2535-40.

[24] Fackler OT, Grosse R. Cell motility through plasma membrane blebbing. J Cell Biol 2008; 181: 879-84.

[25] Muñoz M, Coveñas R. NK-1 receptor antagonists: a new paradigm in pharmacology therapy. Curr Med Chem 2011; 18: 1820-31.

[26] Ho WZ, Cnaan A, Li YH, Zhao H, Lee HR, Song L, *et al.* Substance P modulates human immunodeficiency virus replication in human peripheral blood monocyte- derived macrophages. AIDS Res Hum Retroviruses 1996; 12: 195-8.

[27] Esteban F, González-Moles MA, Castro D, Martín-Jaén M del M, Redondo M, Ruiz-Avila I, *et al.* Expression of substance P and neurokinin-1-receptor in laryngeal cancer: linking chronic inflammation to cancer promotion and progression. Histopathology 2009; 54: 258-60.

[28] González-Moles MA, Mosqueda-Taylor A, Esteban F, Gil-Montoya JA, Díaz- Franco MA, Delgado M, *et al.* Cell proliferation associated with actions of the substance P/NK-1 receptor complex in keratocystic odontogenic tumours. Oral Oncol 2008; 44: 1127-33.

[29] Muñoz M, Martínez-Armesto J, Coveñas R. NK-1 receptor antagonists as antitumor drugs: a survey of the literature from 2000 to 2011. Expert Opin Ther Pat 2012; 22: 735-46.

[30] Muñoz M, González-Ortega A, Rosso M, Robles-Frías MJ, Carranza A, Salinas- Martín MV, *et al.* The substance P/Neurokinin-1 receptor system in lung cancer: focus on the antitumor action of neurokinin-1 receptor antagonists. Peptides 2012; 38: 318-25.

[31] Muñoz M, Pavón A, Rosso M, Salinas MV, Pérez A, Carranza A, *et al.* Immunolocalization of NK-1 receptor and substance P in human normal placenta. Placenta 2010; 31: 649-51.

[32] Muñoz M, Rosso M, Robles-Frías MJ, Salinas-Martín MV, Rosso R, González- Ortega A, *et al.* The NK-1 receptor is expressed in human melanoma and is involved in the antitumor action of the NK-1 receptor antagonist aprepitant on melanoma cell lines. Lab Invest 2010; 90: 1259-69.

[33] Rosso M, Robles-Frías MJ, Coveñas R, Salinas-Martín MV, Muñoz M. The NK-1 receptor is expressed in human primary gastric and colon adenocarcinomas and is involved in the antitumor action of L-733,060 and the mitogenic action of substance P on human gastrointestinal cancer cell lines. Tumor Biol 2008; 29: 245-54.

[34] Moharita A, Harrison, JS, Rameshwar P. Neurokinin receptors and subtypes as potential targets in breast cancer: relevance to bone marrow metastasis. Drug Res Rev 2004; 1: 1-6.

[35] Peng SL. Transcription factors in the pathogenesis of autoimmunity. Clin Immunol 2004; 110: 112-23.

[36] Muñoz M, Rosso M, Coveñas R, Montero I, González-Moles MA, Robles MJ. Neurokinin-1 receptors located in human retinoblastoma cell lines: antitumor action of its antagonist, L-732,138. Invest Ophthalmol Vis Sci 2007; 48: 2775-81.

[37] Brener S, González-Moles MA, Tostes D, Esteban F, Gil-Montoya JA, Ruiz-Avila I, *et al.* A role for the substance P/NK-1 receptor complex in cell proliferation in oral squamous cell carcinoma. Anticancer Res 2009; 29: 2323-9.

[38] Berger M, Neth O, Ilmer M, Garnier A, Salinas-Martín MV, de Agustín Asencio JC, *et al.*. Hepatoblastoma cells express truncated neurokinin-1 receptor and can be inhibited by aprepitant *in vitro* and *in vivo*. J Hepatol 2014; 60: 985-94.

[39] González-Ortega A, Sánchez-Vaderrábanos E, Ramiro S, Salinas-Martín V, Carranza A, Coveñas R, *et al.* Uveal melanoma expresses NK-1 receptors and cyclosporin A induces apoptosis in human melanoma cell lines overexpressing the NK-1 receptor. Peptides 2014; 55: 1-12.

[40] Ernst A, Suhr J, Köhrle J, Bergmann A. Detection of stable N-terminal protachykinin A immunoreactivity in human plasma and cerebrospinal fluid. Peptides 2008; 29: 1201-6.

[41] Rameshwar P, Joshi DD, Yadav P, Qian J, Gascon P, Chang VT, *et al.* Mimicry between neurokinin-1 and fibronectin may explain the transport and stability of increased substance P immunoreactivity in patients with bone marrow fibrosis. Blood 2001; 97: 3025-31.

[42] Hennig IM, Laissue JA, Horisberger U, Reubi JC. Substance-P receptors in human primary neoplasms: tumoral and vascular localization. Int J Cancer 1995; 61: 786-92.

[43] Muñoz M, González-Ortega A, Coveñas R. The NK-1 receptor is expressed in human leukemia and is involved in the antitumor action of aprepitant and other NK-1 receptor antagonists on acute lymphoblastic leukemia cell lines. Invest New Drugs 2012; 30: 529-40.

[44] Muñoz M, Rosso M, González A, Sáenz J, Coveñas R. The broad-spectrum antitumor action of cyclosporin A is due to its tachykinin receptor antagonist pharmacological profile. Peptides 2010; 31: 1643-8.

[45] Muñoz M, Rosso M, Coveñas R. The NK-1 receptor: a new target in cancer therapy. Curr Drug Targets 2011; 12: 909-21.

[46] Esteban F, Muñoz M, González-Moles MA, Rosso M. A role for substance P in cancer promotion and progression: a mechanism to counteract intracellular death signals following oncogene activation or DNA damage. Cancer Metast Rev 2006; 25: 137-45.

[47] Muñoz M, Berger M, Rosso M, González-Ortega A, Carranza A, Coveñas R. Antitumor activity of neurokinin-1 receptor antagonists in MG-63 human osteosarcoma xenografts. Int J Oncol 2014; 44: 137-46.

[48] Nakajima Y, Tsuchida K, Negishi M, Ito S, Nakanishi S. Direct linkage of three tachykinin receptors to stimulation of both phosphatidylinositol hydrolysis and cAMP cascades in transfected Chinese hamster ovary cells. J Biol Chem 1992; 267: 2437-42.

[49] Takeda Y, Blount P, Sachais BS, Hershey AD, Raddatz R, Krause JE. Ligand binding kinetics of substance P and neurokinin A receptors stably expressed in Chinese hamster ovary cells and evidence for differential stimulation of inositol 1, 4, 5-triphosphate and cyclic AMP second messenger responses. J Neurochem 1992; 59: 740-5.

[50] Ames BN, Gold LS. Too many rodent carcinogens: mitogenesis increases mutagenesis. Science 1990; 249: 970-1.

[51] Blaser MJ, Chyou PH, Nomura A. Age at establishment of *Helicobacter pylori* infection and gastric carcinoma, gastric ulcer and duodenal ulcer risk. Cancer Res 1995; 55: 562-5.

[52] Macarthur M, Hold GL, El-Omar EM. Inflammation and cancer II. Role of chronic inflammation and cytokine gene polymorphisms in the pathogenesis of gastrointestinal malignancy. Am J Physiol Gastrointest Liver Physiol 2004; 286: G515-20.

[53] Weitzman SA, Gordon LJ. Inflammation and cancer: role of phagocyte-generated oxidants in carcinogenesis. Blood 1990; 76: 655-63.

[54] Cook GA, Elliott D, Metwali A, Blu AM, Sandor M, Lynch R, *et al.* Molecular evidence that granuloma T lymphocytes in murine Schistosomiasis mansoni express an authentic SP (NK1) receptor. J Immunol 1994; 152: 1830-5.

[55] Keranen U, Jarvinen H, Karkkaine P, Kiviluoto T, Kivilaakso E, Soinila S. Substance P – an underlying factor for pouchitis? Prospective study of substance P and VIP-immunoreactive innervation and mast cells. Dig Dis Sci 1996; 41: 1665- 71.

[56] Keranen U, Jarvinen H, Kiviluoto T, Kivilaakso E, Soinila S. Substance P and VIP-immunoreactive innervation in normal and inflamed pouches after restorative proctocolectomy for ulcerative colitis. Dig Dis Sci 1996; 41: 1658-64.

[57] Walsh DT, Weg VB, Williams TJ, Nourshargh S. Substance P induced inflammatory responses in guinea-pig skin: the effect of specific NK1 receptor antagonists and the role of endogenous mediators. Br J Pharmacol 1995; 114: 1343-50.

[58] Medrano S, Gruenstein E, Dimlich RV. Substance P receptors on human astrocytoma cells are linked to glycogen breakdown. Neurosci Lett 1994; 167: 14- 8.

[59] Warburg O. On the origin of cancer cells. Science 1956; 123: 309-14.

[60] Lang K, Drell TL, Lindecke A, Niggemann B, Kaltschmidt C, Zaenker KS, *et al.* Induction of a metastatogenic tumor cell type by neurotransmitters and its pharmacological inhibition by established drugs. Int J Cancer 2004; 112: 231-8.

[61] Ruhlmann CH, Herrstedt J. Safety evaluation of aprepitant for the prevention of chemotherapy-induced nausea and vomiting. Expt Opin Drug Saf 2011; 10: 449- 62.

[62] Grunberg S, Chua D, Maru A, Dinis J, DeVandry S, Boice JA, *et al.* Single-dose fosaprepitant for the prevention of chemotherapy-induced nausea and vomiting associated with cisplatin therapy: randomized, double-blind study protocol-EASE. J Clin Oncol 2011; 29: 1495-501.

[63] Stiff PJ, Fox-Geiman MP, Kiley K, Rychlik K, Parthasarathy M, Fletcher- Gónzalez D, *et al.* Prevention of nausea and vomiting associated with stem cell transplant: results of a prospective, randomized trial of aprepitant used with highly emetogenic. Biol Blood Marrow Transplant 2013; 19: 49-55.

[64] Olver I, Shelukar S, Thompson KC. Nanomedicines in the treatment of emesis during chemotherapy: focus on aprepitant. Int J Nanomed 2007; 2: 13-8.

[65] Paul B, Trovato JA, Thompson J, Badros AZ, Goloubeva O. Efficacy of aprepitant in patients receiving high-dose chemotherapy with hematopoietic stem cell support. J Oncol Pharm Pract 2010; 16: 45-51.

[66] Bang R, Sass G, Kiemer AK, Vollmar AM, Neuhuber WL, Tiegs G. Neurokinin-1 receptor antagonists CP-96,345 and L-733,060 protect mice from cytokine- mediated liver injury. J Pharmacol Exp Ther 2003; 305: 31-9.

[67] Muñoz M, Rosso M. The NK-1 receptor antagonist aprepitant as a broad-spectrum antitumor drug. Invest New Drugs 2010; 28: 187-93.

[68] Choi MR, Jiles C, Seibel NL. Aprepitant use in children, adolescents, and young adults for the control of chemotherapy-induced nausea and vomiting (CINV). J Pediatr Hematol Oncol 2010; 32: e268-71.

[69] Durand JP, Gourmel B, Mir O, Goldwasser F. Antiemetic neurokinin-1 antagonist aprepitant and ifosfamide-induced encephalopathy. Ann Oncol 2007; 18: 808-9.

[70] Saito H, Yoshizawa H, Yoshimori K, Katakami N, Katsumata N, Kawahara M, *et al.* Efficacy and safety of single-dose fosaprepitant in the prevention of chemotherapy-induced nausea and vomiting in patients receiving high-dose cisplatin: a multicentre, randomised, double-bind, placebo-controlled phase 3 trial. Ann Oncol 2013; 24: 1067-73.

[71] Sánchez RI, Wang RW, Newton DJ, Bakhtiar R, Lu P, Chiu SH, *et al.* Cytochrome P450 3A4 is the major enzyme involved in the metabolism of the substance P receptor antagonist aprepitant. Drug Metab Dispos 2004; 32: 1287-92.

[72] Muñoz M, Coveñas R. Safety of neurokinin-1 receptor antagonists. Expert Opin Drug Saf 2013; 12: 673-85.

[73] Bigioni M, Benzo A, Irrissuto C, Maggi CA, Goso C. Role of NK-1 and NK-2 tachykinin receptor antagonism on the growth of human breast carcinoma cell line MDA-MB-231. Anticancer Drugs 2005; 16: 1083-9.

[74] Guha S, Eibl G, Kisfalvi K, Fan RS, Burdick M, Reber H, *et al.* Broad-spectrum G protein–coupled receptor antagonist, [D-Arg1,DTrp5,7,9,Leu11]SP: a dual inhibitor of growth and angiogenesis in pancreatic cancer. Cancer Res 2005; 65: 2738-45.

[75] Seckl MJ, Higgins T, Widmer F, Rozengurt E. [D-Arg1,Trp5,7,9,Leu11] substance P: a novel potent inhibitor of signal transduction and growth *in vitro* and *in vivo* in small cell lung cancer cells. Cancer Res 1997; 57: 51-4.

[76] Akazawa T, Kwatra SG, Goldsmith LE, Richardson MD, Cox EA, Sampson JH, *et al.* A constitutively active form of neurokinin 1 receptor and neurokinin 1 receptor- mediated apoptosis in glioblastomas. J Neurochem 2009; 109: 1079-86.

[77] Manske JM, Hanson SE. Substance P-mediated immunomodulation of tumor growth in a murine model. Neuroimmunomodulation 2005;12: 201-10.

[78] Prasad S, Mathur A, Jaggi M, Singh AT, Mukherjee R. Substance P analogs containing alpha, alpha-dialkylated amino acids with potent anticancer activity. J Pept Sci 2007; 13: 544-8.

[79] Harford-Wright E, Lewis KM, Vink R, Ghabriel MN. Evaluating the role of substance P in the growth of brain tumors. Neuroscience 2014; 261: 85-94.

[80] Exadaktylos AK, Buggy DJ, Moriarty DC, Mascha E, Sessler DI. Can anesthetic technique for primary breast cancer surgery affect recurrence or metastasis? Anesthesiology 2006; 105: 660-4.

[81] Muñoz M, Rosso M, Casinello F, Coveñas R. Paravertebral anesthesia: how substance P and the NK-1 receptor could be involved in regional block and breast cancer recurrence. Breast Cancer Res Treat 2010; 122: 601-3.

[82] Rodríguez PL, Jiang S, Fu Y, Avraham S, Avraham HK. The proinflammatory peptide substance P promotes blood-brain barrier breaching by breast cancer cells through changes in microvascular endothelial cell tight junctions. Int J Cancer 2014; 134: 1034-44.

[83] Stahl SM. The ups and downs of novel antiemetic drugs, part 1: substance P, 5-HT, and the neuropharmacology of vomiting. J Clin Psychiatry 2003; 64:498-9.

[84] Roila F, Rolski J, Ramlau R, Dediu M, Russo MW, Bandekar RR, *et al.* Randomized, double-blind, dose-ranging trial of the oral neurokinin-1 receptor antagonist casopitant mesylate for the prevention of cisplatin-induced nausea and vomiting. Ann Oncol 2009; 20: 1867-73.

[85] de Jonge ME, Huitema AD, Holtkamp MJ, van Dam SM, Beijnen JH, Rodenhuis S. Aprepitant inhibits cyclophosphamide bioactivation and thiotepa metabolism. Cancer Chemother Pharmacol 2005; 56: 370-8.

[86] Blum RA, Majumdar A, McCrea J, Busillo J, Orlowski LH, Panebianco D, *et al.* Effects of aprepitant on the pharmacokinetics of ondansetron and granisetron in healthy subjects. Clin Ther 2003; 25: 1407-19.

[87] Loos WJ, de Wit WR, Freedman SJ, Van Dyck K, Gambale JJ, Li S, *et al.* Aprepitant when added to a standard antiemetic regimen consisting of ondansetron and dexamethasone does not affect vinorelbine pharmacokinetics in cancer patients. Cancer Chemother Pharmacol 2007; 59: 407-12.

[88] Gore L, Chawla S, Petrilli A, Hemenway M, Schissel D, Chua V, *et al.* Aprepitant in adolescent patients for prevention of chemotherapy-induced nausea and vomiting: a randomized, double-blind, placebo-controlled study of efficacy and tolerability. Pediatr Blood Cancer 2009; 52: 242-7.

[89] Kitchens CA, McDonald PR, Pollack IF, Wipf P, Lazo JS. Synergy between microtubule destabilizing agents and neurokinin 1 receptor antagonists identified by an siRNA synthetic lethal screen. FASEB J 2009; 23: 756.13.

[90] Alfieri AB, Cubeddu LX. Role of NK1 receptors on cisplatin-induced nephrotoxicity in the rat. Naunyn Schmiebergs Arch Pharmacol 2000; 361: 334- 8.

[91] Alfieri AB, Cubeddu LX. Efectos de los antagonistas de los receptores NK1 y de la dexametasona sobre la inflamación neurogénica inducida por ciclofosfamida y por radiación X, en la rata. AVFT 2004; 23: 61-6.

[92] Sendo T, Itoh Y, Goromaru T, Hirakawa T, Ishida M, Nakano H, *et al.* Role of substance P in hypersensitivity reactions induced by paclitaxel, an anticancer agent. Peptides 2004; 25: 1205-8.

[93] Rudd JA, Jordan CC, Naylor RJ. The action of the NK1 tachykinin receptor antagonist CP-99,994 in antagonizing the acute and delayed emesis induced by cisplatin in the ferret. Br J Pharmacol 1996; 119: 931-6.

[94] Ratti E, Bellew K, Bettica P, Bryson H, Zamuner S, Archer G, *et al.* Results from 2 randomized, double-bind, placebo-controlled studies of the novel NK-1 receptor antagonist casopitant in patients with major depressive disorder. J Clin Psychopharmacol 2011; 31: 727-33.

[95] Keller M, Montgomery S, Ball W, Morrison M, Snavely D, Liu G, *et al.* Lack of efficacy of the substance P (neurokinin-1 receptor) antagonist aprepitant in the treatment of major depressive disorder. Biol Psychiatry 2006; 59: 216-23.

[96] Lowenfels AB, Maisonneuve P, Cavallini G, Ammann RW, Lankisch PG, Andersen JR, *et al.* Pancreatitis and the risk of pancreatic cancer. International Pancreatitis Study Group. N Engl J Med 1993; 328: 1433-7.

[97] Spiegel D, Giese-Davis J. Depression and cancer: mechanisms and disease progression. Biol Psychiatry 2003; 54: 269-82.

[98] Hilakivi-Clarke L, Rowland J, Clarke R, Lippman ME. Psychosocial factors in the development and progression of breast cancer. Breast Cancer Res Treat 1994; 29: 141-60.

[99] Okamura M, Yamawaki S, Akechi T, Taniguchi K, Uchitomi Y. Psychiatric disorders following first breast cancer recurrence: prevalence, associated factors and relationship to quality of life. Jpn J Clin Oncol, 2005; 35: 302-9.

[100] Sivam SP, Krause JE, Takeuchi K, Li S, McGinty J, Hong JS. Lithium increases rat striatal β- and γ-preprotachykinin messenger RNAs. J Pharmacol Exp Ther 1989; 248: 1297-301.

[101] Humpel C, Knaus GA, Auer B, Knaus HG, Haring C, Theodorsson E, *et al.* Effects of haloperidol and clozapine on preprotachykinin mRNA tachykinin tissue level release and NK1 receptors in the striatonigral system. Synapse 1990; 6: 1-9.

[102] Shibata K, Haverstick DM, Bannon MJ. Tachykinin gene expression in rat limbic nuclei: modulation by dopamine antagonists. J Pharmacol Exp Ther 1990; 255: 388-92.

[103] Shirayama Y, Mitsushio H, Takashima M, Ichikawa H, Takayashi K. Reduction of substance P after chronic antidepressant treatment in the striatum, substantia nigra and amygdala of the rat. Brain Res 1996; 739: 70-8.

[104] Fehder WP. Alterations in immune response associated with anxiety in surgical patients. CNRA 1999; 10: 124-9.

[105] De Vane CL. Substance P: a new era, a new role. Pharmacotherapy 2001; 21: 1061-9.

CHAPTER 2

Molecular Targeted Drugs under Investigation in Hepatocellular Carcinoma

Mohamed Bouattour*[,1] and Johanna Wassermann[2]

[1]Department of Hepatology, Beaujon University Hospital, Assistance Publique-Hôpitaux de Paris, France; and [2]Department of Medical Oncology, La Pitié Salpêtrière University Hospital, Assistance Publique-Hôpitaux de Paris, France

Abstract: Until no far past, advanced hepatocellular carcinoma (HCC) was considered as an "orphan" disease in terms of effective molecules when compared with other highly prevalent cancers worldwide. Recently, HCC -a tumor renowned to be refractory to systemic chemotherapy- has attracted wide interest as a result of improved understanding of its molecular biology and pathogenesis. HCC is a well-vascularized tumor in which angiogenesis is strongly implicated for aggressiveness and dissemination and targeted drugs (mainly angiogenesis inhibitors) have been tested to block neovessels and various signaling pathways involved in this disease. This approach has been successful, at least for sorafenib -an antiangiogenic and multikinase inhibitor- across 2 large international randomized phase III trials confirming the efficacy and safety of this compound as validated option in patients with advanced-stage HCC.

Approval of sorafenib as the new standard care for advanced HCC raised the interest to investigate plethora of drugs in this pathology and in different setting including earlier stages, and as adjuvant therapy. Currently, several small molecules and antiangiogenic agents are investigated in preclinical and clinical studies with disparate outcomes, with the hope to identify new efficient therapies, thereby opening new prospects but also raising several unmet needs.

This review develops the rational for using these emerging drugs in treatment algorithm of HCC, and highlights the strength and limits of novel compounds with focus on specific challenges for their clinical development.

Keywords: Angiogenesis inhibitors, brivanib, combination therapy, hepatocellular carcinoma, MET inhibitors, mTOR inhibitors, new compounds, regorafenib, sorafenib, sunitinib.

***Corresponding Author Mohamed Bouattour:** Department of Hepatology, Beaujon University Hospital, Assistance Publique-Hôpitaux de Paris, 100 BLD Général Leclerc 92118 Clichy, France;
Tel: +33 1 40 87 55 25; Fax: + 33 1 47 39 61 78; E-mail: mohamed.bouattour@bjn.aphp.fr

Atta-ur-Rahman / M. Iqbal Choudhary (Eds.)

INTRODUCTION

More than thirty years of clinical experience treating patients with advanced/relapsing HCC have been disappointing up to 2007, when finally the sorafenib showed overall survival improvement in two large prospective randomized trials [1, 2]. Before this era, conventional cytotoxic chemotherapies have been an option for patients presenting adequate performance status and liver function [3]. Despite sparse evidence of activity observed in some reports, none of chemotherapy regimen showed overall survival improvement over placebo as first line therapy in randomized trials [4]. Recently, an Asian trial showed that oxaliplatin plus fluorouracil/leucovorin (FOLFOX) regimen improved overall survival in patients with advanced HCC when compared to doxorubicin, a drug potentially difficult to handle in patients with unreliable liver disease [5]. Conventional chemotherapy might still be an alternative in patients upon individual characteristics, especially in the case of disease with rapid kinetics and high proliferation rate and/or resistant to antiangiogenic drugs.

Nevertheless, sorafenib achievements opened wide perspectives in terms of exploring innovative targeted compounds in HCC. Better knowledge of biology and critical signaling pathways in HCC highlighted the need to optimize translational research to select appropriate therapeutic option with regard to individual tumor characteristics.

In this review, we purpose to discuss the rational and challenges for development of molecular targeted drugs in HCC.

ANGIOGENESIS AND MOLECULAR CARCINOGENESIS IN HCC: FROM PIONEERING PROPOSAL TO VALIDATED TARGETED COMPOUNDS

Currently, there is no doubt or controversy concerning the implication of angiogenesis process at all stages in HCC pathogenesis and development. Although HCC displays a heterogeneous and complex carcinogenesis [6], several critical signaling pathways and molecular aberrations implicated in its development and invasion are now well-known. Exhaustive genetic aberrations and disrupted signaling pathways involved in proliferation, survival, differentiation, invasion and metastasis of HCC cells have been obviously detailed elsewhere [7-10]. Advantageously, these dysregulations have offered the opportunity to explore new targets for HCC treatment (Fig. **1**).

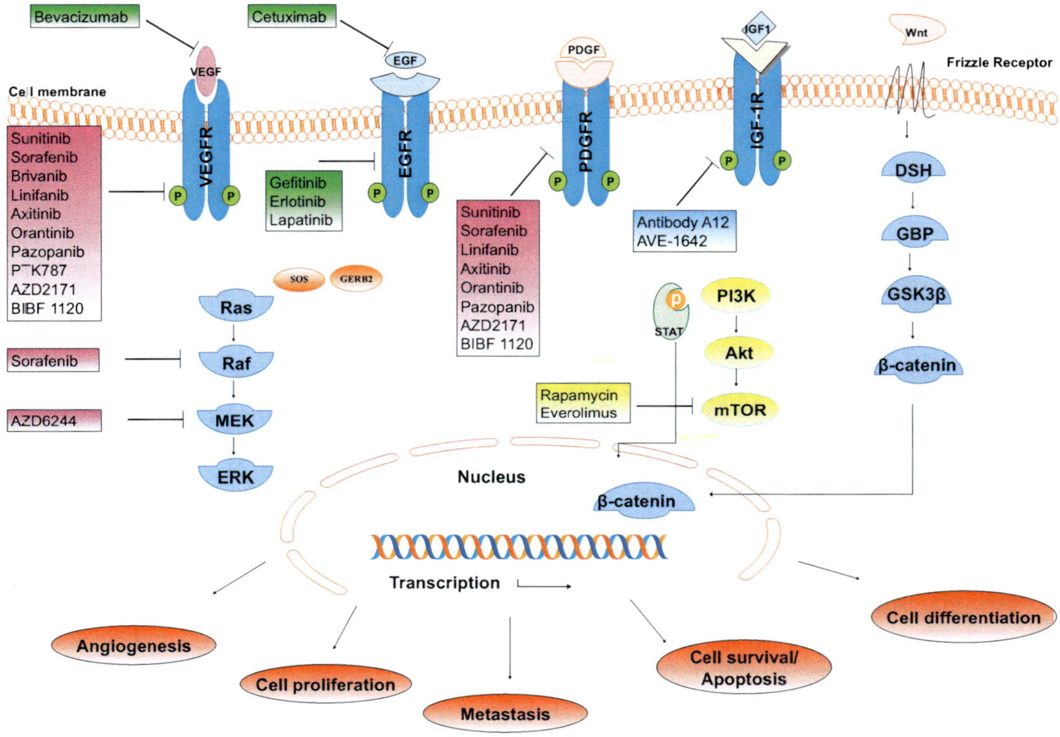

Fig. (1). Representation of molecular targets and signaling pathways involved in HCC and their potential inhibiting compounds (not exhaustive list). VEGF: Vascular Endothelial Growth Factor. PDGFR: Platelet-Derived Growth Factor Receptor. EGFR: Epidermal Growth Factor Receptor. IGF-1R: Insulin-like Growth Factor 1 Receptor. PI3K, Phosphoinositide-3 kinase; AKT, protein kinase B. STAT: Signal Transducer and Activator of Transcription. mTOR: mammalian Target of rapamycin. GRB2: Growth Factor Receptor-Bound protein 2. SOS: Son Of Sevenless. MEK: Mitogen-activated protein kinase/Extracellular signal-regulated Kinase. Wnt: Wingless-type MMTV integration site family member. DAS: Dishevelled. GBP: GSK-3 binding protein. GSK-3: Glycogen Synthase Kinase-3.

HCC is a highly vascularized tumor with a strong predisposition for vascular invasion. The process of tumoral angiogenesis is complex and involves several pro-factors implicated in the new blood vessels development, tumor growth and metastasis. Immunohistochemistry studies showed a significant increasing of the microvessel density correlating with high risk of vascular invasion, metastasis and poor prognosis after resection [11]. Inhibition of angiogenesis induces disruption of the tumor supply in oxygen and its privation of nutrients and consequently suppresses its growth. Therefore, blockade angiogenesis appeared flawlessly suitable as a therapeutic approach for HCC.

Vascular Endothelial Growth Factor (VEGF) is a foremost mediator of angiogenesis in HCC [12-14]. The majority of HCC cells noticeably express VEGF and aberrant expression of VEGF is a major feature of HCC [12-15]. The overexpression of the VEGF has been associated with poor survival [13]. Hence, two approaches appear to be pertinent (Fig. **1**): targeting directly the VEGF (using for example bevacizumab) or ultimately the membrane tyrosine kinases receptors (using for example: sorafenib, sunitinib, brivanib, and others). These compounds had showed some antitumor activity in HCC. Besides the VEGF, the Platelet Growth Factor Receptor (PDGF) and the Basic Fibroblast Growth Factor Receptor (FGFR) were also implicated in angiogenesis, tumor invasion, and metastasis. Furthermore, a high expression of the Epidermal Growth Factor Receptor (EGFR) was observed in 40% to 70% of HCC. The activation of the EGFR by the Transforming Growth Factor-α (TGF-α) or the Epidermal Growth Factor (EGF) induced HCC-cells proliferation [16]. Hence, targeting EGFR appears as a rational option for HCC treatment. Two approaches are possible either using direct antibodies anti-EGFR (for example: cetuximab or panitumumab) or EGFR tyrosine kinases inhibitors (for example: gefitinib, erlotinib and lapatinib). In preclinical models, such compounds induced HCC-cells inhibition [17, 18].

The Phosphatidylinositol 3-Kinase (PI3K)/Akt/mammalian Target Of Rapamycin (mTOR) (PI3K/Akt/m-TOR), another essential survival pathway in HCC, is located downstream of several tyrosine kinases receptors (Fig. **1**). Aberrant m-TOR signaling pathway was observed in about half of patients with HCC [19]. In HCC, the activation of this pathway correlates also with poor prognosis [20]. Currently, mainly m-TOR inhibitors are available such as rapamycin or its analogues (everolimus, temsirolimus).

Thereby, targeting such disrupted signaling pathways in HCC appears to be strongly justified, either using multitargeted agents (*i.e.* sorafenib, sunitinib and brivanib) blocking several kinases, or by combining them with single-target agents (*i.e.* erlotinib, gefitinib, rapamycin). The gold aims were to hinder the activity of the growth factor receptors or related signaling pathways.

Currently, plethora of agents interfering with these biological targets and others (Table **1** and Fig. **1**), are under evaluation in HCC worldwide. An extensive list of these drugs is available and searchable at the website: www.clinicaltrials.gov. In this review we propose to report clinical results from a selected set of innovative compounds developed in HCC. We provide insights on possible advantages and limitations challenging the development of those drugs.

SORAFENIB THE STANDARD THERAPY FOR ADVANCED HCC

Sorafenib (Nexavar®; Bayer And Onyx Pharmaceuticals, International), an oral multi-tyrosine kinases inhibitor targets the intracellular serine/threonine Raf-Kinase, the VEGFR-2-,-3, the PDGFR-β, Fmts-like tyrosine kinase-3 (Flt-3), and stem cell factor receptor (c-Kit). In preclinical models, sorafenib induced apoptosis and inhibited tumor growth with an antiangiogenic effect [21, 22]. Currently, sorafenib is the sole molecule that improved overall survival in patients with advanced HCC based on results of the two large international, blinded, placebo-controlled randomized phase III trials [1, 2]. These trials have been reasonably conducted subsequently the promising results of phase a II study reported by Abou-Alfa *et al.* in 2006 [23]. In the SHARP trial, the sorafenib showed a clinical benefit in the western population since the median overall survival increased to 10.7 months in patients treated with sorafenib compared to 7.9 months for those under placebo (HR = 0.69; 95% CI 0.55-087; p = 0.00058). Almost all patients included in this trial, had a compensated cirrhosis (96.7% Child-Pugh A). The sorafenib yielded extension of the overall survival by 44% and diminution of the relative risk of death by 31% [1]. The same magnitude of benefit was observed in the Asian-Pacific population in which hepatitis B infection was the major etiology of cirrhosis and disease generally was more advanced [2]. In this population, the median overall survival was 6.5 months in the sorafenib group *versus* 4.2 months in the placebo group (HR = 0.68; 95% CI 0.50-093; p = 0.014) [2].

Table 1: Summary of Molecular Targeted Therapies Developed by Pharmaceutical Companies in HCC

Drugs	Company	Main Targets	Current Approval	Trials	Survival Results	Authors
Sorafenib	Bayer, Onyx Pharmaceuticals	VEGFR-2,-3, PDGFR-β,Flt-3), c-Kit	HCC RCC Refractory thyroid cancer	Phase III (SAHRP) sorafenib *vs* P	Median OS: 10.7 *vs* 7.9 months	Llovet *et al.* [1]
				Phase III (Asia-Pacific) sorafenib *vs* P	Median OS: 6.5 *vs* 4.2 months	Cheng *et al.* [2]
Sunitinib	Pfizer	VEGFR-1,-2, PDGFR-α,-β, c-Kit, Flt-3, RET	RCC imatinib-resistant GIST PET	Phase II: open-label	Median OS: 8 months	Faivre *et al.* [29]
				Phase II: open label	Median OS: 9.8 months	Zhu *et al.* [30]
				Phase II: open label	Median OS: 9.3 months	Keorbel *et al.* [31]
				Phase III: sunitinib *vs* sorafenib	Median OS: 7.9 *vs* 10.2 months	Cheng *et al.* [31]
Brivanib	Bristol-Meyers Squibb	VEGFR-2,-3, FGFR-2,-3		Phase II: open-label (first line)	Median OS: 10 months	Park *et al.* [39]
				Phase II: open-label (second line)	Median OS :9.79 months	Finn *et al.* [40]
				Phase III (BRISK-FL) brivanib *vs* sorafenib	Median OS: 9.5 *vs* to 9.9 months	Johnson *et al.* [41]
				Phase III (BRISK-PS) brivanib *vs* P	Median OS: 9.4 *vs* 8.2 months	Llovet *et al.* [42]
Linifanib	Abbott	VEGFR-1-2,-3 PDGFR-β, Flt-3		Phase II: open-label	Median OS: 9.7 months	Toh *et al.* [46]
				Phase III: linifanib *vs* sorafenib	Median OS: 9.1 *vs* 9.9 months	Cainap *et al.* [47]
Regorafenib	Bayer	VEGFR-1-2-3, PDGFR-β, FGFR, TIE2, KIT, RET, RAF	CRC GIST	Phase II: open label	Median OS: 13.8 months	Bruix *et al.* [51]
Cediranib	AstraZeneca	VEGFR-1-2-3, PDGFR, c-KIT		Phase II: open-label	Median OS: 5.8 months	Alberts *et al.* [55]
				Phase II: open-label	Medina OS: 11.7 months	Zhu *et al.* [56]
Orantinib	Taiho Pharmaceutical Co	VEGFR-2, PDGFR, FGFR		phase I/II phase II: open-label	Median OS: 13.1 months Median OS:	Kanai *et al.* [57]
Vandetanib	AstraZenica	VEGFR-2, EGFR, RET	medullary thyroid cancer	Phase II: placebo-controlled	Median OS: 5.75- 5.95 *vs* 4.27 months	Hsu *et al.* [62]

(Table 1) contd.....

Drugs	Company	Main Targets	Current Approval	Trials	Survival results	Authors
Tivantinib	Daiichi Sankyo ArQule	MET		Phase II: placebo-controlled	Median OS: 6·6 *vs* 6.2months Median OS: 7.2 *vs* 3.8 months (High MET)	Santoro *et al.* [72]
Bevacizumab	Genentech Inc	VEGF	CRC Lung cancer Breast cancer RCC	Phase II: open-label	Median OS: 12.4 months	Siegle *et al.* [82]
				Phase II: open-label	Median OS: 8 months	Boige *et al.* [83]
Ramucirumab	ImClone	VEGFR-2		Phase II: open-label	Median OS: 12 months	Zhu *et al.* [89]
Cetuximab	ImClone	EGFR	CRC Head and neck cancer	Phase II: open-label	Median OS: 9.6 months	Zhu *et al.* [70]
Erlotinib	Genentech	EGFR/HER1	Lung cancer Pancreatic cancer	Phase II: open-label	Median OS: 13 months	Philip *et al.* [94]
				Phase II: open-label	Median OS: 10.75 months	Thomas *et al.* [95]
				Phase III (SEARCH) erlotinib+sorafenib *vs* P+sorafenib	Median OS: 9.5 *vs* 8.5 months	Zhu *et al.* [96]
Gefitinib	AstraZeneca	EGFR	Lung cancer	Phase II: open-label	Median OS was 6.5 months	O'Dwyer *et al.* [100]
Lapatinib	GlaxoSmithKline	EGFR, HER-2/NEU	Breast cancer	Phase II: open-label	Median OS: 12.6 months	Bekaii-Saab *et al* [105].
				Phase II: open-label	Median OS: 6.2 months	Ramanathan *et al.* [106]

OS: overall survival, TTRP: time to radiological progression, TTP: time to progression, P: placebo, HCC: hepatocellular carcinoma, RCC: renal cell carcinoma, GIST: gastrointestinal stromal tumor, PET: pancreatic endocrine tumor, CRC: colorectal cancer.

Tolerability of sorafenib in these two trials was overall acceptable and toxicities were manageable. Less than 10% of patients treated in sorafenib arm experienced adverse events ≥ 3 (especially diarrhea and hand-foot skin syndrome). Noticeably, the incidence of hemorrhage was similar in the sorafenib and placebo arms [1].

Regarding these positive results, the FDA, the EMA and other regulatory authorities worldwide granted approval to sorafenib for advanced HCC. Currently, sorafenib is largely prescribed in routine for patients with advanced HCC. The international phase IV, open-label, non-interventional prospective study (GIDEON) evaluated sorafenib under real-life conditions in more than 3000 patients with advanced HCC enrolled from 39 countries [24, 25]. The first preliminary results concerning 500 patients showed that 76% of patients were treated with the approved initial dose of 800 mg/day of sorafenib and 75% of them received treatment for more than 4 weeks. A geographic variations concerning treatment duration and dosing were observed (lower in Asian regions). In the first interim analyses, the overall safety spectrum of sorafenib was consistent with already known in previous clinical studies and no unexpected adverse events were reported [24]. The second interim analyses were conducted when data of 1571 patients were available. About two-third of patients (61%) had Child-Pugh A status and 23% of them had Child-Pugh B. In this study 74% of patients received the approved initial dose of 800 mg of sorafenib. The median daily dose across all patients was 693 mg. Overall, 64% of patients included in this study experienced adverse events related to sorafenib. The majority of adverse events were grade 1-2 and only 9% of them were considered as serious [25]. The final data analyses for the overall included patients are still expected.

Thereby, the proof-of-concept of angiogenesis inhibition in HCC is well yet established. The encouraging results obtained with sorafenib claimed the unmet need to focus in this way in order to stumble on future efficient compounds for patients with advanced HCC, especially whose disease has progressed on or after sorafenib and for patients intolerant to treatment.

SMALL MOLECULES REACHING PHASE III TRIALS IN ADVANCED HCC

Sunitinib (Sutent®; SU011248, Pfizer Inc., New York City, USA)

Sunitinib malate, another oral multi-tyrosine kinase; targets the VEGFR-1,-2, PDGFR-α,-β, c-Kit, Flt-3 and RET [26]. Sunitinib has already been approved for treatment of other well-vascularized tumors including renal cell carcinoma, gastrointestinal stromal tumors and pancreatic endocrine tumors [27]. In preclinical models of HCC, sunitinib showed a potent inhibition of tumor growth through increasing apoptosis, decreasing microvessels density and inhibition of cell proliferation [28].

Three independent phase II studies had previously showed encouraging results regarding efficiency and tolerability of first line sunitinib in patients with advanced HCC [29-31]. In the first study, a minimal response rate was achieved as well as observed with sorafenib, contrasting with interesting antitumor activity. In fact, on 50 mg/day of sunitinib given sequentially (4 weeks on followed by 2 weeks off), 35% of patients achieved stable disease for over 3 months corresponding to disease control rate of 37.8% [29]. Comparable results were observed in a parallel second phase II study evaluating sunitinib at the sequential dose of 37.5 mg/day. In this trial, half of patients experienced stable disease [30]. The median overall survival in these two studies was 8 months and 9.8 months respectively [29, 30]. Subsequently, results of the last phase II Swiss study were reported using continuous sunitinib at the dose of 37.5 mg/day in patients with advanced HCC. About third of patients (33%) included in the study, experienced progression-free survival at 12 weeks and the median overall survival was 9.3 months [31] so similar to the prior two studies.

The initial promising results reported in these phase II studies were not confirmed by the multicenter randomized phase III trial of sunitinib compared to sorafenib as first line in patients with advanced HCC [32]. The study that enrolled 1,073 patients was early halted based on the recommendations of the independent data monitoring committee due to futility and safety reasons [32]. Indeed, despite apparent similarities in term of progression-free survival and time-to-progression, the median overall survival in patients treated with sunitinib was significantly shorter than those treated with sorafenib (7.9 months *vs* 10.2 months, HR = 1.30; 95% CI: 1.13-1.50, p = 0.0014) [32]. Patients treated with sunitinib experienced significantly higher incidence of serious adverse events. Grade ≥ 3 adverse events occurred in 82.1% of patients in the sunitinib arm and in 74.2% of patients in the sorafenib arm. Under sunitinib, the most frequent serious adverse events were thrombocytopenia (29.7%) and neutropenia (25.7%). As expected, hand-foot skin syndrome was the most common severe adverse event in patients treated with sorafenib (21.2%). Severe adverse events yielded discontinuation of sunitinib and sorafenib in 13.3% and 12.7% respectively [32].

These negative results emphasize the importance of cautious interpretation of phase II studies results testing different agents. In the case of sunitinib, its administration seems to be quite problematic in patients with HCC [33] and no reliable dosing scheme was used in phase II studies [34]. The underlying liver disease generates a narrow therapeutic index and the dose of 50 mg/ day routinely given in other cancers appears to be not appropriate for population of patients with advanced HCC [35]. Patients with cirrhosis, even very well compensated, are more vulnerable to toxicities related to drugs [36]. Furthermore, continuous administration without interruption may be better to optimize exposure to sunitinib [33]. Therefore, specific phase I studies dedicated to HCC patients, could redefine the adequate dose and schedule for patients with advanced HCC (Fig. **3**).

Brivanib (BMS-582664; Bristol-Meyers Squibb, USA)

Brivanib alaninate is an orally potent and selective tyrosine kinase inhibitor targeting the VEGFR-2,-3, and FGFR-2,-3. In preclinical models, brivanib induced tumor growth suppression, microvessel density reduction and apoptosis increase [37]. The same finding was observed in a wide variety of human tumor xenografts, including models of chemo-resistant cancer. Evaluation of angiogenesis by dynamic contrast enhanced-magnetic resonance imaging demonstrated a significant diminution of tumor vascular density and tumoral blood flow [38]. Continuous brivanib at the dose of 800 mg/day, was evaluated in a first-line and a second-line setting, through two independent phase II open-label studies in HCC patients with advanced disease [39, 40]. At the first line approach, 55 patients were treated with brivanib and tumoral response was assessed by the modified World Health Organization (WHO) criteria. The 6 month progression-free survival rate was 21.1% (95% CI: 9.6%-35.2%) and the median progression-free survival was 2.7 months (95% CI: 1.4-3.0) according to the independent analysis. The median overall survival was 10 months (95% CI: 6.8-15.2) [39]. Similar promising results were reported in patients previously treated with other antiangiogenic agent. As a second line therapy, brivanib showed exciting clinical benefit with a median overall survival of 9.79 months and a time-to-progression of 2.7 months [40]. Based on these encouraging data and the possible additional inhibition of the FGF-related pathways, brivanib was tested in two large randomized phase III studies (BRISK studies) [41, 42]. In the first study, 1,155 patients with advanced HCC were included and randomized to receive either brivanib or sorafenib treatment as first-line (BRISK-FL) [41]. The primary endpoint of overall survival non-inferiority for brivanib compared to sorafenib was not reached in this study. In the brivanib arm, the median overall survival was 9.5 months compared to 9.9 months in the sorafenib arm (HR = 1.06, 95% CI: 0.93-122, p = 0.3730). Disease control rates were similar between the two groups (65% with sorafenib and 66% with brivanib; 95% CI: 0.80-1.30, p = 0.8739). In term of safety, brivanib appeared to be less well-tolerated than sorafenib, since overall incidence of serious adverse events and rate of treatment discontinuation due to toxicity were higher in the brivanib group compared to the sorafenib group (56% *vs* 48% and 43% *vs* 33% respectively). Disappointing results were also observed with brivanib when used as a second line approach. In a large phase III study, 395 patients with advanced HCC and previously treated with sorafenib were randomized to receive either brivanib or placebo (BRISK-PS). The median overall survival in the brivanib cohort was 9.4 months compared to 8.2 months in the placebo cohort (HR = 0.89; 95% CI: = 0.69-1.15, p = 0.330) [42].

Negative results of this compound stress, once again, the need to improve the selection of the target population [43, 44]. As pointed out by Qi *et al.* [44], around 20% of patients included in these trials have early stage HCC while sorafenib was initially tested and approved in advanced HCC. Patients with early stage HCC had better prognosis, thus, it seems more difficult to achieve easily a significant difference regarding benefit between the two groups.

Linifanib (ABT6869, Abbott, New York, USA)

Linifanib is a new orally tyrosine kinase inhibitors targeting VEGF and PDGF receptor families. In the phase I study, doses of linifanib ≤ 0.25 mg/kg daily were identified as tolerable in 33 patients with solid tumors. In two patients with HCC, a sustained stable disease of 17 months was reported. Assessment with dynamic radiology tools, indicated a decrease in tumor vascular permeability and vascularity in correlation with the drug exposure [45].

Linifanib was tested in a phase II study that enrolled 44 patients (the majority were Asian) with advanced HCC and Child-Pugh A-B classes [46]. Linifanib was administrated at a daily dose of 0.25 mg/kg in Child-Pugh A patients and every other day in Child-Pugh B patients. For all the cohort, the 16 weeks progression-free rate was 31.8% (95% CI: 8.8%-47.6%). The median time-to-progression was 3.7 months (95% CI: 1.9-5.5 months) and the median overall survival was 9.7 months (95% CI: 6.0-12.2 months). The most frequent toxicities grade ≥ 3 were hypertension (25%) and fatigue (13.6%). One case of death possibly related to drug toxicity was reported. Regarding these early promising results, the efficacy and tolerability of linifanib at the dose of 17.5 mg/day was evaluated *versus* sorafenib in a large international randomized no-blinded phase III trial. In this study 1,035 patients with advanced HCC and well compensated cirrhosis were enrolled [47]. The trial was halted by the independent data monitoring committee since the primary endpoints of superiority and non-inferiority were not reached added to a significant high toxicity rate in the linifanib arm. Despite an objective response rate higher with linifanib compared to sorafenib (13% *vs* 6.9%), the median overall survival was lower in the linifanib arm (9.1 months *vs* 9.9, HR = 1.06, 95% CI: 0.93-1.22; p = 0.373). Treatment discontinuation, dose interruption and reduction due to severe toxicities were significantly higher in the linifanib group compared to sorafenib group.

Regorafenib (Stivarga®, BAY 73-4506, Bayer HealthCare, Leverkusen, Germany)

Regorafenib, a sorafenib analog (Fluoro-Sorafenib), is novel oral mulikinase inhibitor targeting VEGF1-3, PGFFR-β, FGFR, TIE-2, KIT, RET and RAF [48]. In preclinical *in vivo* models, regorafenib displayed antitumor activity in a broad range of tumor xenografts [48]. Recently, regorafenib showed a significant clinical benefit in patients with metastatic colorectal carcinoma who failed previous therapies [49] and in patients with gastro-intestinal stromal tumors who failed imatinib and sunitinib [50]. Regorafenib is currently approved by the FDA and EMA for these settings. The safety and efficacy of 160 mg/day of regorafenib (3 weeks on, 1 week off), was evaluated in a phase II study in HCC patients with progressive disease after sorafenib [51]. In this study, 36 patients were evaluable, the median time-to-progression was 4.3 months (95% CI: 2.9-13.1 months) and the median overall survival was 13.8 months (95% CI: 9.3-18.3 months). Common adverse events due to treatment were hand-foot skin syndrome, diarrhea, fatigue and anorexia. Noticeably, almost all patients (97%) experienced dose modification during the study.

Based on these promising early results, an international randomized, double blinded, phase III study, comparing regorafenib to placebo after sorafenib in patients with advanced HCC is currently conducted (NCT01774344).

EMERGING SMALL MOLECULES CURRENTLY EVALUATED IN PHASE II STUDIES

Axitinib (AG-013736; Pfizer, New York, NY, USA)

Axitinib is an oral small molecule tyrosine kinase inhibitor targeting VEGFR, PDGFR and KIT. Axitinib had been shown to display a robust preclinical activity in various models with selectivity and potency for VEGFR [52]. Noticeably, no cross-resistance between axitinib and other molecules was found since antitumor activity of axitinib was reported in patients with metastatic renal carcinoma who failed prior sunitinib, sorafenib and cytokines therapies [53]. Thus, it seems interesting to evaluate this compound in patients with advanced HCC following failure of one prior antiangiogenic therapy. A phase II trial testing axitinib as second line therapy is currently planned (NCT01273662).

Cediranib (Recentin®, AZD2171, AstraZeneca, Cambridge, UK)

AZD2171 is a potent oral tyrosine kinase inhibitor targeting VEFGR-1,-3, PDGFR and c-KIT. This small molecule showed antitumor activity in several human tumor xenograft models. In a phase I study, a daily dose of 45 mg or less of cediranib was suggested and showed encouraging antitumor effect in board range of advanced solid tumors [54]. Cediranib was evaluated in a two-stage phase II study in 28 patients with unresectable or metastatic HCC [55]. The 6 months survival rate was of 42.9% and the median overall survival was 5.8 months (95% CI: 3.4-7.3 months). The median time-to-progression was 2.8 months (95% CI: 2.3-4.4 months). The incidence of serious adverse events related to cediranib was particularly high in this trial. Almost all patients (93%) experienced adverse events grade ≥ 3 including fatigue (46%), anorexia (25%), hypertension (21%) and elevated transaminases (18%). The poor tolerability of this drug could be explained in part by a compromised metabolism due to the liver disease dysfunction. Thereby, another phase II study with a lower dose of cediranib (30 mg/day) was conducted in patients with advanced HCC and good hematologic, hepatic, and renal functions [56]. Even at this dose, cediranib was unable to achieve an antitumor activity with an acceptable safety profile. The median progression-free survival was 5.3 months (95% CI: 3.5-9.7) and the median overall survival was 11.7 months (95% CI: 7.5-13.6 months). Hepatic dysfunction did not seem to affect the steady-state pharmacokinetic of cediranib. However, as well as the first phase II study [55], the incidence of severe toxicities was high including hypertension (29%), hyponatremia (29%), and hyperbilirubinemia (18%) [56]. Therefore the high incidence of toxicity and the minimal clinical benefit will probably circumscribe the development of this molecule in HCC patients.

Orantinib (TSU-68, SU6668, Taiho Pharmaceutical Co., LTD. Japan)

TSU-68 is an oral tyrosine kinas inhibitor targeting the VEGFR-2, PDFGR and FGRF. In a coupled phase I/II Japanese study, TSU-68 was tested in HCC Child Pugh A and B patients [57]. Twice daily 200 mg of TSU-68 was the dosing recommended. Severe toxicities were observed in 11.4% of patients including transaminases elevation, and thrombocytopenia. The rate of objective response was 9.6% (2.9%: complete response and 5.7%: partial response: (5.7%) and stable disease achieved in less than half of patients (42.8%). The median progression-free survival was of 2.1 months contrasting with a surprising median overall survival of 13.1 months [57]. These optimistic results should be somehow interpreted with caution since some patients were not cirrhotic or did not have tumor poor prognosis factors (97% of patients without macrovascular invasion and about half of them with no extrahepatic spread). TSU-68 was also evaluated in a multicenter, open-label, randomized phase II study in patients with HCC and treated with a single session of trans-arterial chemoembolization. In this exploratory study, 103 patients were enrolled. TSU-68 tended to improve progression-free survival but without reaching significance compared to control group (157.0 days, 95% CI: 124-230 days in the experimental group and 122 days, 95% CI: 73.0-170 days in the control group; HR = 0.699, 95% CI: 0450-1.088). The most common severe toxicities were transaminases elevation, thrombocytopenia and fatigue. As mentioned by expert consensus [58, 59], the progression-free survival in this setting was not a relevant endpoint and time to progression should be preferred.

A randomized, double-blinded, placebo-controlled phase III trial of TSU-68 in combination with trans-arterial chemoembolization was planned but not yet recruiting (NCT01465464).

Lenvatinib (E7080, Eisai Co., Ltd, Tokyo, Japan)

Lenvatinib is another oral small molecule multikinase inhibitor targeting VEGFR-1-3, FGFR-1-4, RET, KIT and PDGFRβ. Recently, preliminary data from a phase I-II study evaluating lenvatinib in 49 HCC patients were reported [60]. The modified RECIST criteria (mRECIST) were used to assess the tumor response. Regarding the investigator assessment, 33% of patients achieved partial response. The most common severe toxicities were hypertension (48%), thrombocytopenia (19%) and proteinuria (14%).

Vandetanib (ZD6474, Zactima®, AstraZenica, London, UK)

Vandetanib is an orally potent inhibitor of VEGFR, EGFR and RET tyrosine kinases. In preclinical models and experimental setting, vandetanib showed an inhibitor effects on HCC cell proliferation adhesion, migration and invasion [61]. The efficacy and safety of vandetanib (300 mg and 100 mg once daily) were evaluated in 76 patients with advanced HCC enrolled in a II study [62]. Despite a good safety and tolerability profile, vandetanib showed very limited clinical activity in HCC.

"The future landscape for randomized phase II and III clinical trials of these compounds will be based on head-to-head comparison with sorafenib."

OTHER INNOVATIVE COMPOUNDS SELECTED IN PRECLINICAL MODELS AND UNDER EARLY EVALUATION

Pazopanib (Votrient®, GW786034, GlaxoSmithKline, Brentford, UK)

Pazopanib is an oral, second-generation multi-targeted tyrosine kinase inhibitor targeting VEGFR, PDGFR and c-KIT. Recently, this drug was endorsed by the FDA for treatment of patients with advanced renal carcinoma [63]. Pazopanib was tested in a phase I study with a modified 3+3 design in patients with advanced HCC [64]. The recommended dose was 600 mg twice daily in patients with advanced HCC. The most common related-adverse events ≥ grade 3, were hypertension (25%), transaminases elevation (22%) and diarrhea (4%). Among evaluable patients, partial response or stable disease was reported in 73% of patients. Therefore, pazopanib appears as a promising active drug and that shall deserve further clinical development in HCC.

Vatalanib (PTK787/ZK222584, Novartis-Bayer Schering Pharma, International)

Vatalanib is an orally potent and selective tyrosine kinase inhibitor of VEGFR and also blockades PDGFR and KIT at higher concentration. Vatalanib induced tumor cell apoptosis and decreased vessel formation. The hypoxia induced by ligation of the hepatic artery, enhanced the effect of vatalanib [65] which could support a potential role in combination with trans-arterial chemoembolization. In the phase I study, the suggested dose was 750 mg/day and a half of patients achieved stable [66]. The combination of vatalanib with doxorubicin for advanced HCC was evaluated in a phase I-II study [67]. In this study, the proportion of patients with Child-Pugh B was high (92.6%). The overall response rate was high reaching 26%, but this interesting result did not translate into a remarkable overall survival benefit (median overall survival: 7.3 months, range 0.8-23.6 months). Common serious adverse events were mucositis, alopecia and neutropenia. The development of vatalanib was not carried in HCC for pharmacological and marketing reasons.

BIBF 1120 (Vargatef, Boehringer Ingelheim; Ingelheim-Am-Rhein, Germany)

BIBF 1120 is an orally multikinase inhibitor targeting VEGFR, FGFR and PDGFR which showed antitumor activity by inducing growth arrest and reduced cell survival in cultures [68]. Because of the additional inhibition of FGFR over the VEGFR, the use of BIBF 1120 could be attractive to broader its activity. BIBF 1120 is currently compared to sorafenib in two independent phase II studies for advanced HCC in patients from Europe (NCT1004003) from Asia (NCT00987935).

HEPATOCYTE GROWTH FACTOR (HGF)/C-MET AXIS INHIBITORS

Tivantinib (ARQ 197, Daiichi Sankyo ArQule, Inc, Tokyo, Japan)

The MET pathway (c-MET and its ligand HGF) is disturbed in HCC and MET overexpression correlates with advanced tumor stage and poor prognosis [69].

Tivantinib is an orally small molecule, selective inhibitor of the MET receptor tyrosine kinase. In preclinical models, tivantinib showed antitumor activity in murine xenograft models and its efficacy was confirmed in a board of HCC cell lines [70, 71].

In a multicenter, single-arm, phase 1-b study in pretreated patients with advanced HCC, tivantinib showed preliminary antitumor activity and acceptable toxicity profile [72]. Recently, two doses of tivantinib were evaluated in a randomized, double-blind, placebo-controlled, phase II study including 107 patients with advanced HCC that have progressed on sorafenib. The time-to-progression with tivantinib was 1.6 months *vs* 1.4 months with placebo (HR = 0.64, 90% CI: 0.43-0.94, p = 0.04). The benefit of tivantinib was clearly noticeable in patients with overexpression of c-MET by immunohistochemistry analysis. In fact, patients with high-MET expression tumor showed longer median time-to-progression on tivantinib compared to patients on placebo (2.7 months *vs* 1.4 months; HR = 0.43, 95% CI: 0.19-097, p = 0.03). The median overall survival was 7.2 months on tivantinib while it was 3.8 months on placebo (HR = 0.38, 95% CI: 0.18-0.81; p = 0.01). Interestingly, tivantinib did not show any benefit in patient with low-MET expression tumor. The most common serious toxicities related to tivantinib were neutropenia and anemia [73].

This trial stresses the importance of biomarkers- selection patients to improve results of directed targeted therapy in HCC. Tivantinib is currently evaluated in an international, double-blind, randomized Phase III study in patients with advanced HCC and high-MET expression tumor in the second line setting (NCT01755767).

Foretinib (GSK1363089, EXEL-2880; XL-880, GlaxoSmithKline, Brentford, England)

Foretinib is also another selective inhibitor of c-MET and also inhibits VEGFR-2 tyrosine kinase. Dysregulation of c-MET pathway and its ligand HGF have been shown in HCC. Thus, targeting c-MET pathway seems to be an interesting option [74]. Likewise, in HCC specimens, the overexpression of c-MET correlates with more aggressive disease [75]. The precise role of this pathway in the pathogenesis of HCC is currently incompletely elucidated. In orthotropic transplant of HCC models, inhibition of the HGF/c-MET pathway induced tumor growth suppression and reduction of angiogenesis [76]. Foretinib also showed potential activity in HCC preclinical models since it induced inhibition of tumor angiogenesis, tumor cell proliferation and metastasis [77]. While numerous inhibitors of MET are under development [78], only a few number is under recent investigation in patients with advanced HCC.

Cabozantinib (XL184; Exelixis, Inc. USA)

Cabozantinib is a small molecule tyrosine kinases inhibitor targeting c-MET and VEGFR-2. This compound showed some efficacy in a phase II study that enrolled 41 patients with advanced HCC [79, 80]. Among evaluable patients, most common severe adverse events due to treatment were hand-foot reaction, diarrhea and thrombocytopenia. The overall disease control rate at week 12 was 71% and the median progression-free survival was 4.2 months. Unlike the tivantinib-trial, MET expression was not reported in this study. Cabozantinib is currently evaluated in a phase III, randomized, double-blind, controlled study for patients with advanced HCC in a second-line setting (NCT01908426).

MONOCLONAL ANTIBODY ANTI-VEGF AGENT: BEVACIZUMAB

Bevacizumab (Avastin® Genentech Inc., South San Francisco, CA) is a recombinant, humanized monoclonal antibody targeting directly the VEGF. Bevacizumab was currently approved for treatment of colorectal cancer, renal cell carcinoma, breast carcinoma and non-small cell lung cancer. In orthotopic mouse model, bevacizumab reduced significantly microvessel density and disease progression [81].

Two phase II studies assessed bimonthly intravenous bevacizumab at the dose of 5mg/kg or 10 mg/kg in patients with advanced HCC [82, 83]. Siegle *et al.,* reported a partial response rate of 13% (95% CI: 3%-23%) and disease stabilization for at least 6 months of 65%. In this study, the median progression-free survival was 6.9 months (95% CI: 6.5-9.1 months). The median overall survival was 12.4 months (95% CI: 9.4-19.9 months) and almost quarter of patients (23%) had prolonged survival over 3 years [82]. Similar results were reported the French study [83], since 14% and 42% of included patients experienced respectively partial response and stable disease ≥ 16 weeks. The median progression-free survival was 3 months (95% CI: 2-4 months) and the median overall survival was 8 months (95% CI: 4-9 months). The 6 months and 12 months overall survival rates were 63% and 30%, respectively [83]. Interestingly, high baseline levels of IL-8 and IL-6 impact negatively on patient's prognosis in this study.

These exciting results should be lessened since patients with advanced HCC with poor prognosis factors (CLIP score > 3 [83], tumor liver involvement > 50%, vascular invasion and metastatic [82]) were excluded. Therefore, outcome and natural history of the included patients in these trials could be intrinsically better. Moreover, serious adverse events including bleeding (11%), arterial thromboembolism (6%) and hypertension (15%) were observed.

Bevacizumab associated to standard chemotherapies was also tested in phase II studies [84-86]. Combined to gemcitabine and oxaliplatine (GEMOX), Bevacizumab yielded an objective response rate of 20% among 33 patients enrolled in a phase II study. The median overall survival time 9.6 months [84]. Noticeably, GEMOX alone had shown nearby results in the multicenter French experience with response rate of 22% and median overall survival time of 11 months [87]. Therefore, probably adding bevacizumab to GEMOX did not improve dramatically survival with advanced HCC.

A recent systemic review showed evidence of antitumor activity of bevacizumab in HCC [88], but these early results should be confirmed carefully by further large studies. Probably for marketing reasons, nowadays no phase III studies were conducted to evaluate bevacizumab in HCC worldwide.

MONOCLONAL ANTIBODIES AGAINST VEGFR-2: RAMUCIRUMAB

Ramucirumab (IMC61121b, Cyramza®, ImClone LLC, New Jersey, USA) is a recombinant human monoclonal antibody blocking specifically VEGFR-2. This compound has been tested in a phase II trial enrolling 42 naïve patients with advanced HCC [89]. Ramucirumab was associated with an objective response rate of 9.5%, a median progression-free survival of 4.0 months (95% CI: 2.6-5.7 months) and a median overall survival of 12.0 months (85% CI: 2.6-5.7 months). Ramucirumab showed safe profile and the most common severe adverse events were hypertension (14%), gastrointestinal bleeding (7%), infusion-related reactions (7%) and fatigue (5%). Interestingly and consistent with other anti-VEGF agents, ramucirumab increased the circulating levels of VEGF and PlGF in patients with HCC [89].

MONOCLONAL ANTIBODIES ANTI-EGFR: CETUXIMAB

Cetuximab (Erbitux®, C225, ImClone LLC, New Jersey, USA) is a chimeric monoclonal antibody inhibitor of EGFR. This compound is currently approved for treatment of colorectal cancer and head and neck cancer. Cetuximab alone has been evaluated in patients with HCC across two phase II trials [90, 91]. Zhu *et al.*, [90] reported a median overall survival of 9.6 months and a median progression-free survival of 1.4 months. Independently, the second study showed that 44.4% of patients experienced stable disease for at least 8 weeks with a median progression-free survival of 1.8 months [91]. Results of these two trials are contradictory and the place of cetuximub in HCC treatment remains unclear. Cetuximab was also evaluated in combination to cytotoxic chemotherapy: capecitabine plus oxaliplatine (CAPOX) and GEMOX regimens. These combinations did not show any additional efficacy [92, 93]. Therefore, Cetuximab will never be developed in patients with advanced HCC.

EGFR TYROSINE KINASES INHIBITORS: ERLOTINIB, GEFITINIB, LAPATINIB

Erlotinib (Tarceva®, OSI-774, Genentech, South San Francisco, USA) is an orally potent and specific tyrosine kinase inhibitor of EGFR/HER1. This compound was evaluated alone for patients with advanced HCC in two phase II studies. In the first study, 59% of patients experienced disease control and the median overall survival was 13 months. Most common related adverse-events were cutaneous rash, diarrhea and fatigue [94]. These optimizing results should be temporized since 42% of patients enrolled had no underlying liver disease [94]. In the second study, a progression-free survival at 4 months was observed in 43% of patients and the median overall survival was 10.75 months. In this trial, the authors did not observe any correlation between EGFR expression and overall survival [95].

The SEARCH study, an international randomized placebo-controlled, double-blind phase III trial evaluated the combination of erlotinib and sorafenib compared to sorafenib and placebo as first-line option in patients with advanced HCC. Results of this large trial were disappointing since no benefit was observed when erlotinib was added to sorafenib. In this study, a total of 720 patients with advanced HCC and good liver function were enrolled. The overall survival in patients treated with the combining therapy was 9.5 months compared to 8.5 months in the control group (HR = 0.93, 95% CI: 0.78-1.11, p = 0.204). No statistically significant difference was observed regarding time to progression between the two arms (3.2 months in the sorafenib plus erlotinib group *vs* 4.0 months in the control group, HR = 1.14, 95% CI: 0.94-1,37, p = 0.91) [96].

In a phase II trial, bevacizumab combined to erlotinib showed provocative results since the median time-to-progression, was 9 months and the median overall survival was 15.6 months. The most common adverse events were fatigue (20%), hypertension (15%) and gastrointestinal hemorrhage (12.5%) [97]. These exciting results could be somehow explained by the enrollment of patients with less advanced HCC [3]. Similar results of another phase II study were reported in 59 patients treated with weekly bevacizumab plus daily erlotinib. The median progression-free survival was 7.2 months (95% CI: 5.6-8.3) and median overall survival was 13.7 months (95% CI: 9.6-19.7) [98]. However, Philipp *et al.* [99] showed recently that the combination erlotinib and bevacizumab had moderate activity in patient with advanced HCC, since the median time-to-disease progression was 3.0 months (95% CI: 1.8-7.1) and the median overall survival was 9.5 months. Erlotinib combined to bevacizumab are currently compared to sorafenib as first line in a phase II study (NCT00881751) and also evaluated as second line therapy (NCT01180959).

Gefitinib (Iressa®, ZD1839, AstraZeneca, London, UK) is another tyrosine kinase inhibitor of EGFR. This compound was also evaluated in patients with advanced HCC in a phase II trial [100]. In the first stage of the study, 31 patients were recruited, 3% and 22.6% of patients experienced objective response and stable disease objective respectively. The median progression-free survival was 2.8 months and the median overall survival was 6.5 months. Gefitinib as single agent seems to be not effective in patients with advanced HCC [100], because of a probable crosstalk between the IGF-1R and the EGF signaling pathways [101]. One explanation of resistance to gefitinib seems to be a possible activation of alternative pathways leading tumor survival and proliferation [101, 102]. Combining IGF-1R to EGFR inhibitors could be an option to circumvent the resistance mechanism [103, 104].

Lapatinib (TYKERB®, GW572016, GlaxoSmithKline, Brentford, UK) is an orally inhibitor of the EGFR and the Human EGFR type 2 (HER-2/NEU). In a phase II study, lapatinib at the dose of 1,500 mg/day was evaluated in patients with advanced HCC [105]. Among 25 patients evaluable for response, stable disease was observed in 10 patients (40%) including prolonged tumor stabilization more than 1 year for 8% of patients. The median progression-free survival and overall survival were 1.9 months and 12.6 months respectively. Grade-3 drug-related toxicities including diarrhea, rash and acute renal failure were reported in 11.5% of patients. In this study, skin rash probably correlated with better outcome [105]. A second phase II study tested continuously 1,500 mg/day of lapatinib in patients with HCC and advanced biliary cancer. In the HCC patients group, the objective response rate was 5% and 35% of patients achieved stable disease. The median progression-free survival was 2.3 months and median overall survival was 6.2 months. Treatment was generally well tolerated and the most frequent adverse events were diarrhea (7%), asthenia (6%) and transaminase elevation (9%) [106].

Mammalian Target of Rapamycin Signaling and other Potential Pathways

Rapamycin (sirolimus, Pfizer, Inc, New York, USA) is an inhibitor of m-TOR kinase with potent immunosuppressive and antiproliferative properties and direct and indirect antiangiogenic effects. Several levels of the PI3K/AKT/m-TOR pathway might be blockaded but the most interesting target remains the m-TOR. In rat and xenograft models of HCC, inhibition of the m-TOR pathway by rapamycin or **everolimus** (RAD001, Novartis, Basel, Switzerland)) induced reduced HCC growth and stressed the important role of this pathway in angiogenesis [107, 108]. Moreover, rapamycin displayed an acceptable safety profile and achieved long disease stabilization in selected patients with advanced HCC heavily pretreated [109]. Sirolimus as a single agent was evaluated in two pilot studies [110, 111].

In the first study, 21 and 9 patients with advanced HCC and cholangiocarcinoma respectively were treated with a median dose of 1 mg/day of sirolimus [110]. In the HCC patient's cohort, only one patient experienced partial response and 5 patients achieved tumor stabilization more than 3 months. Following sirolimus introduction, the median, overall survival was 6.5 months (0.2-35.8 months). The treatment was overall well tolerated and no toxicities grade $\geq$3 were reported in HCC patients [110]. In the other phase II study, 25 patients received orally sirolimus (at the dose of 20 mg/week for one month and then 30 mg/week) [111]. Based on RECIST criteria, objective response and disease stabilization were observed in 89% and 32% of patients respectively. In this study, the median time-to-radiological progression and the median overall survival were 15.3 week (8.2-173.9 weeks) and 26.4 weeks (8.2-173.9 weeks) respectively. The most frequent severe toxicities related to sirolimus were infections (8%) thrombocytopenia (8%), interstitial pneumopathy (4%) and mucositis (4%) [111].

Zhu *et al.* [112] tested everolimus in patients with advanced HCC across a phase I-II study and suggested that 10 mg/day was the safe dose. Following this recommended dose, 25 patients with advanced HCC were enrolled. Only one patient in this cohort achieved partial response. Everolimus yielded a median progression-free survival of 3.8 months (85% CI: 2.1-4.6 months) and median overall survival of 8.4 months (95% CI: 3.9-21.1 months) [112].

Recently, disappointing results of the large randomized, placebo-controlled phase III trial (EVOLVE-1), testing the everolimus in patients with advanced HCC as a second line approach after sorafenib, were reported. Everolimus did not improve overall survival in patients whose disease progressed on or after sorafenib or who were intolerant to sorafenib [113]. In fact, the median overall survival on everolimus was 7.56 months compared to 7.33 months on placebo (HR = 1.05, 95% CI: 0.86-1.27, p = 0.675). No significant difference was also detected regarding the median time-to-progression (2.96 months *vs* 2.60 months, HR = 0.93, 95% CI: 0.75-1.15).

TARGETING THE RAF/MEK/ERK SIGNALING PATHWAY

The Raf/MEK/ERK pathway is an important cellular signaling pathway for the development and preservation of HCC [114, 115]. This pathway has been shown to be active in more than 50% of human HCC [116]. In preclinical models of human HCC, selumetinib (AZD6244, AstraZeneca, London, UK), a specific MEK inhibitor, combined to rapamycin induced a potent tumor growth suppression and angiogenesis [117]. Additionally, in orthotopic and ectopic HCC models, the antitumor activity of sorafenib was enhanced by the AZD6244, supporting a potential advantage to combine these agents [118]. However; in clinical setting, selumetinib alone failed to improve the outcome of patients with advanced HCC. Indeed, results of the phase II study testing selumetinib in HCC patients were unreliable since median-time-to progression was 8 weeks [119]. Shen *et al.*, suggested that selected inhibition of MAPK pathway could be insufficient and ineffective for the treatment of advanced HCC [114].

INSULIN-LIKE GROWTH FACTOR-1 RECEPTOR (IGF-1R) INHIBITORS

Investigating the IGFR inhibitors in HCC appears to be interesting. Indeed, it was shown that the IGF axis was disturbed in HCC and implicated in the hepatocarcinogenesis [120, 121]. Overexpression and increased activation of the IGF-1R was described in 33% and about half of HCC, respectively [103]. In Human HCC cell lines, inhibition of the IGF-1R induced tumor growth suppression [104, 122]. Several agents targeting IGF-1R are currently under early clinical development. AVE 1642 combined to sorafenib in a phase I study showed a safe profile in 13 patients with advanced HCC and yielded prolonged disease stabilization in 11 patients [123].

TARGETING WNT-β-CATENIN PATHWAY

The Wnt-ß-catenin pathway is particularly implicated in HCC. Laurent-Puig *et al.* [124] showed that activation of the Wnt/wingless pathway was present in 20% to 30% of HCC and ß-catenin mutation was found in about 20% of HCC [124]. Some drugs targeting the Wnt-ß-catenin pathway are currently tested in early clinical studies but no one is enough developed. Blockade the Wnt-ß-catenin by efficient molecules seems to be rather complex [125].

TRANSFORMING GROWTH FACTOR-BETA (TGF-β)

TGF-ß signaling was associated with progression of HCC and was involved in epithelial to mesenchymal transformation (EMT), cancer stem cells and T-regulatory cells [126, 127]. Usually, in normal liver, TGF-ß is not active, however its level was stimulated due to acute damage and chronic liver disease and the level increase proportionally to the disease severity [128]. TGF-ß signaling may be present in 25% of early HCC [127]. In a recent review, Giannelli *et al.* [129] showed that showed that TGF-ß regulates in HCC numerous steps in tumor progression, angiogenesis and immune suppression regulates numerous steps in tumor progression, angiogenesis, and immune suppression. High levels of TGF-β correlate with aggressive and metastatic HCC [129].

Therefore, inhibition of TGF-β signaling could prevent proliferation, invasion, metastasis and progression. Recently, Faivre *et al.* [130] communicated results of the phase II study exploring LY2157299, a selective inhibitor of TGF-β receptor-1, in patients with HCC previously treated with sorafenib. In this study, 109 patients were enrolled and randomized to receive intermittent dosing of LY2157299 for 14 days followed by 07 days off (37 patients with daily dosing of 160 mg and 72 patients with daily dosing of 300 mg). The treatment was well tolerated and the most frequent serious toxicities related to the drug were: neutropenia (2.8%), anemia (2.8%) and fatigue (1.8%). In 24% of patients, serum AFP levels were decreased by more than 20% compared with baseline. Treatment benefit appears more evident in this sub-group of patients compared to those with no AFP response since time-to-progression was 18.6 weeks and median overall survival was 91.3 weeks compared to 6.6 week and 29.6 weeks [130]. Further investigations were needed to identify the role of TGF-β signaling inhibitors in HCC treatment.

FUTURE PERSPECTIVES OF EMERGING THERAPIES IN HCC

Resistance to Sorafenib: A Real Concern

Despite sorafenib represents a major accomplishment in treatment of advanced HCC after several years of "therapeutic desert", practitioners are confronted daily to the problem of primary or acquired resistance to sorafenib. Treatment resistance affects obviously all malignancies, but it is particularly problematic in the case of HCC because of the lack of validated alternative treatment. Mechanisms of resistance are various including genetic and epigenetic dysregulations, reactive resistance, and stimulation of alternative signaling pathways [115, 131]. Intratumor heterogeneity could also explain mechanism of acquired resistance to sorafenib or other targeted therapy in tumors [132]. In case of disease progression on sorafenib, Americans and Europeans experts suggest either supportive care or inclusion in clinical trials evaluating new drugs [133, 134]. In real-life condition, it seems more difficult for patients and practitioner to propose best supportive care, especially for patients with good performance status and compensated cirrhosis. For these selected patients, a second line therapy is generally required and the participation in clinical trials appears more appropriate. After failure of sorafenib, standard chemotherapies such GEMOX could be an option as showed by some groups [135, 136]. Continuing sorafenib even in case of confirmed progression could be another option in selected patients [131, 137]. Pressiani *et al.* [138] evaluated 1200 mg/day of sorafenib *versus* best supportive care in 101 patients treated with standard dosing of sorafenib and experienced disease progression. In this study, continuing higher dose of sorafenib compared to best supportive care did not show any clinical benefit. In fact, the median overall survival was similar between the two groups (6.1 *versus* 6.0 months; 95% CI: 0.47-1.11, $p = 0.14$) [138].

Combining Therapies: From Concept to Clinical Scale

Regarding the low objective response achieved with single agent targeted therapy, the combined approach either by using several target therapies or with conventional cytotoxic drugs aims to improve clinical response. Albeit, this approach remains a complex matter, to circumvent tumor resistance and to reach additive/synergistic effects without adding concerning interactions or toxicities [139]. Preclinical data support this hypothesis and provide strong rational for clinical investigation of those combinations in HCC patients. Works of Huynh and colleagues provided several preclinical illustrations by impairing the antiangiogenic activity of rapamycin when associated to sorafenib [22], to the MEK inhibitor AZD6244 [117], or bevacizumab [140]. These combinations expanded inhibition of HCC growth in animal models when compared to single agent therapies. Furthermore, several pathways such AKT, IGF and HGF/c-MET pathways frequently compensate the effect of antiangiogenic therapies and this could lead, at least partially, to the development of drug resistance [141].

Currently, it is clearly established that crosstalk exist between various levels of different signaling pathways implicated in HCC. Resistance to targeted molecules could be reversed by simultaneous inhibition of alternative pathways. Therefore, combination strategies mainly aim optimizing inhibition of the more relevant signaling pathway or inhibiting several alternative signaling pathways [115, 142], either by horizontal blockade toward different pathways or by vertical blockade toward the same pathway. Horizontal blockade *via* parallel may target VEGF and FGF signaling pathways (*i.e.* combining brivanib with vandetanib), or VEGF and EGFR signaling pathways (*i.e.* combining bevacizumab with erlotinib) or VEGR and IGF-1R inhibitors (*i.e.* combining sorafenib with AVE1664) or IGF-1R and EGFR. Vertical blockade that targets Raf and MAKP with sorafenib combined to AZDD6244 may be beneficial *via* both parallel (antiangiogenesis and MAPK inhibition) and vertical (simultaneous targeting of Raf and MAPK) [114]. As described above, promising results were observed in patients with HCC when the VEGF and EGFR axis were targeted [97]. Several small studies evaluating sorafenib in combination with other treatments did not show excessive toxicity [143]. As described above, the combination of erlotinib to sorafenib did not show any clinical benefit in patients with advanced HCC [96].

Although combination approach in patients with HCC patients is theoretically feasible, caution is warranted especially in this population weakened by the underlying liver disease. Combination approach warrants further elucidation in well-designed clinical studies.

Combining Targeted Therapy and Locoregional Therapies: Rationale and Purposes

Combining molecularly targeted drugs and locoregional therapies, such as trans-arterial chemoembolization (TACE), hinge on strong rationale [144]. Indeed, in orthotopic HCC models, combining artery ligation and VEGF inhibitor improved significantly the outcome through ischemic hypoxia and inhibition of angiogenesis preventing tumor regrowth [65]. In patients with advanced HCC, elevated levels of VEGF after TACE were shown associated with distant metastasis and short survival [145]. Moreover, several proangiogenic factors such as VEGF and b-FGF have been shown to be transitory increased after TACE though embolization-induced hypoxia [146, 147]. Based on these data, adding targeted therapy may inhibit proangiogenic factors raised by the loco-regional treatment and therefore enhance its outcome [115]. These hypothesizes are currently being analyzed through several clinical trials evaluating sorafenib, brivanib and sunitinib in association to locoregional therapy.

In a prospective mono-center phase II study, combination of sorafenib to TACE using doxorubicin-eluting beads (DEB-TACE) yielded interesting results in term of efficacy. Response assessment by RECIST criteria showed disease control and objective response in 95% and 58% of patients respectively. However, in this study, sorafenib dose adaptation (either reduction or interruption) was generally needed to manage toxicities [148]. In another prospective, single-arm phase II, evaluating sorafenib combined to conventional TACE, sorafenib dosing was reduced in 70% of patients because of toxicities drug-related. This combination showed also some promising results since the median time-to-progression was 7.1 months (95% CI: 4.8-7.5 months) and the 6 months progression-free survival rate was 52% (95% CI: 37.3-66.1%) [149]. A phase III trial assessed the efficacy and safety of sorafenib combined to TACE *versus* TACE alone in Japanese and Korean patients with non-resectable HCC. The combination did not demonstrate any benefit for this population [150]. Overall, the combination approach for patients with advanced HCC seems to be benefit in terms of time-to-progression but not regarding overall survival [151]. Some considerations were not yet resolved concerning this combination such as the timing of sorafenib introduction, the adequate schedule and sequence of the combination and the appropriate assessment tools [152]. Therefore, further well-designed randomized controlled trials are needed to endorse the efficacy of molecular targeted drugs associated to loco-regional therapies.

Targeted Therapies in Advanced Liver Disease

The sorafenib obtained FDA and EMA approval with no precise restriction regarding the Child-Pugh class. In the clinical experience and published data, the efficacy of this compound is clearly compromised when liver function is altered mainly in patients with Child-Pugh C cirrhosis. Although tolerability seems to be similar in patients Child-Pugh A or B [23], the clinical benefit appears lower in patients with advanced liver disease [153-155]. In a first retrospective study, 59 patients (Child-Pugh A-B,-C: 26, 23, 10 respectively) with advanced HCC, have been treated initially with standard dose of sorafenib. In the intention to treat, median overall survival for patients Child-Pugh A, B, and C were 8.3, 4.3 and 1.5 months 1.5 respectively ($p = 0.0001$). The authors advised against the use of sorafenib in patients with very advanced liver disease [153]. In the other retrospective cohort, among 50 patients with HCC treated with sorafenib, 17 (34%) were Child-Pugh B. This subgroup of patients benefited less of sorafenib since the median overall survival was 2 months compared to 8.9 months in patients Child-Pugh A ($p = 0.004$) [154]. The lower exposure to sorafenib may explain the lack of benefit since the duration of treatment was lower in Child-Pugh B patients due to worse tolerability (1.8 *vs* 5 months, $p = 0.02$). Finally, in a third report, 120 patients with advanced HCC were treated with sorafenib. The overall survival time was significantly higher in patients Child-Pugh A compared to those Child-Pugh B (13 *vs* 4.5 months, $p = 0.0008$). Therefore, treatment with sorafenib could be considered with caution in patients Child-Pugh B since they have naturally worse prognosis [155]. It is noticeable that sorafenib and almost targeted therapies are metabolized by the liver, predominantly by CYP3A4, and liver dysfunction may alter their pharmacokinetic features and may affect their tolerability by interacting with non-tumor liver. Otherwise, no significant differences in sorafenib pharmacokinetics were detected between patients Child

Pugh A and B classes [23, 156]. Taken the example of sunitinib, limited inter-patients variability was generally observed. However, inter-individual variation could be detected that could explain in some cases the under/overexposures to sunitinib and thus minimal activity and higher toxicities [26].

Miller *et al.* [156] recommended a reduction of sorafenib dosing at 400mg/day for patients with bilirubin plasma levels > 1.5 times but ≤ 3 times the upper limit of normal (ULN). For patients with bilirubin plasma levels > 3 times, even 200 mg every three days was not tolerated.

Additionally, sorafenib and several targeted therapy are bound to plasma protein with high affinity (*i.e.* 99.5% for sorafenib). Therefore, hypoalbuminemia may affect its bioavailability and then its exposure and its tolerability. The tolerance of sorafenib is expected to be worse in patients with albumin plasma levels lower than 2.5 g/l [156].

Based on these results, sorafenib use in patients with advanced liver dysfunction should be handled with precaution and balanced by the lack of efficiency. Severe adverse events will probably enforce dose reduction, adaptation of schedule, treatment interruption, and management of complications. Thereby, the expected drug efficacy will be impaired. Unfortunately, as the prognosis of the disease depends in a vast proportion on liver deterioration and decompensation, large prospective study in this setting seems superfluous at least for patients Child-Pugh C and advanced Child-Pugh B.

Perspectives from Targeted Therapy in Adjuvant and Neo-Adjuvant Settings

Patients with early HCC stage could benefit from curative treatment however; the outcome can be hampered by recurrences (30-40%) or secondary primary tumors (60-70%) [157]. Recurrence rates after resection may reach 50% and 80% at 2 and 5 years respectively [158], with a 5-year survival limited to 50% [159] even in the case of early stage without portal venous invasion or satellite nodules [160]. Since recurrences compromise dramatically overall survival [161], preventing or delaying relapse after curative treatments has become a major challenge. Previously, several approaches using transarterial chemotherapy, systemic chemotherapy, retinoids, interferon, adoptive immunotherapy, and intra-arterial radioactive lipiodol [157] have been explored as adjuvant therapies in clinical trials with the aim of reducing relapses. The overall benefit was almost anecdotal, thus none of these agents has been adopted as adjuvant treatment in routine practice. As described above, angiogenesis was shown to play a major role in HCC tumorigenesis including growth and metastasis [11, 13], and high VEGF levels have been associated with tumor cell proliferation, venous invasion, and poor prognosis following resection [13, 162]. Positive results obtained with sorafenib in patients with advanced HCC [1, 2] raised the expectation of using this agent in early HCC stage following local ablation and surgery. The synergistic effect of sorafenib with local ablation was observed in nude mice bearing human xenografts. Sorafenib showed a dramatic decrease of microvascular density along with an increase of the area of radiofrequency-induced coagulation necrosis. The extent of radiofrequency-induced necrosis was thought to prevent hyperemia resulting from the inflammation surrounding necrosis, and therefore to limit the occurrence of relapses at the periphery of treated lesions [163].

The hypothesis that sorafenib could reduce tumor recurrence after resection or local ablation was investigated through an international randomized, placebo-controlled phase III trial (STORM, NCT00692770) evaluating 4-year sorafenib *versus* placebo. The primary objective of this trial is recurrence-free survival, secondary objectives being overall survival and safety. Recently, Bruix *et al.* [164] communicated results of the STORM trial at the ASCO 2014. Overall 1,114 patients were randomized to receive either sorafenib or placebo at adjuvant therapy. The study did not met its primary and secondary endpoints since no differences were observed regarding recurrence-free survival (33.4 *vs* 33.8 months; HR = 0.94; 95% CI: 0.78-1.13, p = 0.26), time to recurrence (38.6 vs 35.8 months; HR = 0.89, 95% CI: 0.73-1.08) and overall survival (not reached *vs* not reached, HR = 0.99, 95% CI: 0.76-1.30, p = 0.48) [164].

Expectations in preventing HCC recurrence using targeted therapies may appear as a real challenge since several signaling inhibitors have recently failed showing benefit when used in adjuvant setting in other cancers [165] (*i.e.* bevacizumab or cetuximab in combination with standard chemotherapy as adjuvant setting in colorectal cancers).

Exploring sorafenib and future novel targeted therapies in adjuvant setting requires large randomized clinical trials including patients stratified for high or low risks of recurrence. Additionally, results should be analyzed to distinguish early local recurrence from new primary and metastasis. The cost-effectiveness of such strategy should be balanced by the overall clinical benefit of targeted molecules in this setting. Finally, the better knowledge of HCC biology will certainly help designing trials with future targeted therapies by identifying critical signaling pathways driving tumor growth and angiogenesis.

Likewise, little data were reported regarding sorafenib or others targeted therapies in neoadjuvant setting for HCC. Trials with targeted therapies in advanced setting frequently mitigate the feasibility of efficient translational research [166]. Factors preventing performing such translational research are technical limitation and ethically concerns in performing repeated tumor biopsies in large heterogeneous tumors with potential area of necrosis in patients with restricted life expectancy [167]. Tumor heterogeneity at later stages may be associated with multiple crosstalk and redundant pathways yielded confusing results. Subsequently, a substitute strategy would be to assess new agents in a preoperative "window" setting [166] immediately prior to surgical resection for patient who shall undergo curative surgery (Fig. **2**). This approach allows obtaining paired biopsy samples before treatment and at the moment of diagnosis and to reevaluate the effects of therapies by investigating biological changes occurring in tumor tissues at time of surgery. This setting allows also assessing predictive biomarkers of response that may help to identify subgroups of patients most likely to respond to these therapies as well as patients likely developing primary resistance [167].

The safety of liver resection following sorafenib administration was reported in a French multicenter study including 23 patients with HCC [168]. The incidence of postoperative complications was similar between patients treated with sorafenib and a control group (44 % *vs* 59 %, $p = 0.307$). Similarly, safety data of neoadjuvant sorafenib treatment were reported in 30 patients with renal cell carcinoma [169]. In this cohort, two patients met RECIST criteria for partial response and no patients achieved complete response. However, evaluation of tumor viability using a modification of the Choi criteria showed a decrease in intratumor density of a median of 13% in 88% of evaluable patients. Surgery has been feasible for all patients with no surgical complications related to sorafenib [169]. Currently, the antitumor effect of sorafenib is evaluated in a phase II study including patients with operable HCC (NCT01182272).

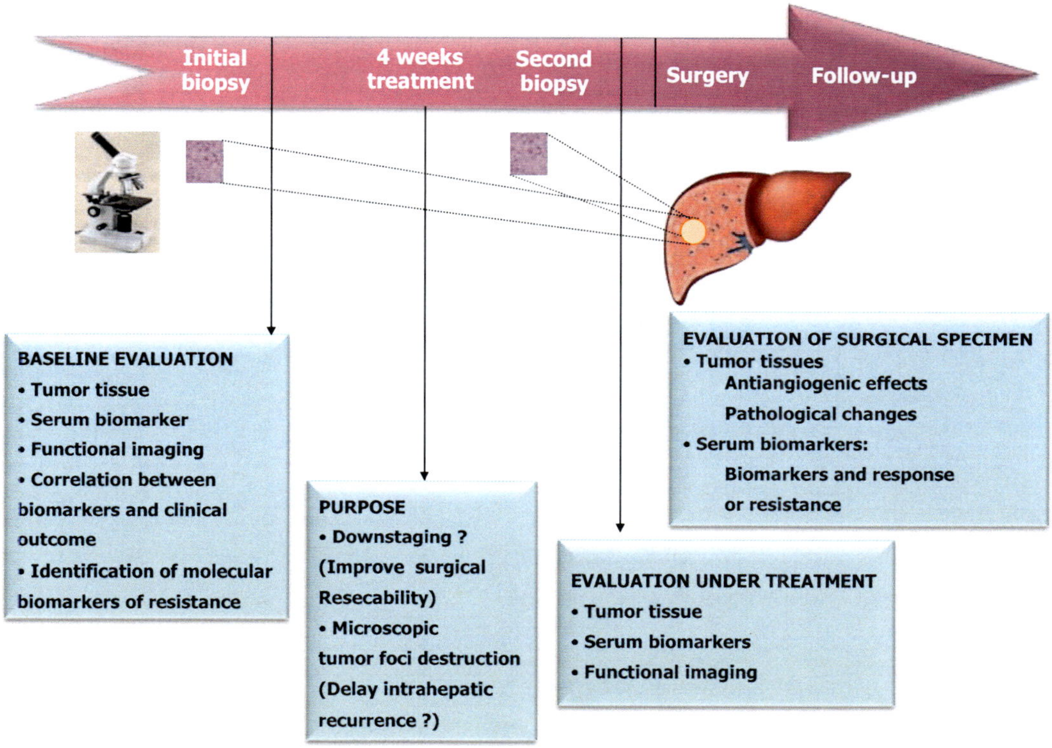

Fig. (2). Schematic illustration and proposal approach for translational research. Sorafenib has been selected because it is currently evaluated before surgery in patients with resectable HCC.

Neoadjuvant therapy aims eventually to reduce the tumor mass, to facilitate technical surgery procedure and to destroy microscopic foci responsible of intrahepatic recurrences [170]. Downstaging the primary tumor is an attractive objective to improve tumor resecability. Despite sorafenib is not always expected to induce tumor-size reduction, it might however participate to a better disease-control before surgery resulting from tumor growth inhibition. Furthermore, it is expected that sorafenib may induce a decrease in intratumor vessels and blood flow in the central part of the tumor, subsequently inducing central tumor necrosis according to its antiangiogenic propriety. Moreover, it is possible that sorafenib may prevent tumor cell dissemination during liver surgery since the liver is being manipulated during surgical procedure. Since the mechanisms of action of sorafenib are complex, it seems interesting to identify the respective role of direct antitumor effects on HCC cells *versus* antiangiogenic effects. This could be achieved by comparing morphological and biological changes in tissue sample prior and after treatment. This setting also allows assessing predictive biomarkers of response that may identify subgroups of patients most likely to respond to treatment as well as patients likely to develop-primary resistance.

The Fig. (**2**) summarizes the conceptual approach of translational research, inspired from the phase II study evaluating sorafenib in patients with resectable HCC (NCT01182272).

Challenges and Limits for Development of New Compounds in HCC

Based on preliminary data of earlier clinical trials, innovative multitargeted agents in development appear to be active in HCC, although, for many, the clinical importance of this activity has not been so far proved. This evolution is promising but the challenge currently is to guarantee that the full potential of multi-targeted agents is achieved by recognizing the most active and safe dose and schedules administration necessarily in suitably selected patients. In the last five years, 80% of phase III clinical trials with targeted agents tested in HCC were negative [132]. It is noteworthy that some of these compounds have shown antitumor activities in HCC animal models. Despite the advantages of these models, they may not reflect accurately human HCC and underlying disease such as chronic inflammatory and fibrosis environment. Given the complexity of faithful reproduction of signaling pathways of HCC, the disease is often addressed at advanced stage with large and multifocal tumor. Furthermore, several molecular aberrations are implicated in HCC. Reproduction of all these specific abnormalities in preclinical models is very complex if even achievable [171]. On the other hand, underlying liver disease could be impaired by several drugs that have potential hepatotoxicity. Liver enzyme perturbations and/or liver dysfunction under targeted therapy are

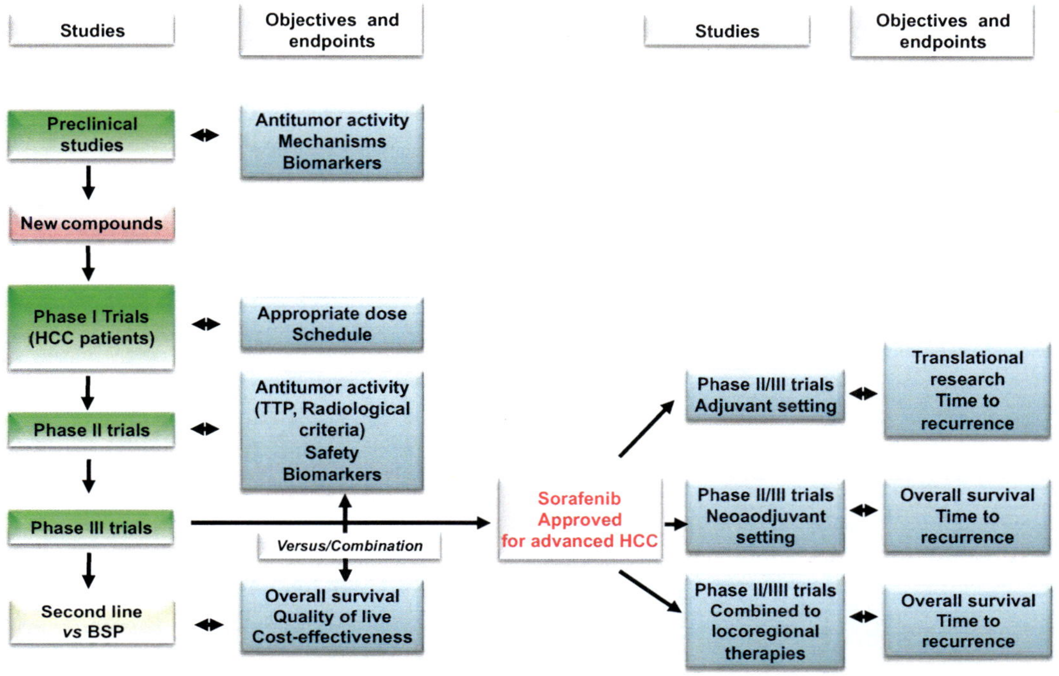

Fig. (3). Summary of trials designs for sorafenib and new compounds under development in hepatocellular carcinoma. List of abbreviations: BSC: best supportive care.

under targeted therapy are troublesome for clinicians. It seems tremendously tricky to establish a relationship between liver disorders and drug toxicities, severity of underlying liver disease, cirrhosis decompensation or tumor-related factors of progression. In HCC and as well as other cancers, drug development has become very complex; multiorganization-based and financially-orientated [172]. Among all drugs under early development, only few will reach further development [173]. Discrepancies can be observed regarding clinical benefit of different emerging drugs in HCC. Heterogeneity of selected patients and disease, (for example patients enrolled in Asian clinical trials testing systemic therapies have often more advanced diseases [174]) imposed standardized guidelines from a panel expert in HCC [58, 59]. The purposes were to homogenize the studied population, to define advanced disease stage and to standardize the trial designs and endpoints. Novel drugs explored in phase II studies should consider time-to-progression as first endpoint; nevertheless, overall survival represents the final endpoint to assess efficiency of targeted therapy investigated in phase III trials. The personalized medicine should be stressed to conduct appropriate phase III trials testing new compounds based on tumor activation or their expected targets [36, 132]. One of the best examples of this approach in HCC is the phase III trial evaluating brivanib in HCC patients with tumoral overexpression of MET.

Finally, sorafenib could be proposed as the control arm for new compounds evaluated in future phase III studies. Some proposals for development of new compounds in patients with HCC are illustrated in Fig. (**3**).

CONCLUSION

Sorafenib was considered as a foremost breakthrough in the field of HCC management. It is the dawn of an exciting new era, with wide open fields of horizons and challenges. Broadening the place of this compound in diverse settings and positioning other innovative agents is fascinating physicians. The competition spirit for all these new agents will be undeniably very beneficial enlarging the therapeutic armamentarium for HCC in a near future. It is wanted that undergoing studies will elucidate some of the issues related to potential combinations and novels compounds. Challenge should be accepted and new drugs should satisfy equilibrium between cost-effectiveness, quality of life, tolerability and safety.

EXECUTIVE SUMMARY

HCC is known to be highly vascularized tumor in which angiogenesis is crucial for its development, survival and progression. Several distrusting signaling pathways affecting cell growth and differentiation are involved in the tumorigenesis of HCC. Thus, this disease offers a large field to investigate plethora of drugs blocking different molecular and vascular disorders.

Sorafenib -an antiangiogenic and antiproliferative compound- had created an authentic revolution in the management of advanced HCC. The approval of sorafenib emphasized the validated concept for targeting molecular receptors and upset signaling pathways involved in this disease. Moreover, the encouraging results of sorafenib opened the competition for other innovative compounds, implicating a majority if not all pharmacological firms, intending to gain their implication in HCC.

Despite this breakthrough, many challenging features for sorafenib and other innovative drugs remain unsolved. First, several disturbed pathways are implicated in hepatocarcinogenesis; and further works are needed to identify key targets for streamline treatment in HCC. The better knowledge of HCC biology will undoubtedly help designing trials with future targeted therapies by identifying critical signaling pathways driving tumor growth and angiogenesis. Second, the effectiveness of concomitant or sequential combination of these compounds to block several targets requires confirmation alongside preclinical models and early clinical evaluation. Moreover, using these compounds in patients with advanced liver disease should be well defined in further studies.

Third, exploring sorafenib and future novel targeted therapies in adjuvant setting requires large randomized clinical trials including patients stratified for high or low risks of recurrence. Results should be analyzed to distinguish early local recurrence from new primary and metastasis. The cost-effectiveness and the development of new compounds in assorted strategies should be balanced by the overall clinical benefit of targeted molecules in different landscapes.

Fourth, there is an unmet need to identify surrogate biomarkers that distinguish subgroups of patients who will benefit from such therapies, to delimit the optimum biological dose and to identify early resistance to treatment. Ideally, "à la carte" therapy may be proposed for patients with advanced HCC in the future. Since sensibility and resistance to these therapies are insufficiently known, translational research will undeniably play a major role for future optimization of these promising therapies. Objective responses according to RECIST criteria are particularly low with such drugs, therefore new radiological methods especially functional imaging warrant validation in further large trials.

Finally, due to the complexity of HCC, treatment decisions need multidisciplinary team including hepatologists, oncologists, interventional radiologists and liver surgeons [175]. This multidisciplinary approach aims to improve management and outcome of patients with HCC [176]. Furthermore, only well-designed phase II and III clinical studies, as described in this chapter, may resolve some urgent requests in this population.

LIST OF ABBREVIATIONS

c-Kit	=	Stem-cell factor receptor
EGF	=	Epidermal-Growth Factor
EGFR	=	Epidermal-Growth Factor Receptor
EMA	=	European Medicines Agency
FDA	=	Food and Drug Administration
FGF	=	Fibroblast-Growth Factor
Flt-3	=	Fmts-Like Tyrosine kinase-3
HCC	=	Hepatocellualar Carcinoma
HER	=	Human Epidermal growth factor Receptor
HGF	=	Hepatocyte-Growth Factor
IGF	=	Insulin-like Growth Factor
IGF-1R	=	Insulin-like Growth Factor-1 Receptor (IGF-1R)
PDGF	=	Platelet-Growth Factor Receptor
PI3K/AKT/mTOR	=	Phosphatidylinositol 3-Kinase/Akt/mammalian Target of Rapamycin
RECIST	=	Response Evaluation Criteria in Solid Tumors
RET	=	Rearranged during Transfection
TACE	=	Trans-Arterial Chemo-Embolization
TGF-α	=	Transforming-Growth Factor-α
TGF-ß	=	Transforming-Growth Factor-ß
VEGF	=	Vascular Endothelial-Growth-Factor
VEGFR	=	Vascular Endothelial-Growth Factor Receptor

ACKNOWLEDGEMENTS

None declared.

CONFLICT OF INTEREST

Mohamed Bouattour has received occasional honoraria for speaking and travel grants from Bayer Pharma.

REFERENCES

[1] Llovet JM, Ricci S, Mazzaferro V, *et al.* Sorafenib in advanced hepatocellular carcinoma. N Engl J Med 2008; 359: 378-90.

[2] Cheng A-L, Kang Y-K, Chen Z, *et al.* Efficacy and safety of sorafenib in patients in the Asia-Pacific region with advanced hepatocellular carcinoma: a phase III randomised, double-blind, placebo-controlled trial. Lancet Oncol 2009; 10: 25-34.

[3] Faivre S, Bouattour M, Raymond E. Novel molecular therapies in hepatocellular carcinoma. Liver Int 2011; 31 Suppl 1: 151-60.

[4] Mathurin P, Rixe O, Carbonell N, *et al.* Review article: Overview of medical treatments in unresectable hepatocellular carcinoma--an impossible meta-analysis? Aliment Pharmacol Ther 1998; 12: 111-26.

[5] Qin S, Bai Y, Lim HY, *et al.* Randomized, multicenter, open-label study of oxaliplatin plus fluorouracil/leucovorin *versus* doxorubicin as palliative chemotherapy in patients with advanced hepatocellular carcinoma from Asia. J Clin Oncol 2013; 31: 3501-8.

[6] Farazi PA, DePinho RA. Hepatocellular carcinoma pathogenesis: from genes to environment. Nat Rev Cancer 2006; 6: 674-87.

[7] Pang RWC, Poon RTP. From molecular biology to targeted therapies for hepatocellular carcinoma: the future is now. Oncology 2007; 72 Suppl 1: 30-44.

[8] Hoshida Y, Toffanin S, Lachenmayer A, Villanueva A, Minguez B, Llovet JM. Molecular classification and novel targets in hepatocellular carcinoma: recent advancements. Semin Liver Dis 2010; 30: 35-51.

[9] Llovet JM, Bruix J. Molecular targeted therapies in hepatocellular carcinoma. HEPATOLOGY 2008; 48: 1312-27.

[10] Thomas MB, Abbruzzese JL. Opportunities for targeted therapies in hepatocellular carcinoma. J Clin Oncol 2005; 23: 8093-108.

[11] Poon RT-P, Ng IO-L, Lau C, *et al.* Tumor microvessel density as a predictor of recurrence after resection of hepatocellular carcinoma: a prospective study. J Clin Oncol 2002; 20: 1775-85.

[12] Yoshiji H, Kuriyama S, Yoshii J, *et al.* Vascular endothelial growth factor tightly regulates *in vivo* development of murine hepatocellular carcinoma cells. HEPATOLOGY 1998; 28: 1489-96.

[13] Poon RTP, Ho JWY, Tong CSW, Lau C, Ng IOL, Fan S-T. Prognostic significance of serum vascular endothelial growth factor and endostatin in patients with hepatocellular carcinoma. Br J Surg 2004; 91: 1354-60.

[14] Moon WS, Rhyu KH, Kang MJ, *et al.* Overexpression of VEGF and angiopoietin 2: a key to high vascularity of hepatocellular carcinoma? Mod Pathol 2003; 16: 552-7.

[15] Chow NH, Hsu PI, Lin XZ, *et al.* Expression of vascular endothelial growth factor in normal liver and hepatocellular carcinoma: an immunohistochemical study. Hum Pathol 1997; 28: 698-703.

[16] Harada K, Shiota G, Kawasaki H. Transforming growth factor-alpha and epidermal growth factor receptor in chronic liver disease and hepatocellular carcinoma. Liver 1999; 19: 318-25.

[17] Huether A, Höpfner M, Baradari V, Schuppan D, Scherübl H. EGFR blockade by cetuximab alone or as combination therapy for growth control of hepatocellular cancer. Biochem Pharmacol 2005; 70: 1568-78.

[18] Höpfner M, Sutter AP, Huether A, Schuppan D, Zeitz M, Scherübl H. Targeting the epidermal growth factor receptor by gefitinib for treatment of hepatocellular carcinoma. J Hepatol 2004; 41: 1008-16.

[19] Villanueva A, Chiang DY, Newell P, *et al.* Pivotal role of mTOR signaling in hepatocellular carcinoma. Gastroenterology 2008; 135: 1972-83.

[20] Schmitz KJ, Wohlschlaeger J, Lang H, *et al.* Activation of the ERK and AKT signalling pathway predicts poor prognosis in hepatocellular carcinoma and ERK activation in cancer tissue is associated with hepatitis C virus infection. J Hepatol 2008; 48: 83-90.

[21] Liu L, Cao Y, Chen C, *et al.* Sorafenib blocks the RAF/MEK/ERK pathway, inhibits tumor angiogenesis, and induces tumor cell apoptosis in hepatocellular carcinoma model PLC/PRF/5. Cancer Res 2006; 66: 11851-8.

[22] Huynh H, Ngo VC, Koong HN, *et al.* Sorafenib and rapamycin induce growth suppression in mouse models of hepatocellular carcinoma. J Cell Mol Med 2009; 13: 2673-83.

[23] Abou-Alfa GK, Schwartz L, Ricci S, *et al.* Phase II study of sorafenib in patients with advanced hepatocellular carcinoma. J Clin Oncol 2006; 24: 4293-300.

[24] Lencioni R, Kudo M, Ye S-L, *et al.* First interim analysis of the GIDEON (Global Investigation of therapeutic decisions in hepatocellular carcinoma and of its treatment with sorafeNib) non-interventional study. Int J Clin Pract 2012; 66: 675-83.

[25] Lencioni R, Kudo M, Ye S-L, *et al.* GIDEON (Global Investigation of therapeutic DEcisions in hepatocellular carcinoma and of its treatment with sorafeNib): second interim analysis. Int J Clin Pract 2013; 68: 609-17.

[26] Faivre S, Demetri G, Sargent W, Raymond E. Molecular basis for sunitinib efficacy and future clinical development. Nat Rev Drug Discov 2007; 6: 734-45.

[27] Raymond E, Dahan L, Raoul J-L, *et al.* Sunitinib malate for the treatment of pancreatic neuroendocrine tumors. N Engl J Med 2011; 364: 501-13.

[28] Huynh H, Ngo VC, Choo SP, *et al.* Sunitinib (SUTENT, SU11248) suppresses tumor growth and induces apoptosis in xenograft models of human hepatocellular carcinoma. Curr Cancer Drug Targets 2009; 9: 738-47.

[29] Faivre S, Raymond E, Boucher E, *et al.* Safety and efficacy of sunitinib in patients with advanced hepatocellular carcinoma: an open-label, multicentre, phase II study. Lancet Oncol 2009; 10: 794-800.

[30] Zhu AX, Sahani DV, Duda DG, *et al.* Efficacy, safety, and potential biomarkers of sunitinib monotherapy in advanced hepatocellular carcinoma: a phase II study. J Clin Oncol 2009; 27: 3027-35.

[31] Koeberle D, Montemurro M, Samaras P, *et al.* Continuous Sunitinib treatment in patients with advanced hepatocellular carcinoma: a Swiss Group for Clinical Cancer Research (SAKK) and Swiss Association for the Study of the Liver (SASL) multicenter phase II trial (SAKK 77/06). Oncologist 2010; 15: 285-92.

[32] Cheng A-L, Kang Y-K, Lin D-Y, *et al.* Sunitinib *versus* sorafenib in advanced hepatocellular cancer: results of a randomized phase III trial. J Clin Oncol 2013; 31: 4067-75.

[33] Faivre SJ, Bouattour M, Dreyer C, Raymond E. Sunitinib in hepatocellular carcinoma: redefining appropriate dosing, schedule, and activity end points. J Clin Oncol 2009; 27: e248-250.

[34] Finn RS. Emerging targeted strategies in advanced hepatocellular carcinoma. Semin Liver Dis 2013; 33 Suppl 1: S11-19.

[35] Sablin M-P, Dreyer C, Colichi C, *et al.* Benefits from pharmacological and pharmacokinetic properties of sunitinib for clinical development. Expert Opin Drug Metab Toxicol 2010; 6: 1005-15.

[36] Villanueva A, Hernandez-Gea V, Llovet JM. Medical therapies for hepatocellular carcinoma: a critical view of the evidence. Nat Rev Gastroenterol Hepatol 2013; 10: 34-42.

[37] Huynh H, Ngo VC, Fargnoli J, *et al.* Brivanib alaninate, a dual inhibitor of vascular endothelial growth factor receptor and fibroblast growth factor receptor tyrosine kinases, induces growth inhibition in mouse models of human hepatocellular carcinoma. Clin Cancer Res 2008; 14: 6146-53.

[38] Bhide RS, Lombardo LJ, Hunt JT, *et al.* The antiangiogenic activity in xenograft models of brivanib, a dual inhibitor of vascular endothelial growth factor receptor-2 and fibroblast growth factor receptor-1 kinases. Mol Cancer Ther 2010; 9: 369-78.

[39] Park J-W, Finn RS, Kim JS, *et al.* Phase II, open-label study of brivanib as first-line therapy in patients with advanced hepatocellular carcinoma. Clin Cancer Res 2011; 17: 1973-83.

[40] Finn RS, Kang Y-K, Mulcahy M, *et al.* Phase II, open-label study of brivanib as second-line therapy in patients with advanced hepatocellular carcinoma. Clin Cancer Res 2012; 18: 2090-8.

[41] Johnson PJ, Qin S, Park J-W, *et al.* Brivanib *versus* sorafenib as first-line therapy in patients with unresectable, advanced hepatocellular carcinoma: results from the randomized phase III BRISK-FL study. J Clin Oncol 2013; 31: 3517-24.

[42] Llovet JM, Decaens T, Raoul J-L, *et al.* Brivanib in patients with advanced hepatocellular carcinoma who were intolerant to sorafenib or for whom sorafenib failed: results from the randomized phase III BRISK-PS study. J Clin Oncol 2013; 31: 3509-16.

[43] Kelley RK. Brivanib and FOLFOX in hepatocellular carcinoma: finding the common themes among negative trials. J Clin Oncol 2013; 31: 3483-6.

[44] Qi X, Jia J, Fan D, Han G. Brivanib for Hepatocellular Carcinoma Trials: Selection Bias From Barcelona Clinic Liver Cancer Stage? J Clin Oncol 2014; 32: 968.

[45] Wong C-I, Koh T-S, Soo R, *et al.* Phase I and biomarker study of ABT-869, a multiple receptor tyrosine kinase inhibitor, in patients with refractory solid malignancies. J Clin Oncol 2009; 27: 4718-26.

[46] Toh HC, Chen P-J, Carr BI, *et al.* Phase 2 trial of linifanib (ABT-869) in patients with unresectable or metastatic hepatocellular carcinoma. Cancer 2013; 119: 380-7.

[47] Cainap C, Qin S, Huang W-T, *et al.* Phase III trial of linifanib *versus* sorafenib in patients with advanced hepatocellular carcinoma (HCC). J Clin Oncol 2013; 31: Abstract 249.

[48] Wilhelm SM, Dumas J, Adnane L, *et al.* Regorafenib (BAY 73-4506): a new oral multikinase inhibitor of angiogenic, stromal and oncogenic receptor tyrosine kinases with potent preclinical antitumor activity. Int J Cancer 2011; 129: 245-55.

[49] Grothey A, Van Cutsem E, Sobrero A, *et al.* Regorafenib monotherapy for previously treated metastatic colorectal cancer (CORRECT): an international, multicentre, randomised, placebo-controlled, phase 3 trial. Lancet 2013; 381: 303-12.

[50] Demetri GD, Reichardt P, Kang Y-K, *et al.* Efficacy and safety of regorafenib for advanced gastrointestinal stromal tumours after failure of imatinib and sunitinib (GRID): an international, multicentre, randomised, placebo-controlled, phase 3 trial. Lancet 2013; 381: 295-302.

[51] Bruix J, Tak W-Y, Gasbarrini A, *et al.* Regorafenib as second-line therapy for intermediate or advanced hepatocellular carcinoma: Multicentre, open-label, phase II safety study. Eur J Cancer 2013; 49: 3412-9.

[52] Hu-Lowe DD, Zou HY, Grazzini ML, *et al.* Nonclinical antiangiogenesis and antitumor activities of axitinib (AG-013736), an oral, potent, and selective inhibitor of vascular endothelial growth factor receptor tyrosine kinases 1, 2, 3. Clin Cancer Res 2008; 14: 7272-83.

[53] Rini BI, Wilding G, Hudes G, *et al.* Phase II study of axitinib in sorafenib-refractory metastatic renal cell carcinoma. J Clin Oncol 2009; 27: 4462-8.

[54] Drevs J, Siegert P, Medinger M, *et al.* Phase I clinical study of AZD2171, an oral vascular endothelial growth factor signaling inhibitor, in patients with advanced solid tumors. J Clin Oncol 2007; 25: 3045-54.

[55] Alberts SR, Fitch TR, Kim GP, *et al.* Cediranib (AZD2171) in patients with advanced hepatocellular carcinoma: a phase II North Central Cancer Treatment Group Clinical Trial. Am J Clin Oncol 2012; 35: 329-33.

[56] Zhu AX, Ancukiewicz M, Supko JG, *et al.* Efficacy, safety, pharmacokinetics, and biomarkers of cediranib monotherapy in advanced hepatocellular carcinoma: a phase II study. Clin Cancer Res 2013; 19: 1557-66.

[57] Kanai F, Yoshida H, Tateishi R, *et al.* A phase I/II trial of the oral antiangiogenic agent TSU-68 in patients with advanced hepatocellular carcinoma. Cancer Chemother Pharmacol 2011; 67: 315-24.

[58] Thomas MB, Jaffe D, Choti MM, *et al.* Hepatocellular carcinoma: consensus recommendations of the National Cancer Institute Clinical Trials Planning Meeting. J Clin Oncol 2010; 28: 3994-4005.

[59] Llovet JM, Di Bisceglie AM, Bruix J, *et al.* Design and endpoints of clinical trials in hepatocellular carcinoma. J Natl Cancer Inst 2008; 100: 698-711.

[60] Okita K, Kumada H, Ikeda K, *et al.* Phase I/II study of E7080 (lenvatinib), a multitargeted tyrosine kinase inhibitor, in patients (pts) with advanced hepatocellular carcinoma (HCC): Initial assessment of response rate. J Clin Oncol 2012; 30: Abstract 320.

[61] Giannelli G, Azzariti A, Sgarra C, Porcelli L, Antonaci S, Paradiso A. ZD6474 inhibits proliferation and invasion of human hepatocellular carcinoma cells. Biochem Pharmacol 2006; 71: 479-85.

[62] Hsu C, Yang T-S, Huo T-I, *et al.* Vandetanib in patients with inoperable hepatocellular carcinoma: a phase II, randomized, double-blind, placebo-controlled study. J Hepatol 2012; 56: 1097-103.

[63] Motzer RJ, Hutson TE, Cella D, *et al.* Pazopanib *versus* sunitinib in metastatic renal-cell carcinoma. N Engl J Med 2013; 369: 722-31.

[64] Yau T, Chen P-J, Chan P, *et al.* Phase I dose-finding study of pazopanib in hepatocellular carcinoma: evaluation of early efficacy, pharmacokinetics, and pharmacodynamics. Clin Cancer Res 2011; 17: 6914-23.

[65] Yang ZF, Poon RTP, Liu Y, *et al.* High doses of tyrosine kinase inhibitor PTK787 enhance the efficacy of ischemic hypoxia for the treatment of hepatocellular carcinoma: dual effects on cancer cell and angiogenesis. Mol Cancer Ther 2006; 5: 2261-70.

[66] Koch I, Baron A, Roberts S, *et al.* Influence of hepatic dysfunction on safety, tolerability, and pharmacokinetics (PK) of PTK787/ZK 222584 in patients (Pts) with unresectable hepatocellular carcinoma (HCC). J Clin Oncol 2005; 23: Abstract 4134.

[67] Yau T, Chan P, Pang R, Ng K, Fan ST, Poon RT. Phase 1-2 trial of PTK787/ZK222584 combined with intravenous doxorubicin for treatment of patients with advanced hepatocellular carcinoma: implication for antiangiogenic approach to hepatocellular carcinoma. Cancer 2010; 116: 5022-9.

[68] Hilberg F, Roth GJ, Krssak M, *et al.* BIBF 1120: triple angiokinase inhibitor with sustained receptor blockade and good antitumor efficacy. Cancer Res 2008; 68: 4774-82.

[69] Kondo S, Ojima H, Tsuda H, *et al.* Clinical impact of c-Met expression and its gene amplification in hepatocellular carcinoma. Int J Clin Oncol 2013; 18: 207-13.

[70] Munshi N, Jeay S, Li Y, *et al.* ARQ 197, a novel and selective inhibitor of the human c-Met receptor tyrosine kinase with antitumor activity. Mol Cancer Ther 2010; 9: 1544-53.

[71] Previdi S, Abbadessa G, Dalò F, France DS, Broggini M. Breast cancer-derived bone metastasis can be effectively reduced through specific c-MET inhibitor tivantinib (ARQ 197) and shRNA c-MET knockdown. Mol Cancer Ther 2012; 11: 214-23.

[72] Santoro A, Simonelli M, Rodriguez-Lope C, *et al.* A Phase-1b study of tivantinib (ARQ 197) in adult patients with hepatocellular carcinoma and cirrhosis. Br J Cancer 2013; 108: 21-4.

[73] Santoro A, Rimassa L, Borbath I, *et al.* Tivantinib for second-line treatment of advanced hepatocellular carcinoma: a randomised, placebo-controlled phase 2 study. Lancet Oncol 2013; 14: 55-63.

[74] Takami T, Kaposi-Novak P, Uchida K, *et al.* Loss of hepatocyte growth factor/c-Met signaling pathway accelerates early stages of N-nitrosodiethylamine induced hepatocarcinogenesis. Cancer Res 2007; 67: 9844-51.

[75] Osada S, Kanematsu M, Imai H, Goshima S. Clinical significance of serum HGF and c-Met expression in tumor tissue for evaluation of properties and treatment of hepatocellular carcinoma. Hepatogastroenterology 2008; 55: 544-9.

[76] Son G, Hirano T, Seki E, *et al.* Blockage of HGF/c-Met system by gene therapy (adenovirus-mediated NK4 gene) suppresses hepatocellular carcinoma in mice. J Hepatol 2006; 45: 688-95.

[77] Qian F, Engst S, Yamaguchi K, *et al.* Inhibition of tumor cell growth, invasion, and metastasis by EXEL-2880 (XL880, GSK1363089), a novel inhibitor of HGF and VEGF receptor tyrosine kinases. Cancer Res 2009; 69: 8009-16.

[78] Comoglio PM, Giordano S, Trusolino L. Drug development of MET inhibitors: targeting oncogene addiction and expedience. Nat Rev Drug Discov 2008; 7: 504-16.

[79] Cohn AL, Kelley RK, Yang T-S, *et al.* Activity of cabozantinib (XL184) in hepatocellular carcinoma patients (pts): Results from a phase II randomized discontinuation trial (RDT). J Clin Oncol 2012; 30: Abstract 261.

[80] Verslype C, Cohn AL, Kelley RK, *et al.* Activity of cabozantinib (XL184) in hepatocellular carcinoma: Results from a phase II randomized discontinuation trial (RDT). J Clin Oncol 2012; 30: Abstract 4007.

[81] Finn RS, Bentley G, Britten CD, Amado R, Busuttil RW. Targeting vascular endothelial growth factor with the monoclonal antibody bevacizumab inhibits human hepatocellular carcinoma cells growing in an orthotopic mouse model. Liver Int 2009; 29: 284-90.

[82] Siegel AB, Cohen EI, Ocean A, *et al.* Phase II trial evaluating the clinical and biologic effects of bevacizumab in unresectable hepatocellular carcinoma. J Clin Oncol 2008; 26: 2992-8.

[83] Boige V, Malka D, Bourredjem A, *et al.* Efficacy, safety, and biomarkers of single-agent bevacizumab therapy in patients with advanced hepatocellular carcinoma. Oncologist 2012; 17: 1063-72.

[84] Zhu AX, Blaszkowsky LS, Ryan DP, *et al.* Phase II study of gemcitabine and oxaliplatin in combination with bevacizumab in patients with advanced hepatocellular carcinoma. J Clin Oncol 2006; 24: 1898-903.

[85] Sun W, Sohal D, Haller DG, *et al.* Phase 2 trial of bevacizumab, capecitabine, and oxaliplatin in treatment of advanced hepatocellular carcinoma. Cancer 2011; 117: 3187-92.

[86] Hsu C-H, Yang T-S, Hsu C, *et al.* Efficacy and tolerability of bevacizumab plus capecitabine as first-line therapy in patients with advanced hepatocellular carcinoma. Br J Cancer 2010;102:981-6.

[87] Zaanan A, Williet N, Hebbar M, *et al.* Gemcitabine plus oxaliplatin in advanced hepatocellular carcinoma: a large multicenter AGEO study. J Hepatol 2013; 58: 81-8.

[88] Fang P, Hu J, Cheng Z, Liu Z, Wang J, Jiao S. Efficacy and safety of bevacizumab for the treatment of advanced hepatocellular carcinoma: a systematic review of phase II trials. PloS One 2012; 7: e49717.

[89] Zhu AX, Finn RS, Mulcahy M, *et al.* A phase II and biomarker study of ramucirumab, a human monoclonal antibody targeting the VEGF receptor-2, as first-line monotherapy in patients with advanced hepatocellular cancer. Clin Cancer Res 2013; 19: 6614-23.

[90] Zhu AX, Stuart K, Blaszkowsky LS, *et al.* Phase 2 study of cetuximab in patients with advanced hepatocellular carcinoma. Cancer 2007; 110: 581-9.

[91] Gruenwald V, Wilkens L, Gebel M, *et al.* A phase II open-label study of cetuximab in unresectable hepatocellular carcinoma: Final results. J Clin Oncol 2007; 25: 4598.

[92] Asnacios A, Fartoux L, Romano O, *et al.* Gemcitabine plus oxaliplatin (GEMOX) combined with cetuximab in patients with progressive advanced stage hepatocellular carcinoma: results of a multicenter phase 2 study. Cancer 2008; 112: 2733-9.

[93] Sanoff HK, Bernard S, Goldberg RM, *et al.* Phase II Study of Capecitabine, Oxaliplatin, and Cetuximab for Advanced Hepatocellular Carcinoma. Gastrointest Cancer Res 2011; 4: 78-83.

[94] Philip PA, Mahoney MR, Allmer C, *et al.* Phase II study of Erlotinib (OSI-774) in patients with advanced hepatocellular cancer. J Clin Oncol 2005; 23: 6657-63.

[95] Thomas MB, Chadha R, Glover K, *et al.* Phase 2 study of erlotinib in patients with unresectable hepatocellular carcinoma. Cancer 2007; 110: 1059-67.

[96] Zhu AX, Rsomorduc, Olivier, Evans J, *et al.* SEARCH: a phase III, randomized, double-blind, placebo-controlled trial of sorafenib plus erlotinib in patients with hepatocellular carcinoma (HCC). Ann Oncol 2012; 23: Abstract LBA2.

[97] Thomas MB, Morris JS, Chadha R, *et al.* Phase II trial of the combination of bevacizumab and erlotinib in patients who have advanced hepatocellular carcinoma. J Clin Oncol 2009; 27: 843-50.

[98] Kaseb AO, Garrett-Mayer E, Morris JS, *et al.* Efficacy of bevacizumab plus erlotinib for advanced hepatocellular carcinoma and predictors of outcome: final results of a phase II trial. Oncology 2012; 82: 67-74.

[99] Philip PA, Mahoney MR, Holen KD, *et al.* Phase 2 study of bevacizumab plus erlotinib in patients with advanced hepatocellular cancer. Cancer 2012; 118: 2424-30.

[100] O'Dwyer PJ, Giantonio BJ, Levy DE, Kauh JSW, Fitzgerald DB, Benson AB. Gefitinib in advanced unresectable hepatocellular carcinoma: Results from the Eastern Cooperative Oncology Group's Study E1203. J Clin Oncol 2006; 24: Abstract 4143.

[101] Desbois-Mouthon C, Cacheux W, Blivet-Van Eggelpoël M-J, *et al.* Impact of IGF-1R/EGFR cross-talks on hepatoma cell sensitivity to gefitinib. Int J Cancer 2006; 119: 2557-66.

[102] Wheeler DL, Dunn EF, Harari PM. Understanding resistance to EGFR inhibitors-impact on future treatment strategies. Nat Rev Clin Oncol 2010; 7: 493-507.

[103] Desbois-Mouthon C, Baron A, Blivet-Van Eggelpoël M-J, *et al.* Insulin-like growth factor-1 receptor inhibition induces a resistance mechanism *via* the epidermal growth factor receptor/HER3/AKT signaling pathway: rational basis for cotargeting insulin-like growth factor-1 receptor and epidermal growth factor receptor in hepatocellular carcinoma. Clin Cancer Res 2009; 15: 5445-56.

[104] Höpfner M, Huether A, Sutter AP, Baradari V, Schuppan D, Scherübl H. Blockade of IGF-1 receptor tyrosine kinase has antineoplastic effects in hepatocellular carcinoma cells. Biochem Pharmacol 2006; 71: 1435-48.

[105] Bekaii-Saab T, Markowitz J, Prescott N, *et al.* A multi-institutional phase II study of the efficacy and tolerability of lapatinib in patients with advanced hepatocellular carcinomas. Clin Cancer Res 2009; 15: 5895-901.

[106] Ramanathan RK, Belani CP, Singh DA, *et al.* A phase II study of lapatinib in patients with advanced biliary tree and hepatocellular cancer. Cancer Chemother Pharmacol 2009; 64: 777-83.

[107] Semela D, Piguet A-C, Kolev M, *et al.* Vascular remodeling and antitumoral effects of mTOR inhibition in a rat model of hepatocellular carcinoma. J Hepatol 2007; 46: 840-8.

[108] Huynh H, Chow KHP, Soo KC, *et al.* RAD001 (everolimus) inhibits tumour growth in xenograft models of human hepatocellular carcinoma. J Cell Mol Med 2009;13:1371-80.

[109] Bouattour M, Wassermann J, Dreyer C, *et al.* Rapamycin in patients with advanced hepatocellular carcinoma progressing on prior antiangiogenic therapy. J Clin Oncol 2012; 30: Abstract 356.

[110] Rizell M, Andersson M, Cahlin C, Hafström L, Olausson M, Lindnér P. Effects of the mTOR inhibitor sirolimus in patients with hepatocellular and cholangiocellular cancer. Int J Clin Oncol 2008;13: 66-70.

[111] Decaens T, Luciani A, Itti E, *et al.* Phase II study of sirolimus in treatment-naive patients with advanced hepatocellular carcinoma. Dig Liver Dis 2012; 44: 610-6.

[112] Zhu AX, Abrams TA, Miksad R, *et al.* Phase 1/2 study of everolimus in advanced hepatocellular carcinoma. Cancer 2011; 117: 5094-102.

[113] Zhu AX, Kudo M, Assenat E, *et al.* EVOLVE-1: Phase 3 study of everolimus for advanced HCC that progressed during or after sorafenib. J Clin Oncol 2014; 32: Abstract 172.

[114] Shen Y-C, Hsu C, Cheng A-L. Molecular targeted therapy for advanced hepatocellular carcinoma: current status and future perspectives. J Gastroenterol 2010; 45: 794-807.

[115] Shin JW, Chung Y-H. Molecular targeted therapy for hepatocellular carcinoma: current and future. World J Gastroenterol WJG 2013; 19: 6144-55.

[116] Calvisi DF, Ladu S, Gorden A, *et al.* Ubiquitous activation of Ras and Jak/Stat pathways in human HCC. Gastroenterology 2006; 130: 1117-28.

[117] Huynh H. AZD6244 (ARRY-142886) enhances the antitumor activity of rapamycin in mouse models of human hepatocellular carcinoma. Cancer 2010; 116: 1315-25.

[118] Huynh H, Ngo VC, Koong HN, *et al.* AZD6244 enhances the anti-tumor activity of sorafenib in ectopic and orthotopic models of human hepatocellular carcinoma (HCC). J Hepatol 2010;52:79-87.

[119] O'Neil BH, Goff LW, Kauh JSW, *et al.* Phase II study of the mitogen-activated protein kinase 1/2 inhibitor selumetinib in patients with advanced hepatocellular carcinoma. J Clin Oncol 2011;29:2350-6.

[120] Scharf J-G, Braulke T. The role of the IGF axis in hepatocarcinogenesis. Horm Metab Res 2003; 35: 685-93.

[121] Tovar V, Alsinet C, Villanueva A, *et al.* IGF activation in a molecular subclass of hepatocellular carcinoma and pre-clinical efficacy of IGF-1R blockage. J Hepatol 2010; 52: 550-9.

[122] Cantarini MC, de la Monte SM, Pang M, *et al.* Aspartyl-asparagyl beta hydroxylase over-expression in human hepatoma is linked to activation of insulin-like growth factor and notch signaling mechanisms. HEPATOLOGY 2006; 44: 446-57.

[123] Faivre SJ, Fartoux L, Bouattour M, *et al.* A phase I study of AVE1642, a human monoclonal antibody-blocking insulin-like growth factor-1 receptor (IGF-1R), given as a single agent and in combination with sorafenib as first-line therapy in patients with advanced hepatocellular carcinoma (HCC). J Clin Oncol 2011; 29: 270.

[124] Laurent-Puig P, Legoix P, Bluteau O, *et al.* Genetic alterations associated with hepatocellular carcinomas define distinct pathways of hepatocarcinogenesis. Gastroenterology 2001; 120: 1763-73.

[125] Moon RT, Kohn AD, De Ferrari GV, Kaykas A. WNT and beta-catenin signalling: diseases and therapies. Nat Rev Genet 2004; 5: 691-701.

[126] Thiery JP. Epithelial-mesenchymal transitions in tumour progression. Nat Rev Cancer 2002; 2: 442-54.

[127] Giannelli G, Villa E, Lahn M. Transforming Growth Factor-β as a Therapeutic Target in Hepatocellular Carcinoma. Cancer Res 2014; 74: 1890-94.

[128] Meindl-Beinker NM, Matsuzaki K, Dooley S. TGF-β signaling in onset and progression of hepatocellular carcinoma. Dig Dis Basel Switz 2012; 30: 514-23.

[129] Giannelli G, Mazzocca A, Fransvea E, Lahn M, Antonaci S. Inhibiting TGF-β signaling in hepatocellular carcinoma. Biochim Biophys Acta 2011; 1815: 214-23.

[130] Faivre SJ, Santoro A, Kelley RK, *et al.* A phase 2 study of a novel transforming growth factor-beta (TGF-{beta}1) receptor I kinase inhibitor, LY2157299 monohydrate (LY), in patients with advanced hepatocellular carcinoma (HCC). J Clin Oncol 2014; 32: LBA173.
[131] He AR, Goldenberg AS. Treating hepatocellular carcinoma progression following first-line sorafenib: therapeutic options and clinical observations. Ther Adv Gastroenterol 2013; 6: 447-58.
[132] Villanueva A. Rethinking future development of molecular therapies in hepatocellular carcinoma: a bottom-up approach. J Hepatol 2013; 59: 392-5.
[133] Bruix J, Sherman M, American Association for the Study of Liver Diseases. Management of hepatocellular carcinoma: an update. Hepatol Baltim Md 2011; 53: 1020-2.
[134] Verslype C, Rosmorduc O, Rougier P, ESMO Guidelines Working Group. Hepatocellular carcinoma: ESMO-ESDO Clinical Practice Guidelines for diagnosis, treatment and follow-up. Ann Oncol Off J Eur Soc Med Oncol ESMO 2012; 23 Suppl 7: vii41-48.
[135] Patrikidou A, Sinapi I, Regnault H, *et al.* Gemcitabine and oxaliplatin chemotherapy for advanced hepatocellular carcinoma after failure of anti-angiogenic therapies. Invest New Drugs 2014. [Epub ahead of print].
[136] Mir O, Coriat R, Boudou-Rouquette P, *et al.* Gemcitabine and oxaliplatin as second-line treatment in patients with hepatocellular carcinoma pre-treated with sorafenib. Med Oncol Northwood Lond Engl 2012; 29: 2793-9.
[137] Woo HY, Heo J, Yoon KT, *et al.* Clinical course of sorafenib treatment in patients with hepatocellular carcinoma. Scand J Gastroenterol 2012; 47: 809-19.
[138] Pressiani T, Rimassa L, Boni C, *et al.* Phase II randomized trial on dose-escalated sorafenib (S) *versus* best supportive care (BSC) in patients with advanced hepatocellular carcinoma (HCC) with disease progression on prior S treatment. J Clin Oncol 2011; 29: Abstract 4115.
[139] Dancey JE, Chen HX. Strategies for optimizing combinations of molecularly targeted anticancer agents. Nat Rev Drug Discov 2006; 5: 649-59.
[140] Huynh H, Chow PKH, Palanisamy N, *et al.* Bevacizumab and rapamycin induce growth suppression in mouse models of hepatocellular carcinoma. J Hepatol 2008; 49: 52-60.
[141] Semenza GL. Targeting HIF-1 for cancer therapy. Nat Rev Cancer 2003; 3: 721-32.
[142] Bouattour M, Dreyer C, Faivre S, Raymond E. New antiangiogenic compounds and strategies in clinical development. Present Future Angiogenic Ther. Cancer, Permanyer Publications; 2010: 63-84.
[143] Bertino G, Di Carlo I, Ardiri A, *et al.* Systemic therapies in hepatocellular carcinoma: present and future. Future Oncol 2013; 9: 1533-48.
[144] Dufour J-F, Bargellini I, De Maria N, De Simone P, Goulis I, Marinho RT. Intermediate hepatocellular carcinoma: current treatments and future perspectives. Ann Oncol Off J Eur Soc Med Oncol ESMO 2013; 24 Suppl 2: ii24-29.
[145] Shim JH, Park J-W, Kim JH, *et al.* Association between increment of serum VEGF level and prognosis after transcatheter arterial chemoembolization in hepatocellular carcinoma patients. Cancer Sci 2008; 99: 2037-44.
[146] Sergio A, Cristofori C, Cardin R, *et al.* Transcatheter arterial chemoembolization (TACE) in hepatocellular carcinoma (HCC): the role of angiogenesis and invasiveness. Am J Gastroenterol 2008; 103: 914-21.

[147] Xiao E-H, Guo D, Bian D-J. Effect of preoperative transcatheter arterial chemoembolization on angiogenesis of hepatocellular carcinoma cells. World J Gastroenterol 2009; 15: 4582-6.

[148] Pawlik TM, Reyes DK, Cosgrove D, Kamel IR, Bhagat N, Geschwind J-FH. Phase II trial of sorafenib combined with concurrent transarterial chemoembolization with drug-eluting beads for hepatocellular carcinoma. J Clin Oncol 2011; 29: 3960-7.

[149] Park J-W, Koh YH, Kim HB, *et al.* Phase II study of concurrent transarterial chemoembolization and sorafenib in patients with unresectable hepatocellular carcinoma. J Hepatol 2012; 56: 1336-42.

[150] Kudo M, Imanaka K, Chida N, *et al.* Phase III study of sorafenib after transarterial chemoembolisation in Japanese and Korean patients with unresectable hepatocellular carcinoma. Eur J Cancer 2011; 47: 2117-27.

[151] Liu L, Chen H, Wang M, *et al.* Combination Therapy of Sorafenib and TACE for Unresectable HCC: A Systematic Review and Meta-Analysis. PloS One 2014; 9: e91124.

[152] Abou-Alfa GK. TACE and sorafenib: a good marriage? J Clin Oncol 2011; 29: 3949-52.

[153] Pinter M, Sieghart W, Graziadei I, *et al.* Sorafenib in unresectable hepatocellular carcinoma from mild to advanced stage liver cirrhosis. Oncologist 2009; 14: 70-6.

[154] Ozenne V, Paradis V, Pernot S, *et al.* Tolerance and outcome of patients with unresectable hepatocellular carcinoma treated with sorafenib. Eur J Gastroenterol Hepatol 2010; 22: 1106-10.

[155] Hollebecque A, Cattan S, Romano O, *et al.* Safety and efficacy of sorafenib in hepatocellular carcinoma: the impact of the Child-Pugh score. Aliment Pharmacol Ther 2011; 34: 1193-201.

[156] Miller AA, Murry DJ, Owzar K, *et al.* Phase I and pharmacokinetic study of sorafenib in patients with hepatic or renal dysfunction: CALGB 60301. J Clin Oncol 2009; 27: 1800-5.

[157] Schwartz JD, Schwartz M, Mandeli J, Sung M. Neoadjuvant and adjuvant therapy for resectable hepatocellular carcinoma: review of the randomised clinical trials. Lancet Oncol 2002; 3: 593-603.

[158] Imamura H, Matsuyama Y, Tanaka E, *et al.* Risk factors contributing to early and late phase intrahepatic recurrence of hepatocellular carcinoma after hepatectomy. J Hepatol 2003; 38: 200-7.

[159] Belghiti J, Kianmanesh R. Surgical treatment of hepatocellular carcinoma. HPB 2005; 7: 42-9.

[160] Adachi E, Maeda T, Matsumata T, *et al.* Risk factors for intrahepatic recurrence in human small hepatocellular carcinoma. Gastroenterology 1995; 108: 768-75.

[161] Rougier P, Mitry E, Barbare J-C, Taieb J. Hepatocellular carcinoma (HCC): an update. Semin Oncol 2007; 34: S12-20.

[162] Yamaguchi R, Yano H, Iemura A, Ogasawara S, Haramaki M, Kojiro M. Expression of vascular endothelial growth factor in human hepatocellular carcinoma. Hepatol Baltim Md 1998; 28: 68-77.

[163] Hakimé A, Hines-Peralta A, Peddi H, *et al.* Combination of radiofrequency ablation with antiangiogenic therapy for tumor ablation efficacy: study in mice. Radiology 2007; 244: 464-70.

[164] Bruix J, Takayama T, Mazzaferoo V, *et al.* STORM: A phase III randomized, double-blind, placebo-controlled trial of adjuvant sorafenib after resection or ablation to prevent recurrence of hepatocellular carcinoma (HCC). J Clin Oncol 2014; 32, Abstract 4006.

[165] Allegra CJ, Yothers G, O'Connell MJ, *et al.* Phase III trial assessing bevacizumab in stages II and III carcinoma of the colon: results of NSABP protocol C-08. J Clin Oncol 2011; 29: 11-6.

[166] Le Tourneau C, Faivre S, Siu LL. Molecular targeted therapy of head and neck cancer: review and clinical development challenges. Eur J Cancer Oxf Engl 1990 2007; 43: 2457-66.

[167] Bouattour M, Dreyer C, Raymond E, Faivre S. Evaluation of antiangiogenic effects: Biomarkers and functional imaging. Present Future Angiogenic Ther. Cancer, Permanyer Publications; 2010: 35-51.

[168] Barbier L, Fuks D, Pessaux P, *et al.* Safety of liver resection for hepatocellular carcinoma after sorafenib therapy: a multicenter case-matched study. Ann Surg Oncol 2013; 20: 3603-9.

[169] Cowey CL, Amin C, Pruthi RS, *et al.* Neoadjuvant clinical trial with sorafenib for patients with stage II or higher renal cell carcinoma. J Clin Oncol 2010; 28: 1502-7.

[170] Zhou W-P, Lai ECH, Li A-J, *et al.* A prospective, randomized, controlled trial of preoperative transarterial chemoembolization for resectable large hepatocellular carcinoma. Ann Surg 2009; 249: 195-202.

[171] Newell P, Villanueva A, Friedman SL, Koike K, Llovet JM. Experimental models of hepatocellular carcinoma. J Hepatol 2008; 48: 858-79.

[172] Jayson G, Harris J. How participants in cancer trials are chosen: ethics and conflicting interests. Nat Rev Cancer 2006; 6: 330-6.

[173] Gan HK, You B, Pond GR, Chen EX. Assumptions of expected benefits in randomized phase III trials evaluating systemic treatments for cancer. J Natl Cancer Inst 2012; 104: 590-8.

[174] Hsu C, Shen Y-C, Cheng C-C, Hu F-C, Cheng A-L. Geographic difference in survival outcome for advanced hepatocellular carcinoma: implications on future clinical trial design. Contemp Clin Trials 2010; 31: 55-61.

[175] Peck-Radosavljevic M, Greten TF, Lammer J, *et al.* Consensus on the current use of sorafenib for the treatment of hepatocellular carcinoma. Eur J Gastroenterol Hepatol 2010; 22: 391-8.

[176] Bouattour M, Ozenne V, Goutte N, *et al.* A high rate of potentially curative therapy for hepatocellular carcinoma in referral centers. HEPATOLOGY 2009; 50: Abstract 1750.

CHAPTER 3

Ruthenium Compounds Targeting Cancer Therapy

Denise de Oliveira Silva*

Department of Fundamental Chemistry, Institute of Chemistry, University of São Paulo, Av. Prof. Lineu Prestes, 748, 05508-000, São Paulo, SP, Brazil

Abstract: The contribution of metal compounds to oncology is well-known due to the clinical relevance of cisplatin drug and its analogues in current *Platinum Cancer Chemotherapy*. The undesirable drawbacks, *e.g.*, limited range of treatable cancers, tumor resistance and serious side-effects, associated to the use of platinum drugs, nevertheless, account for the developing of new alternative metal-based anticancer drugs. A number of promising ruthenium compounds exerting anticancer/antitumor activities has been reported in the last decades and significant progress was achieved with the entrance of the anti-metastatic NAMI-A and the cytotoxic KP1019 (and its analogue KP1339) Ru(III) compounds into human clinical trials. Selected Ru-based drugs considering the diversity of structures and oxidation states as well as the distinctly different chemical, biochemical and pharmacological activities (*e.g.*, anti-metastatic or cytotoxic activities in tumors) are discussed in this chapter, updating the 2010 review by the same author. The two classical Ru(III)-based drugs and different families of Ru(II)-organometallics are presented. The chapter includes also the novel class of diruthenium(II,III)-(pharmaceuticals) metallodrugs, with focus on Ru_2(II,III) metal-metal bonded cores coordinated to ligands derived from pharmaceuticals such as non-steroidal anti-inflammatory drugs or the γ-linolenic acid, targeting glioma cancer therapy.

Keywords: Anticancer, antitumor, cytotoxicity, diruthenium(II,III), glioma, γ-linolenic acid, metal-based drugs, non-steroidal anti-inflammatory drugs, ruthenium(II), ruthenium(III).

INTRODUCTION

Metal-based drugs, although still in an early stage of development compared to non-metal (or purely organic drugs) have received increased attention in the field of medicinal chemistry in recent years. In terms of requirements, metal-based

***Corresponding Author Denise de Oliveira Silva:** Department of Fundamental Chemistry, Institute of Chemistry, University of São Paulo. Av. Prof. Lineu Prestes, 748, 05508-000, São Paulo, SP, Brazil;
Tel: +55 11 30919124; Fax: +55 11 3815-5640; E-mail: deosilva@iq.usp.br

Atta-ur-Rahman / M. Iqbal Choudhary (Eds.)

candidates to drug formulation have to meet basically the same criteria, *i.e.*, medically beneficial effects and minimal side-effect toxicities, of non-metal drugs [1, 2]. Therefore, the major challenge to the design of metal-based drugs, similarly to that of organic drugs, consists in achieving the desired balance between biological activity and minimal toxicity. Although the use of metal and metal compounds as therapeutic agents can be traced back to several thousands of years, as exemplified by the ancient uses of gold (2500 BC), copper and iron (1500 BC) [3], their role and mode of action as pharmaceuticals are still not well-known. Nevertheless, the relevance of metallotherapeutic drugs exhibiting a diversity of biological and biomedical properties is indubitably recognized nowadays, as can be seen by the fast development of related scientific fields, such as bioinorganic chemistry, biological inorganic chemistry and medicinal inorganic chemistry [1-7].

Metal ions exerting important physiological functions have been incorporated by mammals through evolution. Essential metal ions such as iron, zinc, copper, cobalt and molybdenum play crucial role in the body biochemistry. The human health depends on these metal ions and, consequently, certain pathologies may be associated to their unbalanced (*i.e.*, either lack or excess) quantities. For example, deficiency of iron can cause anemia while iron overloading is associated to hereditary haemochromatosis [8-10]. Metals and their compounds, in a variety of forms, *e.g.*, metal salts or oxides, but especially as coordination complexes, show a diversity of functions. They play key role as essential elements, as protein/enzyme regulators and enzyme mimics, and they are involved in transporting, signaling and genomic coding [3, 4]. In clinic, applications range from contrast agents to radiopharmaceuticals and therapeutic drugs. Examples of medical problems and metabolic disorders treatable with metallodrugs are bipolar disorders, gastrointestinal diseases, arthritis, diabetes, cancer, parasitic infections (malaria), bacterial and viral (particularly HIV) diseases, neurological diseases (Parkinson's, Alzheimer's), cardiovascular and age-related inflammatory diseases, among others [3, 4, 11]. In addition to the approved metallopharmaceuticals (*e.g.*, platinum, arsenium, zinc, copper and technetium drugs) for clinical use, current attention comprises also a number of metallodrugs (including other metal compounds) undergoing clinical trials (from Phase I to Phase IV) [11].

Advantages of using metal-based drugs, alternatively to traditional organic pharmaceuticals, include the possibilities of, *e.g.*, achieving lacking therapeutic treatments, enhancing efficacy, and/or reducing undesirable side-effects. Moreover, metal ions (or metalloenzymes) may be involved in the activation and/or biotransformation of organic drugs, and some drugs may have an effect (direct or indirect) on the metal ion metabolism [4].

The relevance of metal-based drugs as therapeutic agents is well-known in oncology due to the key role of platinum coordination complexes in the current clinical treatment of many types of cancer all over the world. Metal coordination complexes (which are composed by a metal ion forming coordination bonds with the ligands, *i.e.*, organic and/or inorganic molecules or ions), in addition to their relevant role in human biochemical processes, offer a rich and versatile platform to the design of metallopharmaceuticals. Their unique features allow exploiting advantages, *e.g.*, alternative modes of action and novel pharmacological properties, over purely organic drugs. Changes on the type of metal ion and/or on the nature of the coordinated ligands (organic and/or inorganic molecules or ions) can lead to a variety of geometries in distinct structures, providing a diversity of mechanisms of action. Variable metal oxidation states may be accessible in the physiological environment. The chemical reactivity may be fine-tuned for thermodynamics (*e.g.*, by modulating metal-ligand bonds and/or redox potentials) and kinetics (by modulating rates of ligand exchange reactions). The nature of the coordinated ligands may also be relevant to mechanisms involving either ligand centered redox processes or target site recognition associated to the activity of released ligands [12, 13]. Furthermore, the ability of metals to form unique shapes by arranging organic moieties three-dimensionally can be exploited for designing organic-like small-molecule probes and drugs [14].

Platinum Chemotherapeutic Drugs

The main classical example for the relevance of metal-based drugs in medicine is *cisplatin*, the leading platinum chemotherapeutic drug showing unique pharmacological properties to treat cancer. Chemotherapy (used to kill the fast dividing cells and, consequently, to slow or stop the cancer spreading) is one of the three current approaches (*i.e.,* chemotherapy, surgery, and radiation therapy) in oncology clinic, being systemically used in more than 50% patients diagnosed with cancer. In particular, the chemotherapy based on platinum drugs, *i.e.*, the *Platinum Cancer Chemotherapy*, accounts for multibillions of dollars worldwide annual sales associated to oncology treatments.

Relevant aspects of platinum anticancer drugs and their mechanisms of action are extensively discussed at the literature [see, for example, references 15-24]. Thus, only a brief overview is given here with the aim of providing information to explain the development of the ruthenium compounds as potential metal-based anticancer drugs.

Cisplatin, *cis*-diamminedichloridoplatinum(II), is a coordination complex of formula *cis*-$[PtCl_2(NH_3)_2]$ (Fig. **1a**) that became famous as a purely inorganic metal-based drug serendipitously discovered to inhibit the division of bacterial cells [25]. Cisplatin was approved as a drug in 1979 making a significant breakthrough in medical clinic for treatment of cancer. After the treatment with the platinum drug, testicular cancer (which was causing a high number of patient deaths at that time) showed 90% patient cure [26]. Currently, the cisplatin drug is administrated to treat a variety of solid tumors in standard chemotherapy, individually or together with other anticancer drugs or radiotherapy [27]. Routine uses of cisplatin comprise mainly metastatic testicular tumors, ovarian tumors and advanced bladder cancer, although the drug can also be used for non-small cell lung, small cell lung, melanoma, head and neck, and cervical cancers [15, 18]. The drug action process involves several steps such as accumulation into the cells, intracellular activation by hydrolysis, interactions with DNA and other targets, and Pt-DNA adducts cellular processing. Despite the key role in chemotherapy, the applications of cisplatin are considered to be restricted to a small range of types of human cancer; the drug is not effective for common cancers such as breast and colon tumors, and lacks response to metastatic cancers. Another disadvantage is the inherent or developed resistance of certain tumors after the administration of the drug. In addition, patients undergoing treatment with cisplatin may suffer from highly toxic side-effects, *e.g.*, nephrotoxicity (the major dose-limiting toxicity), neurotoxicity and emetogenicity [21].

The first attempts to overcome these limitations were based on finding platinum analogous compounds which could achieve modes of action similar to that of cisplatin, *i.e.,* cytotoxicity associated to DNA-binding ability. The first drug analogues were thus inspired on the square-plane structure represented by the general formula *cis*-$[PtN_nL_m]$, N = *N*-donor ligand (*e.g.*, ammonia or amine group) and L = anionic ligand (*e.g.*, chloride or organic acid derivate anion), and n and m = 1 or 2 for monodentate or bidentate ligand, respectively. The nature of the non-leaving *N*-donor ligands has been related to anticancer properties and formation of DNA adducts, whereas the type of the leaving L anionic ligands may be associated to bio-distribution as well as to side-effects [28]. Thousands of potential platinum drugs developed according to this strategy were found to show poor aqueous solubility, low efficacy and/or high toxicity, consequently, being either abandoned in Phase I or II clinical trials or excluded from cancer therapy applications [21]. Only five compounds from this generation of classical platinum complexes were selected to clinical use. Carboplatin (approved in 1989) and oxaliplatin (2002) (Fig. **1a**) together with cisplatin are the major anticancer platinum-drugs approved by the FDA (Food and Drug Administration). These three drugs are currently sold in the worldwide market to be clinically used in approximately 50% tumor treatments. Carboplatin is mostly used for treatment of advanced ovarian carcinoma and its reduced toxicity makes it suitable for high-dose chemotherapy. Oxaliplatin is effective particularly for metastatic colorectal cancer, showing lower toxicity than carboplatin or cisplatin [29-31]. The other three drugs: nedaplatin (1996, small and non-small cell lung cancer, head and neck tumors, cervix carcinoma, bladder and oesophageal tumors), lobaplatin (2004, testicular, ovarian and gastric carcinomas, small cell lung tumors and metastatic breast cancer) and heptaplatin (2005, gastric cancer) are used only in few countries, respectively, Japan, China and South Korea [21].

Regardless the effects against malignant tumors, these generations of cisplatin-like drugs were not able to achieve the expected significant improvement on clinical efficacy compared to the parent cisplatin. Consequently, alternative strategies to exploit the anticancer properties of platinum compounds started to be developed. Platinum(IV) octahedral complexes that are kinetically more inert than Pt(II) square-plane compounds were found to act as prodrugs that can be converted to the more reactive Pt(II) species [32]. Two examples of promising Pt(IV) anticancer drugs are the compounds with the formula $[PtCl_2(O_2CCH_3)_2(NH_3)(L)]$ where L = cyclohexylamine or adamantylamine. Satraplatin (Fig. **1b**), currently undergoing clinical trials against metastatic prostate cancers, can be orally administrated, in contrast to Pt(II) drugs which are introduced intravenously into the human body [33]. The mechanism of action of these compounds (inside the cell) has been assumed to involve activation by reduction to the correspondent Pt(II) more reactive species, which undergo subsequent aquation and then modify the nuclear DNA causing the cell death. The reduction may proceed by several pathways involving dissociation of axial and/or equatorial ligands, *e.g.,* loss of two axial acetate ligands, loss of one axial acetate and one equatorial chloride, or elimination of two equatorial ligands [34]. Moreover, platinum(IV) drugs can be photo-activated to Pt(II) at the tumor site [35]. Carrier-based approaches have also been investigated for delivering platinum drugs to tumor sites, including the use of polymeric conjugates and suitable carriers such as liposomes, micelles, dendrimers and inorganic solid particles [36]. These strategies may improve the solubility and prolong the half-life of platinum drugs in the human body, among other advantages such as increasing distribution into tumor sites, providing sustained or triggered release in tumors, reducing undesirable side-effects and suppressing development of resistance to the drug [36-38]. Platinum compounds have been attached to cationic and tumor-targeting constructs [17, 39], modified peptides [40], lipid nanocapsules [41-43], carbon nanotubes [44], and nanoparticles based on polymers [45, 46] or functionalized-metals [47]. Platinum drug-carrier delivery systems such as cisplatin-liposome, oxilaplatin-liposome and cisplatin-micelle macromolecular systems are currently undergoing clinical trials [36]. One of the most promising liposomal formulations, already in Phase III, is Lipoplatin [48], a formulation containing ~ 9% cisplatin and ~ 91% lipids (w/w) with particle size about 110 nm [49, 36].

Finally, despite all the drawbacks (*e.g.*, inherent or therapy-induced resistance, dose-limiting toxic side-effects, limited activity range and lack of selectivity) the important role of cisplatin and its analogues in relieving symptoms and increase patient survival still accounts for their worldwide clinical use, either individually or in combination with organic chemotherapeutic drugs. Nevertheless, the search for new alternative metal-based drugs that may show activity against human cancers and overcome platinum-drugs drawbacks is needed. Compounds of ruthenium, osmium, titanium, gold, tin, gallium, arsenic, copper, zinc, bismuth and molybdenum have been studied for antitumor properties, and zinc, iron, ruthenium and lanthanides porphyrins have been investigated for photodynamic therapy [3, 4]. Furthermore, non-classical targeted-therapy approach has emerged as an interesting alternative for designing anticancer metal-based drugs offering perspectives to achieve higher selectivity and minimal adverse side-effects [50].

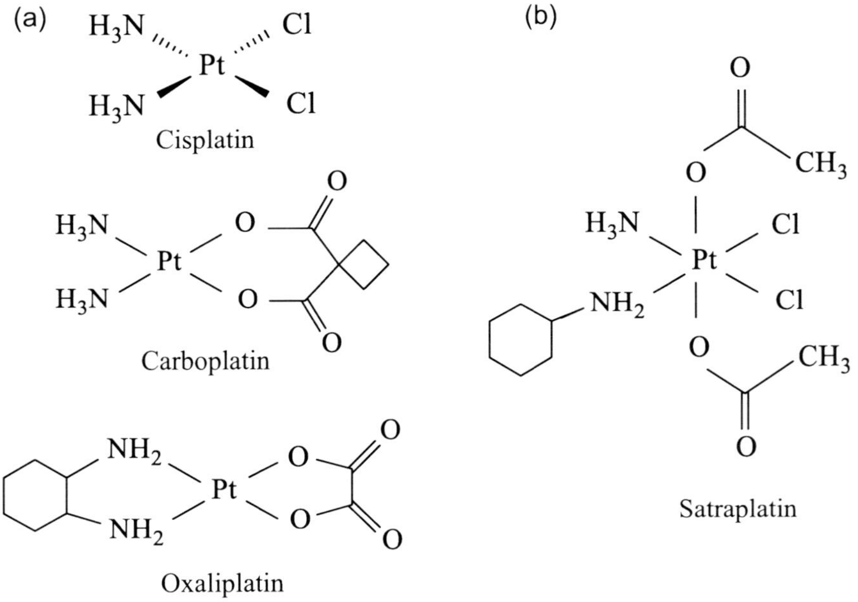

Fig. (1). The three platinum(II) anticancer drugs (cisplatin, carboplatin and oxaliplatin) approved by FDA (**a**) and the platinum(IV) drug (satraplatin) currently in clinical trials (**b**).

Ruthenium-Based Antitumor/Anticancer Drugs

Due to the well-succeed chemotherapeutic properties, cisplatin was considered, at the beginning, as a drug model for developing other alternative metal-based anticancer drugs. The first searches for new metal-drugs were, consequently, mainly focused on mimicking the cisplatin chemical properties. However, since the efforts to broaden the platinum(II) family were to some extent disappointing to the expectations (in particular due to lack of significant improvements in reducing side-effects and tumor resistance), new directions towards to non-platinum chemotherapeutics surfaced as interesting alternative strategies to find novel candidates to anticancer drugs.

In this context, ruthenium compounds soon emerged as the most promising non-platinum drugs displaying antitumor/anticancer activities. Their ability to show alternative mechanisms of action, independent of binding to DNA, was later recognized as important feature to overcome limitations of platinum drugs. It should be noted that the tumor resistance to cisplatin, even though it is cell line-dependent, may involve basically three main mechanisms: "reduced drug uptake and/or increased drug efflux, degradation and deactivation by intracellular thiols and improved repair or tolerance of DNA-cisplatin adducts" [18]. In particular, cisplatin-DNA lesions may be repaired by proteins, *e.g.,* "nucleotide excision repair (NER) proteins, mismatch repair (MMR) proteins and DNA-dependent protein kinase (DNA-PK) protein" [51]. Therefore, alternative modes of action involving other targets than DNA may provide different routes to anticancer activity of metallodrugs disfavoring DNA-repairing mechanisms. Furthermore, in general, ruthenium complexes show chemical and pharmacokinetic behaviors distinct from those of platinum compounds, binding extensively with proteins and excluding DNA as the main target *in vivo.*

Ruthenium compounds, in addition to the role as anti-proliferative agents against cancer cells, have potential also for a diversity of other medicinal applications, *e.g.*, as immune suppressant agents, nitric oxide scavengers, photosensitizers, antimicrobial and antimalarial agents [2, 3].

Studies on ruthenium complexes as potential drug candidates for cancer therapy can be traced back to the late 1980s, even though the first reports on their biological properties date from 1950-1960 [52, 53]. The evolution of the number of publications focusing on antitumor and/or anticancer properties of ruthenium compounds, compared to platinum, is shown in Fig. (**2**). The Thomson Reuters Web of Knowledge^{SM} database [54] was searched individually for the following pairs of keywords: (1) *metal* (Pt or Ru) and *antitumor*; and (2) *metal* (Pt or Ru) and *anticancer*. The data are displayed in three graphics (a), (b) and (c), which show the number of publications for the keyword pairs: *metal + anticancer, metal + antitumor,* and *metal + (anticancer + antitumor*), respectively. Some articles were counted twice in the later, since the repeating cases appearing on the searches were not subtracted from each other. Plot (c) shows that the interest in ruthenium started mainly from the 1990 decade, which is coincident with the highest number of publications for platinum. Plots (a), (b) and (d) - with the last showing publications for the two metals in the current year, up to April 15 - give evidence for the further increased attention on ruthenium, especially in the more recent years (2005 - 2014). Interestingly, in the last nine years, although publications are almost twice times higher for platinum than for ruthenium, reports on ruthenium are growing faster, in contrast to reports on platinum which remained approximately constant along the more recent years.

The recent fast evolution of the reports is a good indicator encouraging the further development of new generations of ruthenium chemotherapeutic drugs. The research studies, however, are still in their beginning compared to platinum, requiring future efforts to increase the number of ruthenium anticancer drugs in clinical trials. The diversity of biological properties shown by a large structural variety of compounds together with diverse information about molecular targets and mechanisms of action still challenge the systematization about anticancer activity of ruthenium-based drugs. On the other hand, the collected data (*e.g.*, chemistry data, reactivity in solution and in biological environment, biochemical and pharmacological properties) up to the present date can be used as valorous guide for future directions towards exploiting either the existing or new classes of complexes with the aim of finding novel ruthenium metallopharmaceuticals. The number of reports on ruthenium compounds as potential anticancer drugs is enormous, comprising distinct metal oxidation states, a variety of structures (including, *e.g.*, mononuclear, dinuclear and polinuclear compounds, traditional coordination complexes and organometallic compounds), as well as a vast diversity of biological activities (*e.g.*, cytotoxicity, induction of apoptosis in cancer cells, antimetastatic properties, interactions with DNA, selective enzyme inhibition) [see, *e.g.*, references 50, 55-71]. Therefore, since it is not possible either to cover all the different types of reported compounds or to discuss all the available data, the present chapter will encompass only representative selected families of ruthenium complexes and the most important features associated to their antitumor/anticancer properties.

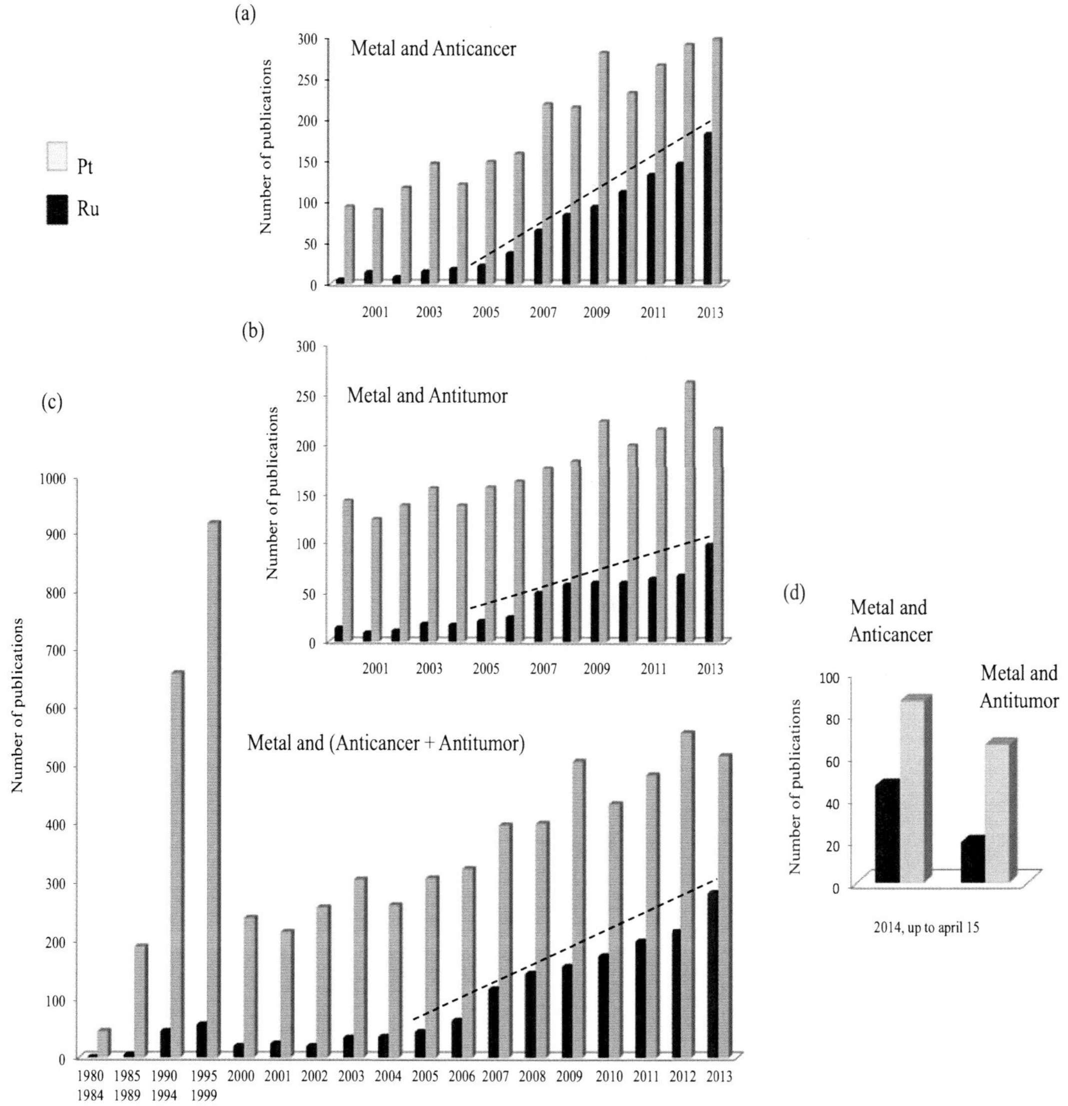

Fig. (2). Number of publications per year (or period) by searching individually the pairs of keywords: metal and anticancer (**a**); metal and antitumor (**b**); metal and (anticancer + antitumor) (**c**); comparison between the two metals for the current year searched up to April 15, 2014 (**d**). Source: *Thomson Reuters Web of Knowledge*^{SM} database.

RUTHENIUM COMPOUNDS TARGETING CANCER THERAPHY

Ruthenium Complexes and Features Related to their Biological Activity

Ruthenium, atomic number 44, is a transition metal located at group 8 and period 5 of the Periodic Table. It belongs to the "platinum group" (Ru, Os, Rh, Ir, Pt, Pd) that includes metals which show similar physical and chemical properties and usually share the same mineral deposits. Ruthenium may exhibit a large variety of oxidation states ranging from −2 to +8. Among numerous applications, its compounds show catalytic activity for chemical transformations and properties that suit towards pharmacological applications. The rich synthetic chemistry can be worked to give a broad diversity of structures, from classical coordination complexes to organometallic compounds. The two most common metal oxidation states are Ru(III) and Ru(II). Ruthenium(II) in classical coordination complexes can easily undergo oxidation to Ru(III) unless the metal is coordinated to good π-acceptor ligands, in contrast to ruthenium(III) complexes which are usually stable in air atmosphere. Both oxidation states, Ru(II) and Ru(III), are accessible in biological fluids under physiologically conditions. Ruthenium(IV) is found in oxo-species and although it may occur as an intermediate in reactions of Ru(III) compounds, no direct association of this higher oxidation state to ruthenium metallodrugs has been reported. Furthermore, high oxidation states are chemically very reactive, and the biological chemistry of *d*-block metals, except for bleomycin and enzymes such as cytochrome P_{450}, has not been related to oxo-ions [2].

In classical coordination complexes, the ruthenium metal center (in both Ru(II) and Ru(III) oxidation states) is usually coordinated to six ligands in an octahedral geometry, in contrast to the square-planar geometry of the four-coordinated Pt(II) complexes (Fig. **3**). The geometry was historically important to the choice of ruthenium for designing new metallodrugs, since octahedral compounds were expected to show different reactivity from that of square-planar compounds.

The mechanisms involved in the activity of metal coordination complexes are not well understood yet and may be associated to a variety of distinct features including those particularly related to the chemical behavior in the biological environment. The metal-drug activity may depend on the type of metal and also on the ligands since the nature of the ligands affect, *e.g.,* the metal coordination geometry and the redox properties, among other features of the complex [72].

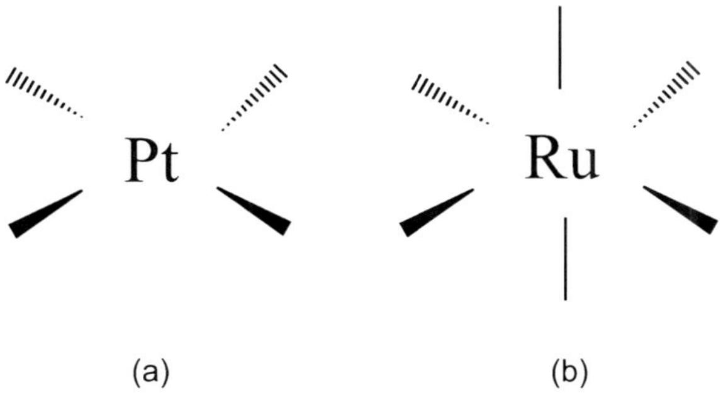

Fig. (3). Square-planar coordination geometry of Pt(II) compounds (**a**), and octahedral coordination geometry of Ru(II) and Ru(III) compounds (**b**).

In general, metal complexes behave as prodrugs undergoing transformations, which may involve ligand substitution reactions and/or redox processes, before they reach the target. Biotransformation is one of the most important processes affecting the activity that will depend on the type of species formed in the biological environment. The major bioactive species are improbable to be the entire original complexes, *i.e.*, the starting complexes having the metal ion coordinated to all the original ligands. In fact, the original complexes have tendency to undergo reactions to give a variety of derived species, *e.g.,* a) complexes having the metal coordinated to only part of the original ligands, b) the individual metal, c) the ligands, d) the metal and some of dissociated ligands [73]. An interesting categorization has been suggested to systematize metal-drug actions according to five classes [73]: (1) Functional compounds (the metal fragment exerts functional role binding directly the biological target); (2) Structural compounds (the metal exerts structural role determining the shape of the compound and leading to non-covalent interactions with the biological target); (3) Metal ion as carriers for active ligands (the metal functions as a carrier for active ligands to be delivered *in vivo*, and may protect the ligands before delivering); (4) Metal complexes as catalysts (the metal complex behaves as catalyst *in vivo*, *e.g.* with production of reactive oxygen species (ROS) causing cell damage); (5) Photoactive metal compounds (the metal compound acts as a photosensitizer). In particular, features associated to the activity of functional compounds are difficult to control in the biological environment. These features comprises thermodynamic parameters, pharmacokinetics and bio-distribution (that are affected by the nature of the non-leaving ligands and may be related to, *e.g.*, lipophilicity, charge, size, solubility and non-covalent interactions) and kinetics of activation (that may be related to the nature of the leaving ligands if activation occurs through ligand exchange, or to the redox potential if an oxidation state change of the metal precedes aquation) [73].

The biological activity of metal-based drugs usually involves their reactions with nucleophiles in the human body. The most common reaction is the ligand substitution in which one of the ligands originally coordinated to the metal center is replaced by a new attacking ligand. Ruthenium and platinum are relatively inert metals that exchange ligands within the range of 1-2 hours, exhibiting ligand exchange rates comparable to the rates found for cellular division processes [74]. The ligand exchange kinetics may play a key role in the anticancer activity of ruthenium complexes. Both ruthenium and platinum compounds exhibiting high anticancer activity were found to undergo ligand substitution reactions to give the correspondent active species in the biological environment. These compounds thus behave as prodrugs that may be activated by aquation (*i.e.*, replacement of one or more coordinated ligands such as chloride by water molecules). The aquation may occur after redox processes, *e.g.*, for Ru(III) complexes, or alternatively ligand substitution may precede redox reactions. Consequently, the direct binding of activated metabolites to biomolecular targets is likely to be involved in the biological activity of ruthenium compounds.

The ligand substitution rates can be compared to the water exchange rate, *i.e.*, the rate at which the complex exchanges coordinated water with the free water existing in solution, according to the reaction represented in equation (1) [2].

$$[M(H_2{}^{16}O)_y]^{n+} + H_2{}^{17}O \rightleftharpoons [M(H_2{}^{16}O)_{y-1}(H_2{}^{17}O)]^{n+} + H_2{}^{16}O \quad \textbf{(1)}$$

The kinetics and the mechanism of ligand exchange reactions depend on the type of metal and its oxidation state as well as on the nature of the coordinated ligands. Ruthenium(II) complexes are usually kinetically more labile to ligand substitution than ruthenium(III) complexes as indicated by the values of water exchange rate constants that are higher for Ru(II) (~ 10^{-2} s^{-1}, 25 °C) than for Ru(III) (~ 10^{-6} s^{-1}, at 25 °C) complexes. In addition to the higher lability, the Ru(II) aqua-species show exchange rate constant value about only an order of magnitude above that of Pt(II) and, consequently, might be more suitable for biological targets reactions than complexes of Ru(III). Different modes of action may also be related to distinct ligand exchange reaction mechanisms. In contrast to the Pt(II) square-planar complexes that exchange their ligands *via* associative process (where the new ligand coordinates the metal ion prior to the releasing of one of the original ligands), Ru(II) octahedral complexes tend to exchange ligand *via* dissociative mechanism (where the dissociation of one of the original ligands generate a five-coordinate intermediate prior to the addition of the new incoming ligand) [2].

Transition metal ions can undergo redox processes switching between oxidation states which are accessible in the living organism physiological conditions. Cancer cells show distinct redox metabolism compared to healthy tissues, usually causing disturbance in the intracellular redox balance. Potential anticancer complexes, *e.g.,* complexes of the metals platinum, gold, arsenic, ruthenium, rhodium, copper, vanadium, cobalt, manganese, gadolinium and molybdenum, were found to have an effect on cellular redox homeostasis [75]. Metal complexes can affect cellular redox chemistry either directly (through metal or ligand centers) or indirectly (by binding to biomolecules participating of cellular redox pathways). Therefore, the strategy of targeting redox balance in cancer cells may also be interesting, for example, to overcome tumor resistance, to expand the range of treatable cancers and to achieve selectivity over normal cells [75]. The control of the activation by redox processes, and/or ligand substitution reactions, is an important challenge to trigger biological response in the right region of tissues and at the optimum time, and can offer unique features (unavailable to purely organic drugs) to the design of metal-based drugs [13, 76].

Oxidation-reduction reactions may have important role in the pharmacology of ruthenium since the Ru(II) and Ru(III) oxidation states can be interconverted by substances in the body. The activity of the kinetically more inert Ru(III) complexes has been explained by the "activation-by-reduction" mechanism [77]. The reduction of Ru(III) prodrugs has been assumed to be the first step of the action mode facilitating ligand substitution reactions and coordination to biological targets such as proteins [75, 78]. Ruthenium(III) may be reduced by endogenous bio-reductants (*e.g.*, glutathione and ascorbic acid) to the more labile Ru(II) species before undergoing ligand substitution reactions to generate aqua-species capable of exchanging labile water ligands with biological targets. Activation of ruthenium complexes by ligand exchange prior reduction may also take place. Processes of reduction and ligand substitutions depend on the ligand coordination environment around the metal ion. The choice of the ligands may be important to achieve biologically accessible metal reduction potentials. Moreover, the reduction potentials of metabolite species may be significantly different from those of the original Ru(III) complexes. The net charge of the complex and the nature of the coordinated ligands affect the kinetics of aquation of Ru(II) and Ru(III) compounds [72]. Additionally, some compounds "without exchangeable ligands may be active *per se* with no need of activation" [56].

The activation-by-reduction may offer selectivity against solid tumor masses. The reducing microenvironment of hypoxic tumors (due to insufficient vascularization, compared to normal tissues) may favor the reduction of Ru(III) to Ru(II) besides disfavoring possible metal re-oxidation by molecular oxygen [64]. The selective activation-by-reduction can also be exploited for designing bio-reductive metal-based prodrugs that might act on redox cycle involving reactive oxygen species (ROS) [72].

It should be noted that the activation-by-reduction processes, despite showing relevance for the mode of action of ruthenium(III)-based drugs, may not be needed for activation of other ruthenium compounds having the metal ion in the lowest Ru(II) oxidation state such as ruthenium(II)-organometallic complexes.

The ligand substitution reaction in metal complexes depends basically on the affinity of the ligand for the metal ion. Platinum(II) ion is classified as soft acid, while both Ru(II) and Ru(III) ions lie in the intermediate line between hard and soft acids, although Ru(II) is softer than Ru(III) [79]. Thus, similarly to platinum, both ruthenium ions exhibit good affinity for nitrogen- and sulfur-containing ligands and can exchange *O*-donor (hard bases) coordinated ligands, such as water, by *N*-donor or *S*-donor (intermediate or soft bases) ligands that are present in the biological environment. The coordination of such ligands has been found to play a key role in the binding of ruthenium drugs to biological molecules, proteins and proteomic targets [80, 81].

The interactions with a number of proteins/enzymes may have essential role in inducing effects, directing biological activities and determining pharmacological and toxicological profiles of metal-based drugs [82]. A variety of potential binding partners having, *e.g.*, nitrogen- or sulfur-donor atoms capable of coordinating to the ruthenium metal ion, are accessible in the blood stream. In particular, the interactions with the two plasma proteins, human serum albumin (HSA, present in human serum at the concentrations of about 40 mg mL^{-1} [83]) and transferrin (3.0 mg mL^{-1} [84]), may be associated to relevant processes such as biodistribution, toxicity and mechanism of action of metallodrugs. Although metal complexes, in general, exhibit lower protein binding constants than organic drugs [85], the serum proteins albumin and transferrin, being the first available targets after the intravenous administration, may have important role in the metallodrug action. In fact, numerous molecules are found to bind and to be transported by HSA, the most abundant plasma protein and primary binding partner when the drug is intravenously administrated.

Ruthenium compounds are usually less toxic to the human body than platinum drugs. Although the low toxicity is not well-elucidated yet, it has been associated in part to the ability of ruthenium (a non-essential and non-endogenous metal) to mimic the early *d*-block endogenous iron (Fe) in binding to biological molecules. The uptake of some ruthenium compounds has also been related to an iron mimetic transferrin-mediated process, offering advantage for drug transportation into tumor cells since the rapidly dividing cells show higher need of iron than health cells. However, it is important to note that the behavior of the Ru and Fe metal ions (which have similar size, oxidation states and coordination geometry) may be quite distinct from those of their correspondent metal complexes which show distinct thermodynamic and kinetic behaviors. The competition of ruthenium complexes for the iron binding sites in proteins and enzymes (*e.g.,* apo-transferrin) thus will depend on their speciation (*i.e.*, the nature of the coordinated ligands, and the species net charge) in the biological environment. Furthermore, the mimetic behavior might result in opposite effect that can interfere in iron pathways involved in cell metabolism, as has been found for gallium [56]. Other important related features are the accumulation of macromolecules resulting of enhanced permeability and retention effect, and the tumor drug enrichment due to higher expression of transferrin receptors at the tumor cells surface since tumors growing fast requires iron [56].

The First Studies on Ruthenium Antitumor Complexes

The biological properties of ruthenium are known for many years and ruthenium red, $[\{Ru(NH_3)_5\}(\mu\text{-}O)\{Ru(NH_3)_4\}(\mu\text{-}O)\{Ru(NH_3)_5\}]^{6+}$, having a $[Ru^{III}(\mu\text{-}O)Ru^{IV}(\mu\text{-}O)Ru^{III}]$ mixed oxidation state core, is maybe the most famous compound in the field. It has application as a biological stain, and it was also found to show properties as tumor growth inhibitor and immunosuppressant [2]. Nevertheless, the first class of ruthenium compounds investigated in detail for antitumor properties was composed by ammine-chlorido-ruthenium(III) complexes, the analogues of the ammine-chlorido-platinum(II) compounds. The $[Ru(NH_3)_3Cl_3]$ complex was the first to have the anticancer activity (in murine tumor models) reported, but the poor solubility was not appropriate for a drug formulation [77, 86]. The chemical inertness of this compound led to the proposal of the activation-by-reduction mechanism in an attempt to explain its biological activity. It was assumed that the hypoxic environment of cancer cells would favor the reduction of Ru(III) to the more labile Ru(II) species in tumors compared to normal tissue [77, 87].

Subsequently, dimethylsulfoxide (dmso) was introduced as a ligand into the ruthenium complexes with the aim of improving their solubility in water [88]. The coordination of this ligand can also be associated to important biological purposes, since dmso shows intrinsic capability to diffuse through phospholipidic membranes and, consequently, can facilitate the cell permeability. As a ligand, dmso exhibits ambidentate character, *i.e.*, it is capable of coordinating metal ions either by the oxygen (*O*-dmso) or the sulfur (*S*-dmso) atom, depending on both electronic and steric factors [89]. In particular, Ru(II) can be stabilized against air-oxidation to Ru(III) by the presence of the moderately good π-acceptor *S*-dmso ligand, while Ru(III) in *S*-dmso complexes are easily reduced to Ru(II). The dmso, being a relatively good leaving-ligand, may undergo exchange reactions with water molecules to form the correspondent aqua-complexes that may act as important reactive metabolites in the biological environment [56].

Historically, the *cis*- and *trans*- geometrical isomers of $[RuCl_2(dmso)_4]$, with the chloride ligands in *cis*- and *trans*-configurations, respectively, were the first Ru(II)-dmso complexes reported to show antitumor properties. The thermodynamically most stable *cis*-isomer has two *S*-dmso ligands in a *trans*-configuration whereas the third *S*-dmso occupies a *trans*-position to the only *O*-dmso ligand. The *trans*-isomer, which can be formed by isomerization of the *cis*-species under irradiation, has four *S*-dmso molecules in a plane perpendicular to the plane of the axial chloride ligands. Both of the isomers undergo aquation reactions that may be involved in their biological activity (activation by hydrolysis), with the higher activity of the *trans*-isomer being associated to a faster hydrolysis reaction and to a higher number of free coordination sites [56]. The *cis*-isomer, examined firstly, was found to be active against primary tumor and metastasis in mice, exhibiting cytoxicity *in vivo* that was approximately three orders of magnitude lower than the cytotoxicity of cisplatin. The high dosages (800 mg kg^{-1}) required for its activity, however, led to the further investigation of the *trans*-isomer which showed antitumor properties (in murine tumor models *in vivo*) and 20-fold higher activity against metastasis. It was effective in reducing spontaneous metastases, in contrast to cisplatin which was more active in reducing the primary tumor. The administrations of the two isomers, however, were limited by the high dosages required to achieve therapeutic effects comparable to that of cisplatin [56, 88, 90].

The discovery of the antimetastatic activity of these complexes encouraged the investigation of the chemical and the biological properties of other ruthenium(II)-dmso compounds [91-93]. The strategy of making structural modifications by the introduction of new L ligands, such as 5-nitrofurylsemicarbazone or metronidazole, to form $[RuCl_2(dmso)_2L_2]$ mixed derivatives, nonetheless, failed to improve the biological activity [94, 95]. This type of mixed compound, on the other hand, was found to exhibit unique chemistry that probably might have an effect on their behavior in the biological environment. The mixed compounds can admit five geometrical isomers with distinct *cis*- or *trans*- configurations for the three ligands, chloride, dmso and the L ligand. *N*-donor heterocyclic bases, for example, were found to be capable of replacing two dmso molecules in the *cis*-$[RuCl_2$(*O*-dmso)(*S*-dmso)$_3]$ to give mixtures of *cis,cis,cis*- and *cis,cis,trans*-$[RuCl_2$(*S*-dmso)$_2L_2]$ geometrical isomers [96-98]. Moreover, these compounds may show photochemical reactions as exemplified by the *cis,cis,trans*-$[RuCl_2$(*S*-dmso)$_2L_2]$, L = 4-*t*-butylpyridine, that undergoes photochemical selective labilization of the *S*-dmso ligand under near-UV irradiation [99]. Light induced reactions might also be an interesting alternative for the biological activity of ruthenium-dmso compounds. The *cis*- and *trans*-$[RuCl_2(dmso)_4]$ isomers exhibit UVA photo-dependent cytotoxicity in human and murine melanoma cells, and their reactivity towards oligonucleotides is related to photochemical pathway [100]. The influence of the anionic ligand nature was studied by exchanging the chlorides with dicarboxylates, but only one of the isolated complexes, the [*fac*-Ru(*S*-dmso)$_3(H_2O)$(cbdc)$]_2$, cbdc =1,1-cyclobutane dicarboxylate, dimer was moderately active against human oral carcinoma and murine cell lines [90]. On the other hand, the *trans,cis,cis*-$[RuCl_2(dmso)_2L_2]$, L = 2-amino-5-methyl-thiazole, was able to strongly inhibiting cathepsin B, "an attractive druggable target for cancer, rheumatoid arthritis and other important diseases" [101]. Most importantly, the contribution of the studies on ruthenium-dmso compounds led to the development of the compound NAMI-A, the first ruthenium-based drug to reach human clinical trials.

Ruthenium(III) Anticancer Drugs in Clinical Studies

The development of ruthenium-based antitumor/anticancer drugs, unquestionably, has received a solid contribution from all the accumulated scientific knowledge over the past 30 years. The recognition of ruthenium compounds as drug candidates for chemotherapy, nevertheless, was particularly driven forward by the entrance into human clinical trials of the two well-known antineoplastic ruthenium(III) drugs: the KP1019, (Hind)$[RuCl_4(ind)_2]$, ind = 1-*H*-indazole), and the NAMI-A, (Him)$[RuCl_4$(dmso)(im)], im = 1-*H*-imidazole (Fig. **4**).

KP1019 belongs to a family of ruthenium compounds having the general structure $[RuCl_4L_2]^-$, L = *N*-donor heterocycle, which was developed in the 1980s. The $[RuCl_4L_2]^-$ anionic framework contains a Ru(III) ion coordinated to four chloride ligands located in an equatorial plane that is perpendicular to the axial plane formed by the two symmetrical neutral *N*-heterocyclic L ligands, in a *trans*-configuration. The electron neutrality of the negative charge is given by a positively charged counter-ion that can be the corresponding protonated *N*-heterocycle ion or another cation such as sodium. The interest in this series of compounds was driven mainly by the findings that KP1019 and the isostructural analogue KP418, (Him)[$RuCl_4(im)_2$], im = 1-*H*-imidazole, were active against several tumor models, including platinum-resistant colorectal autochthonous tumors which resembles human colon cancers [102, 103].

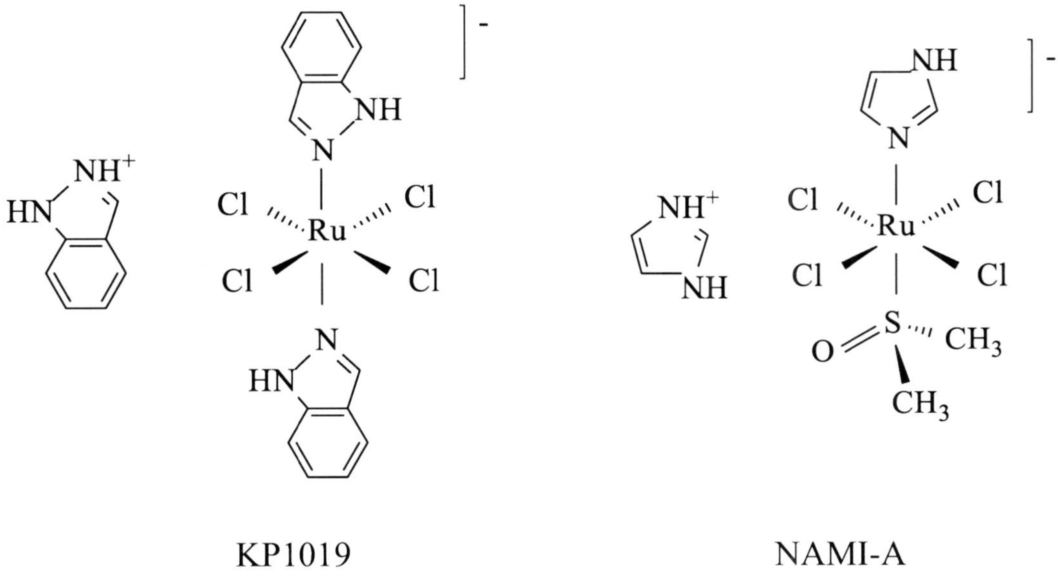

Fig. (4). Structures of KP1019 and NAMI-A.

Another complex, the NAMI, (Na)*trans*-[$RuCl_4$(dmso)(im)], structurally analogous to KP418 but isolated as sodium salt and having one dmso in a *trans*-configuration to the imidazole ligand, was found to be specifically active against metastasizing solid tumors in mice [88]. Its structure was later modified by replacing the sodium ion with the protonated positively charged Him^+ counter-ion to give the NAMI-A, which due to the higher stability in solid state was selected for clinical trials [104].

NAMI-A, currently in Phase I/II stage of development, reached clinical trials in 1999, being the first ruthenium-based drug administered to humans. It was followed by KP1019, which entered clinical Phase I trials in 2004. These two drugs exhibit mild toxicity towards normal healthy cells. Regardless the structural relationships (Fig. **4**) they show distinct behavior concerning to anticancer profiles, possible molecular targets and mechanisms of action. NAMI-A is poorly cytotoxic *in vitro* (> 10^{-4} mol L^{-1}, in almost all cell lines) but shows selective activity *in vivo* towards secondary tumors, inhibiting metastasis formation in lung metastases from several types of solid tumors (mouse, human). It is active in tumors intrinsically resistant to cisplatin, thus being capable of overcoming cisplatin resistance. Interactions with DNA are weak compared to cisplatin. Supposed targets are likely integrins and the mode of action may involve multiple interactions with components of the tumor microenvironment [67]. KP1019 shows cytotoxicity *in vitro* (~ 10^{-5} mol L^{-1}, in colorectal carcinoma cells) and exerts effective cytotoxicity in primary tumors, colorectal cancers (animal, human). It is also active in tumors intrinsically resistant to cisplatin, thus overcoming cisplatin resistance. It interacts with DNA in a similar way to cisplatin, but showing weaker interactions. Supposed targets are likely DNA, and apoptosis may occur *via* the mitochondrial pathway and reactive oxygen species (ROS) formation [67].

Both of the ruthenium(III) compounds can easily undergo reduction in the presence of biological reducing agents, thus they are considered as prodrugs that may be converted *via* reductive metabolism to more labile Ru(II) pharmacologically active species. The Ru(III)/Ru(II) redox potentials of KP1019 and NAMI-A (0.03 and 0.24 V *vs* NHE, pH 7.0, respectively), for example, are within the biologically relevant window [105, 106]. The metal center reduction may be promoted by bio-reducing agents such as ascorbic acid or glutathione and the reduced Ru(II) species can exchange ligands, subsequently interacting with biomolecules [13, 107, 108]. Although the mechanism of action and the biological targets have not been fully elucidated yet, it has been suggested that the ruthenium(III) drugs may act as functional compounds similarly to platinum-drugs. The metal could reach the biological targets either carrying some of the original ligands or not. The original ligands might also help to protect against fast and/or unwanted reactions gradually dissociating from the coordination sphere and leaving the metal ion to reach the target [73].

NAMI-A

NAMI-A is a highly effective inhibitor of the development and growth of pulmonary metastases in solid tumors models *in vivo*, and it was capable of inducing reduction of lung metastases growth in human non-small cell lung cancer xenotransplanted into nude mice. The cytotoxicity on tumor cells *in vitro* was not significant, and the cytotoxicity (mmol L^{-1} concentrations) on animal model primary tumors was negligible compared to cisplatin (μmol L^{-1} concentrations). The activity against metastases was responsible for its entrance into human clinical trials as anticancer candidate against non-small cell lung cancer [104, 109-114]. That was the main reason for the success of the drug since metastases of solid tumors, poorly responding to chemotherapy, result frequently in a higher number of cancer patient deaths compared to primary tumors [59]. The selectivity of NAMI-A for metastatic cells has been associated to the clonal origin of metastatic cells in the lung; moreover, drug metabolites able to bind to collagens of the extracellular matrix were found in the lung [56]. In Phase I, the drug was evaluated in 24 patients previously submitted to surgery and chemotherapy, with radiotherapy or not, showing good tolerability for a range of sub-toxic doses [67, 115]. Negligible hematological toxicity was observed, but a reversible mild renal dysfunction as well as nausea and vomiting occurred at high dose levels; the recommended dose for further clinical studies was 300 mg m^{-2} [115]. More recently, NAMI-A started to be investigated for a second line therapy use, combined with gemcitabine, in non-small-cell lung metastatic carcinoma [67].

The mode of action of NAMI-A still remains unclear. Nevertheless, the diverse biological effects and the possible targets suggest the occurrence of multiple mechanisms acting outside the cells, at the cell membrane, and also inside the cells [67, 116-119]. In contrast to platinum-drugs, the nuclear DNA is unlikely the primary target for NAMI-A, since its ability to bind DNA is weak, both *in vitro* and *in vivo* [109, 120-122]. NAMI-A binds strongly and within minutes to the plasma proteins, human serum albumin and transferrin [107, 123, 124]. The mechanism of action of NAMI-A may comprise several processes such as blockage of the progression of cell cycle at G_2-M pre-mitotic phase [67], interference with tumor cells interactions with extracellular matrix, comprising an increase of actin-dependent cell adhesion [117, 118], inhibition of matrix degradation by matrix metalloproteinase [125], and reduction of cell invasiveness and migration leading to less malignant cell phenotype [113, 125]. The mechanism of controlling metastasis has been related to combined anti-angiogenic and anti-invasive effects on tumor cells and blood vessels [126]. The control of angiogenesis has been associated to scavenging properties of NAMI-A on the NO produced by the endothelial cells [81]. In terms of anti-invasive effects, NAMI-A is capable of reducing spontaneous invasion of matrigel by tumor cells with dose-dependent reduction of gelatinase release and activation of adhesion molecules such as beta-integrins [81, 117, 127].

Studies with serum proteins have shown that an apo-transferrin-NAMI-A adduct was not able to bind specifically to transferrin receptor 1 (TfR1), in contrast to Fe(III)-transferrin that binds strongly to the same receptor. In the absence of excess Fe(III) and albumin, NAMI-A might specifically bind to the Fe(III)-Tf sites, but this binding is unlikely to affect significantly the cellular uptake of the drug *in vivo*. The binding of NAMI-A to albumin was found to affect its interactions with other blood proteins, *e.g.*, immunoglobulins, suggesting that the crosslinking of extracellular proteins by Ru(III) may be involved in the antimetastatic activity of the metallodrug [128]. NAMI-A was crystallized with the hen egg white lysozyme releasing the three original ligands, *i.e.,* the four chloride anions and the neutral dmso and imidazole ligands, to leave the naked ruthenium ion to coordinate the protein at two distinct aspartates. This data is an evidence for the view of NAMI-A behaving as classical prodrug that undergoes activation which results, subsequently, on the metalation of protein targets. The original ligands were suggested to play a role in directing the metal center to the protein surface anchoring sites [129].

NAMI-A, similarly to cisplatin, is cleared by kidneys, but was found to induce renal damage in mice with advanced carcinomas. Recent studies, however, suggest that the clinical signs of renal toxicity caused by the drug may be prevented by appropriate procedures during the curative cycles of treatment [130].

KP1019 and KP1339

KP1019 entered into clinical trials mainly due to the cytotoxic activity against cisplatin-resistant tumors. In contrast to NAMI-A, it was not capable of modifying metastatic cells behavior [131]. However, it was found to show marked effects on autochthonous chemically-induced colorectal cancer in mouse [103, 132], on colorectal cancer cells *in vitro* [133-135] and on chemoresistant colon carcinoma *in vivo* [136]. The drug activity *in vitro* encompassed > 80% specimens in studies including more than 50 primary explanted human tumors [137]. The compound was considered sufficiently stable for intravenous administration, entering into clinical evaluation. Phase I clinical trial in humans was completed with the patients showing disease stabilization, and moderate toxicity accompanying the treatments, but the drug low solubility limited the total dose to 600 mg per patient (twice a week for 3 weeks) [138]. The pharmacokinetic behavior *in vivo* (including humans), taking into account both the protein binding and the half-life time release from the blood, was shown to be very close to that of NAMI-A [67]. To overcome the solubility problems, the more soluble sodium salt KP1339, (Na)[$RuCl_4$(ind)$_2$], currently in Phase I-IIa, was included into clinical studies in humans.

The behavior of KP1019 was shown to be different from that of cisplatin. Its interaction with DNA involves DNA-DNA and DNA-protein crosslinks 15-fold less intense than cisplatin, single strand breaks are enhanced when the drug is reduced by bio-reducing agents, and conformational changes on secondary structure of DNA are weaker than those induced by cisplatin [67]. However, triggering of apoptosis by DNA-binding cannot be excluded, even though the intrinsic mitochondria pathway seems to be predominantly involved in the apoptotic process in colorectal cell lines [138].

The drug shows important interactions with biomolecules reacting with both of the human serum proteins, with the major amount binding to the most abundant albumin and a smaller amount binding to transferrin. While albumin is the thermodynamically preferred partner for KP1019, the reaction with transferrin is favored by kinetics [139]. KP1019, as well as its analogue KP1339, is capable of binding site I and site II of human serum albumin with moderately strong affinity. Considerable displacements of three established site markers, *i.e.,* warfarin, dansylglycine and bilirubin, were observed upon addition of both Ru(III) drugs suggesting their ability to bind to both sites. The lack of preference for either binding site and the similarity of results found for both metal drugs demonstrated no influence of the counter-ion. Moreover, the affinity of the ruthenium drug for the bilirubin binding site is suggested to show possible clinical relevance on the treatment of patients with elevated bilirubin levels [140]. The relatively low toxicity and the apparent tumor selectivity of KP1019 have been associated partially to transferrin-mediated drug transports. KP1019 was found in part to bind specifically to human apo-transferrin. Cellular uptake experiments (in human colon carcinoma) confirmed that the transport of KP1019 into the cell is promoted by transferrin. The cellular accumulation was found to follow the order: KP1019-Fe(III)-transferrin conjugate >> KP1019 > KP1019-transferrin adduct, suggesting that iron binding is needed for protein-receptor interactions [141].

KP1339 was found to show cytotoxic activity moderately lower than that of KP1019, even though a significant correlation based on IC_{50} values for distinct cancer cell models has been found for their cytotoxic profiles. Intracellular distribution patterns suggest that the major targets for both drugs are cytosolic rather than nuclear. KP1019 and KP1339 are capable of binding to multiple small soluble proteins as well as to large complexes/organelles, after rapidly entering into tumor cells. The cytosolic retention was higher for KP1019 which is more cytotoxic suggesting the importance of cytoplasm protein targets for the exerted activity. The pattern of cytosolic protein binding of these ruthenium drugs differs from the cisplatin pattern, supporting unique mode of action distinct from the platinum drugs [142].

The chemistry of the redox-active KP1019 was recently investigated by analyses based mainly on the concept of coordination charge related to possible coordination-oxidations pairs and also on metal model-compounds representing possible coordination motifs and oxidation states *in vivo*. The studies revealed that the mode of action of KP1019 may involve release of chloride to a first coordination shell rich in *O*- and/or *N*- ligands. The dissociation of chloride was also a hint for the possible interaction with the apo-transferrin. Ru(II) and Ru(III) species in a *S*-, *N*-, *Cl*-coordination environment were found in the presence of glutathione. Liver and tumor samples from mice after treatment with KP1019 and KP1339 showed identical first coordination environments. Ruthenium was found to strongly penetrate into the tumor tissue near blood vessels and in the edge regions of the tissue samples [143]. It is worth to mention that the investigation of the changes in the chemical environment of metal centers (*e.g.,* oxidation states, coordination environment, identity and number of adjacent atoms) and of the chemical state of elements within subcellular compartments have been used for other metal-based drugs providing important information to elucidate their interactions with, *e.g.*, reducing agents, biomolecular targets and transport molecules *in vitro* and *in vivo* [144, 145].

The combination of KP1339 with sorafenib, a multi-kinase inhibitor currently used in standard first-line therapy for advanced hepatoma, was found to be promising *in vitro* and *in vivo* against human hepatoma models. Synergistic activities were associated to several mechanisms including enhanced accumulation levels of both drugs resulting in enhanced induction of apoptosis; blocking of KP1339-mediated activation of P38 signaling, abrogation of KP1339-induced G_2-M arrest with check point-independent DNA-synthesis block and loss of mitotic cell populations. The combined KP1339/sorafenib therapy enhanced (by 3.9-fold) the mean survival of Hep3B hepatoma xenograft compared to KP1339 (2.4-fold increase in life span) and sorafenib (induced a 1.9-fold prolonged survival) [146].

Despite the promising clinical activity and low adverse effects, the clinical application of KP1019 is currently limited mainly by the low solubility and stability of the drug in aqueous solution. Nanoparticle systems containing polymer-based micelles loaded with the ruthenium drug has been suggested as strategy for improving both the stability and the activity. They were found to enhance stability in aqueous solution, to facilitate cellular accumulation of KP1019 with lower IC_{50} values, to increase cell cycle arrest in G_2-M phase, to increase DNA damage, and to enhance levels of apoptotic cell death [147].

Ruthenium(II) Organometallics and Anticancer Properties

A second class of ruthenium compounds undergoing interesting biological studies with the aim of finding new metal anticancer drug candidates comprises organometallic compounds, *i.e.*, ruthenium complexes having direct ruthenium-carbon bonds. Differently from the classical ruthenium(III) coordination complexes (NAMI-A, KP1019 and their analogues), the organometallic compounds contain the ruthenium metal ion in the Ru(II) lower oxidation state. A number of ruthenium(II)-organometallics have been found to show properties as potential antitumor and/or antimetastatic drugs [see, *e.g.*, references 1, 62, 63, 65, 68, 70, 71, 148-159].

The first recognized organometallic of ruthenium (reported in 1992) to exhibit biological activity was the compound [Ru(η^6-benzene)(metronidazole)Cl_2] which showed higher cytotoxicity than the metronidazole parent ligand [148]. Few years later, at the end of 1990s, and following the encouraging results shown by the Ru(III) complexes, series of Ru(II)-organometallics started to be examined for anticancer/antitumor properties. Two main classes of ruthenium(II)-arene complexes, the originally named "piano-stool" organometallics and the "RAPTA" complexes (Fig. **5**), emerged, being particularly exploited for chemical, biochemical and biological properties [71]. Representative complexes are, *e.g.*, the RM175 ([Ru(η^6-biphenyl)(en)Cl][PF_6], en = ethylenediamine) [160] and the prototype RAPTA-C ([Ru(η^6-*p*-cymene)(pta)Cl_2], pta = 1,3,5-triaza-7-phosphatricyclo[3.3.1.1]decane) [161] organometallics (Fig. **5**).

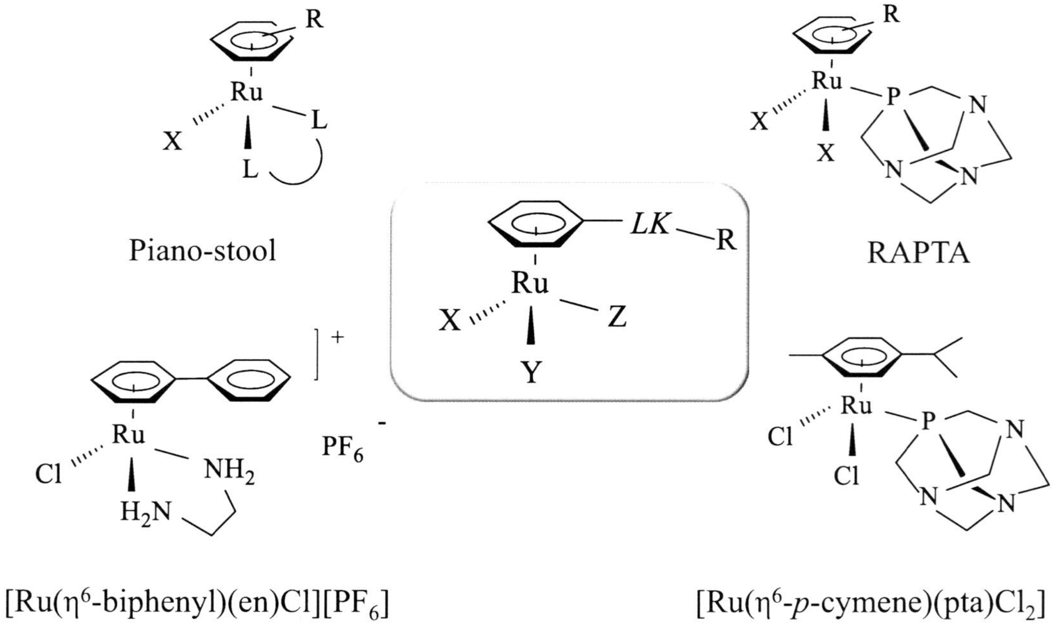

Fig. (5). Generic structure of ruthenium(II)-arene compounds (X, Y and Z can be mono, bis or tris-dentate ligands) (center) [69]; generic structure of the originally named piano-stool (upper left) and respective example (bottom left); generic structure of RAPTA (upper right) and respective example (bottom right).

Ruthenium(II)-Arenes Originally Named "Piano-Stool"

The ruthenium(II)-arenes of the type $[Ru(arene)(LL)(X)]^{n+}$, originally named as "piano-stool" half-sandwich compounds, are formed by three basic building blocks: the arene ligand, a LL bidentate ligand (typically, neutral or monoanionic *N,N*-, *N,O*-, or *O,O*-chelating ligand) and a monodentate X ligand (usually, a halide such as chloride). The positively charged complexes may be isolated as PF_6^- salts but neutral species can also be formed, depending on the nature of the LL ligand. The choice of the arene substituents as well as of the monodentate and the bidentate ligands allows fine-tuning physical, chemical and pharmacological properties of these compounds [162-165]. The analogy with the piano-stool comes from the arrangement of the ligands in the structure, with the arene representing the seat and the X and LL ligands resembling the legs of the piano stool. The presence of the arene provides a hydrophobic face to these organometallics. The six-electron donor ligand shows π-donor/π-acceptor dual characteristic that promotes the stabilization of the metal ion in the Ru(II) low oxidation state. The geometry of the compounds can be described as either pseudo-tetrahedral (if the arene is assumed to occupy one coordination site) or octahedral (for the arene occupying three facial coordination sites). In general, Ru-arene bonds are stable to hydrolysis, but in some cases the arene cleavage may be relevant for the mode of action [164, 166, 167]. The nature of the arene may affect cell uptake and interactions with potential targets, while the nature of the LL bidentate ligand is associated to the anticancer activity and the ligand X may act as an activation site. These piano-stool complexes can be activated by releasing the ligand X to leave a free coordination site for binding DNA or other target biomolecules. The good aqueous solubility of the complexes and the relatively inertia of the arene towards displacement under physiological conditions are advantageous for possible clinical use of the Ru(II)-arene compounds [56, 62, 149, 151].

The compounds of the general formula $[Ru(\eta^6\text{-arene})(en)Cl]PF_6$ keeps analogy with cisplatin having the ethylenediamine in the place of the two NH_3 ligands. They exhibit cytotoxicity at levels similar to cisplatin [56, 151]. RM175, in preclinical studies, shows ability to overcome platinum resistance, as exemplified by its activity against ovarian carcinoma resistant to cisplatin [168]. The presence of larger arene ligands such as biphenyl, tetrahydroanthracene and tetrahydronaphthalene favors higher cytotoxicity. The hydrophobicity of the arene was found to affect the cytotoxic activity. Compounds of *p*-cymene or biphenyl showed IC_{50} values similar to that of carboplatin, while compounds of tetrahydronaphthalene were equipotent with cisplatin against the human ovarian cancer cells [56]. RM175 was found to bind to DNA, resulting in cell death for colorectal HCT116 cells [169]. Additionally, it was active against MCa mammary carcinoma *in vivo* and caused metastasis reduction [67, 170]. Oligonucleotide binding studies revealed that the $[Ru(\eta^6\text{-}p\text{-cymene})(en)Cl]^+$ complex, after activation *via* chloride/water exchange binds to guanine bases [171]. The guanine binding apparently is enhanced by the formation of (N-H) ethylenediamine - (O) guanine hydrogen bonds, in analogy to cisplatin [71]. The $[Ru(\eta^6\text{-arene})(en)]^{2+}$ mode of binding to nucleotide bases, however, depends on the nature of the arene ligand. For larger arene rings such as biphenyl, dihydroanthracene, or tetrahydroanthracene, in contrast to single hydrocarbon rings in the *p*-cymene and benzene, the binding of the Ru-arene fragment seems to be promoted by hydrophobic interactions and by arene-(purine base) π-stacking interactions. Therefore, the Ru(II)-arene DNA interactions, depending on the arene for this class of complexes, may involve both the coordination to guanine-N*7* in double-helical DNA and non-covalent, hydrophobic interactions that can include arene intercalation to DNA and minor groove binding [71, 171-173]. Moreover, the distinct antitumor activity compared to cisplatin has been supported by the fact that removal of Ru(II)-arene adducts from DNA does not occur preferentially by nucleotide excision repair [67]. Nevertheless, the biological activities of ruthenium(II)-arene compounds may be not always related to their DNA-binding ability, but involve multi-targeted mechanisms [174-176]. The mode of action has also been associated to p53 and p21 in the growth arrest, and to p53 and Bax in the apoptotic response [67].

Additionally, these compounds may undergo redox reactions in cells. RM175 was found to react with glutathione to form species that may be involved in a potential redox-mediated pathway to DNA binding [177]. The $[Ru(\eta^6\text{- biphenyl})(en)Cl]PF_6$ participates in competition reactions involving the tripeptide glutathione (*γ*-L-Glu-L-Cys-Gly; GSH), the abundant intracellular thiol, and guanosine 3',5'-cyclic monophosphate, cGMP, in a way dependent of the solution composition. The reaction with GSH in unbuffered (pH ~ 3) solution gave firstly three intermediate adducts (an *S*-bound thiolato complex, [(η^6-biphenyl)Ru(en)(GS-*S*)], and two carboxylate-bound glutathione products), with subsequently dissociation of the ethylenediamine ligand to form [((η^6-biphenyl)Ru)$_2$(GS-μ-*S*)$_3$]$^{2-}$ dinuclear species. Under physiologically relevant conditions, at pH 7, the thiolato complex, instead of forming the dinuclear species, underwent oxidation by dioxygen to generate the [(η^6-biphenyl)Ru(en)(GS(O)-*S*)] sulfenato complex. Competitive reaction of the original complex with GSH and cGMP gave predominantly the [(η^6-biphenyl) Ru(en)(cGMP-N*7*)]$^+$ adduct [178]. The formation of highly charged multinuclear species and the involvement of ligand-based redox processes in reaction pathways of metallodrugs were further elucidated. Ruthenium multinuclear species [{(η^6-biphenyl))Ru(GSO$_2$)}$_4$]$^{2-}$ and [{(η^6-biphenyl)Ru(GSO$_2$)$_2$}$_2$]$^{8-}$containing glutathione sulfinate (GSO$_2$) ligands were identified for the reactions with GSH. In addition, evidences were found for the involvement of water in oxygen atom insertion into S-O bonds in the oxidized glutathione (sulfenate and sulfinate) ligands [179].

Interestingly, studies on biological/biochemical activity were performed for the [Ru(η^6-biphenyl)(en)Cl]$^+$ (that exerts anti-metastatic activity) comparatively to its isostructural osmium(II)-arene (which is not anti-metastatic). Results showed distinct behavior for both of the metal(II)-arene complexes, confirming the relevance of the nature of the metal and thus giving support for the key role of ruthenium metal ion in the anti-metastatic activity [170].

RAPTA Complexes

The ruthenium(II)-arenes of the general formula [Ru(η^6-arene)(pta)X$_2$], known as RAPTA (ruthenium-arene-pta), are typically formed by the pta amphiphilic monodentate ligand, one arene ligand and an anionic X ligand (usually chloride, or a chelating dicarboxylate) (Fig. **5**). The activation of RAPTA compounds may involve dissociation of the chloride ligands. The arene ligand may also be released in some cases, while the pta is strongly bounded to the metal ion. RAPTA derivatives containing dicarboxylate bidentate ligands are more inert towards aquation [56].

The [Ru(η^6-arene)(pta)Cl_2] RAPTA series, despite exhibiting only mild effects on primary tumors, were found to show important antimetastatic properties *in vivo* [161]. RAPTA-C and RAPTA-T, [Ru(η^6-toluene)(pta)Cl_2], proved to be the most active representatives of the series. RAPTA-C, similarly to NAMI-A, is very active *in vivo* inhibiting lung metastases in CBA mice and shows low toxicity. It was found to increase levels of p53, leading to apoptosis, and to be selectively active towards highly invasive cancer cell lines in relation to less aggressive tumors and healthy cells [71, 180]. RAPTA-T exhibits low cytotoxicity *in vitro* (10^{-5} - 10^{-4} mol L^{-1}) and shows some selectivity towards secondary tumors *in vivo* [67]. Even though in lower extension than NAMI-A, it is able to inhibit the formation of lung metastases, without significant effect on the primary tumor, tested on the mouse MCa mammary carcinoma [161, 181]. The mode of action involves modulation of cytoskeleton. It interacts with extracellular matrix components, thus inhibiting some steps of the metastatic process; it selectively inhibits detachment, migration, invasion and reattachment, processes which are associated to the formation of metastatic tumor [71]. However, in spite of the promising activities and pharmacokinetics, the high doses required for effective treatment may be a limitation to the use of RAPTA compounds.

Some RAPTA compounds are capable of inhibiting the enzyme cathepsin B, most likely after activation by aquation. Coordination of Ru(II) to the sulfur atom of the active site of cysteine is implemented by additional contacts with nearby protein residues [182]. There are few evidences for direct DNA damage by these compounds. Nevertheless, differently from cisplatin and other platinum cytotoxic drugs, which preferentially bind to DNA, the prototype RAPTA-C was shown to bind to the protein histone core of nucleosome DNA, replacing the two original chloride ligands with two glutamate residues of the protein to give a crystalline adduct [183]. Proteomic studies have been conducted with the aim of elucidating the mode of action of antimetastatic ruthenium compounds on human cancer cells. RAPTA-T and NAMI-A were found to induce proteomic alterations that were substantially distinct from those of cytotoxic platinum drugs, confirming different mechanisms of actions for the ruthenium complexes compared to the platinum compounds. Furthermore, both ruthenium antimetastatic compounds were found to have 9 common proteomic alterations out of a total of 27 suggesting a high correlation between their mechanisms of action [184].

General Features of Ru-arenes and Other Organometallic Complexes

The ruthenium(II)-arene compounds can be represented by the generalized structure shown at the center of Fig. (**5**). The accumulated studies on chemical, biochemical and biological properties of these compounds during the years enabled the proposition of ways to modify the structure aiming to tune their pharmacological properties [71]. Ruthenium(II) is stabilized by the arene ligand resulting in strong Ru-arene bonds and in a quite stable Ru-arene scaffold which allows rationale structural modification to incorporate functionality that can be directed even to targeted chemotherapy. For example, LK (Fig. **5**) can be a stable or enzyme cleavable linker, and R a bioactive group with a synergistically acting biological role, an enzyme inhibitor, a tumor targeting group, *etc.* The bulky hydrophobic surface provided by the arene is associated to a degree of selectivity for binding biomolecular targets. However, although increasing hydrophobicity may lead to enhanced cytotoxicity, it may not necessarily improve the selectivity (cancer *vs* healthy cells). Polyaromatic rings can be introduced into the arene to favor non-covalent interactions with DNA. The ancillary Y (and Z) ligand can be selected to modulate biological/pharmacological properties of the Ru(II)-arene compounds. The X (and Y) leaving ligand(s) should be sufficiently labile to undergo exchange reactions (*e.g.*, with water, at controlled rates) that will be important for interactions with biomolecular targets. Hydrolysis of the Ru-Cl bond, for example, allows subsequent coordination of the metal ion to relevant targets, with the ruthenium also playing active role. The nature of the labile ligands allows modulating the reaction rate with biomolecular targets [71].

The influence of the nature of the YZ chelating ligand (*e.g., N,N-* or *N,O-* or *O,O-* donor ligands) and of the X leaving-group has been illustrated for Ru(II)-arene compounds [149, 163, 167]. In a series of $[Ru(\eta^6\text{-arene})(YZ)Cl]^{n+}$ complexes, the YZ chelating ligand was found to affect the rate and extent of aquation, the pKa of the aqua-species, as well as the rate and selectivity of nucleobases binding. Complexes such as $[Ru(\eta^6\text{-arene})(en)Cl]^+$ undergo fast hydrolysis in aqueous solution to form aqua-species having pKa values which allow the formation of the complex at physiological pH and its interaction with DNA bases. The replacement of the chelating ligand from a *N,N*-donor such as ethylenediamine (en) with *O,O*-donor such as acetylacetonate (acac) may cause a dramatic effect on the reactivity of the ruthenium-arene with respect to hydrolysis, cytotoxicity and DNA base specificity [149]. Changing the ethylenediamine with the acac ligand in the [Ru(η^6-*p*-cymene)(acac)Cl] leads to an increase on the rate and the extent of hydrolysis, and on the pKa value (from 8.25, en, to 9.41, acac) of the coordinated water in the aqua-species. The acac ligands, being strong σ-donor/π-donor, increase electron density towards ruthenium, thus decreasing the acidity of the ruthenium center and favoring the formation of reactive aqua-species at physiological pH (pH 7.4) more than the en ligand [149]. Replacement of the en ligand with acac also leads to changes on the nucleobase specificity; reactions with nucleobases were found to be dependent on the hydrogen-bond character (donor/acceptor) of the YZ chelating ligand [167]. The complex [Ru(η^6-*p*-cymene)(glycine)$H_2O]^+$ having the *N,O*-donor chelating glycine undergoes very fast hydrolysis and shows water-coordinated pKa equals to 8.25, forming highly stable and reactive aqua-species that may account for the lack of cytotoxicity [149]. Similarly, other *N,O*-chelated complexes (mostly amino acidates) were shown to be inactive against cancer cells, perhaps due to the extensive hydrolysis of the chloride-complex, leading to deactivating reactions with biomolecules [163]. The effect of [Ru(η^6-arene)(YZ)Cl]A complexes, in which A can be PF_6^-, YZ is an *N,N*- (diamine), *N,O*- (*e.g.*, amino acidate), or *O,O*- (*e.g.*, *β*-diketonate) chelating ligand, and the arene ranges from benzene derivatives to fused polycyclic hydrocarbons, was tested in human ovarian cancer cells. The most active complexes were those containing extended polycyclic arenes and where YZ = ethylenediamine. Complexes with the arene having polar substituents or YZ = bipyridyl-ligands exhibited reduced activity while the *O,O*-chelated complexes showed activity that depends on the arene and also on the substituents [163].

More recently, attention has been focused on exploiting ruthenium-arene complexes aiming targeted chemotherapy, even though the studies are still in earlier stage of development [50, 71, 149, 185-188]. The ruthenium(II)-arene unit has been used as a synthon to prepare a diversity of derivatives, including multinuclear compounds and clusters, many of which have already been evaluated for biological properties [see, *e.g.,* references 62, 71]. Examples of modified structures, although not necessarily the most important regarding chemical/biochemical/biological features, are shown in Fig. (**6**) and discussed for main features.

The structural modification with a thio-derivative such as the *N*-substituted 2-pyridinecarbothioamide ligand (Fig. **6a**) led to highly antiproliferative activity, depending on lipophilicity and steric factors, in colon carcinoma and non-small lung cancer cell lines. The behavior in aqueous solution and the stability under acidic conditions suggested potential suitability for oral administration. The quantitative estimates of drug-likeness indicate a drug-likeness similar to those of established anticancer drugs (*e.g.,* erlotinib, tamoxifen, imatinib, sorafenib). The modified complex binds to histone proteins in the nucleosome core particle *via* coordination of the metal center to a histidine side chain of the protein [189]. Complexes modified with phosphite-carbohydrate ligands (Fig. **6b**) replacing the pta ligand show only moderate cytotoxicity [190-193]. A compound containing arene modified with antracene derivative was used to track the uptake of the compound into cancer cells, showing accumulation into the cell cytoplasm [71]. The ruthenium-arene has also been modified with the aim of evaluating the role of the complexes as inhibitor of the Pgp protein that is involved in multidrug resistance. The coordination of the ruthenium-arene unit to an imidazole derivatized with anthracene ligand (Fig. **6c**) led to effectiveness that was higher than those of known inhibitors [71]. The incorporation of a bioactive functionality may also result in interesting synergistic effects with the ruthenium-arene unit [150, 185, 194-197]. For example, the ruthenium-arene derivatized with the ethacrynic acid, an inhibitor of glutathione-*S*-transferase, led to a complex (Fig. **6d**) with increased cytotoxicity. The interaction with the enzyme was found to involve the insertion of the ethacrynic acid into the catalytic site and coordination of the ruthenium to cysteine residues that is followed by releasing of the metal unit with the ethacrynic acid remaining in the catalytic site [150]. Complexes formed by attaching ruthenium-arene units to staurosporine (Fig. **6e**) have been designed as protein kinase inhibitors. The replacement of the sugar in the molecule of staurosporine with the ruthenium unit carrying numerous substituents

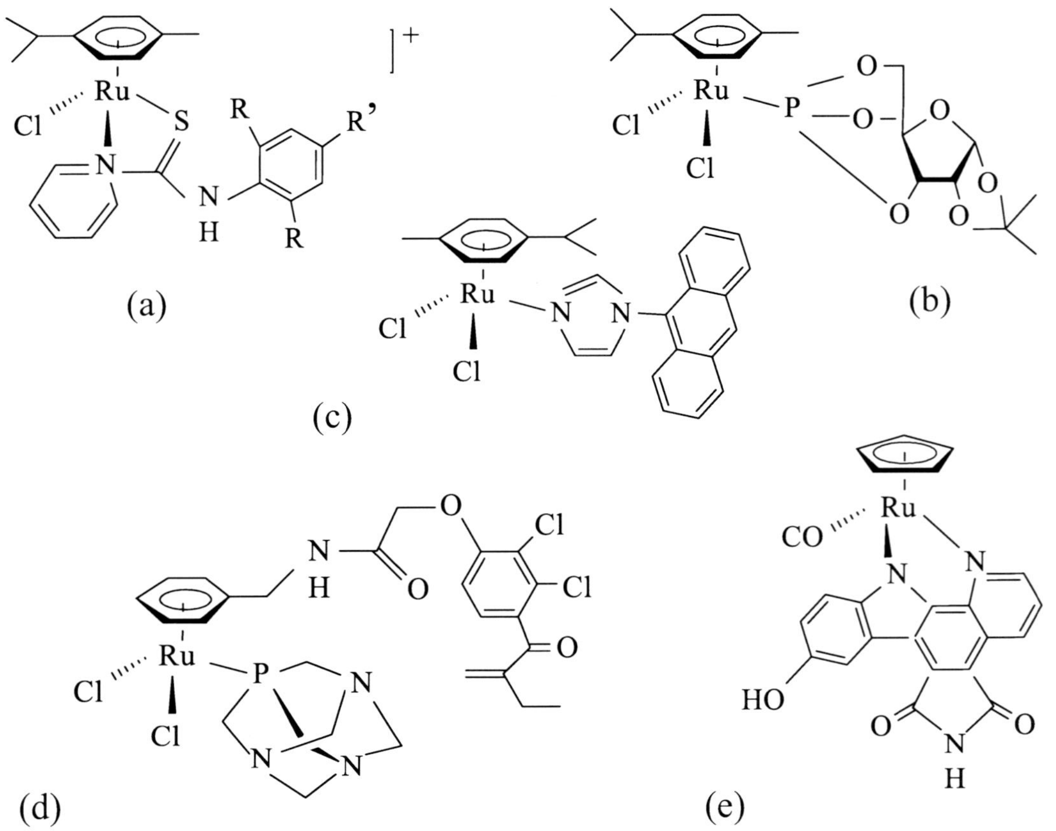

Fig. (6). Structures of ruthenium(II)-arene compounds containing a thio-derivative (**a**), a phosphorous-modified sugar (**b**), an anthracene-modified imidazole (**c**), the glutathione *S*-transferase inhibitor ethacrynic acid (**d**), and Ru-arene kinase inhibitor mimicking staurosporine (**e**).

gave a family of products capable of a significantly increase affinity and selectivity for enzymes [198-200]. In particular, 'Ru(η^5-C_5H_5)'-staurosporine derivatives, tested in human melanoma cells *in vitro*, were able to promote apoptotic cell death mediated by p53 and the mitochondrial pathway [201]. Compounds incorporating natural products, *e.g.,* flavone and maltol derivative ligands have also been investigated. Water-soluble Ru(II)-arene dinuclear compounds with maltol-derived linkers between [Ru(η^6-*p*-cymene)Cl] units show cytotoxic effects in human cancer cell lines, with IC_{50} dependent on the spacer length between the metal centers. The cytotoxicity was correlated with lipophilicity and aqueous solubility [202] and the compounds were found to crosslink DNA duplex and DNA-protein [203].

Other Ru(II)-organometallics having the 'Ru(η^5-C_5H_5)' motif attached to phosphines have also been exploited for modification with chelating ligands. The introduction of *N-N'*- or *N,O*-heteroaromatic ligands, for example, was found to provide stability and good cytotoxicity against several human cell lines [204]. Investigations on the mode of action of these compounds in human tumor cell lines suggested the endosomal/lysosomal system as a possible target for anticancer metal-based drugs [205].

Diruthenium(II,III) Metal-Metal Bonded Complexes

Properties and Biological Activity

The third class of potential antitumor/anticancer drugs presented here consists of complexes having the mixed-valence diruthenium(II,III) metal-metal multiply bonded core. Compounds which contain the [Ru_2] dinuclear core stabilized by multiple bonds between the two metal atoms have attracted theoretical and experimental interest since the 1960s decade [206]. Dinuclear tetracarboxylatos of the formula $[Ru_2(O_2CR)_4L_m]^{n+}$ (m = 1 or 2; n = 0 - 2), in which R is derivative of, *e.g.*, alkyl, aryl, alcoxyl group or metallocene, and L is an axial ligand, *e.g.*, a Lewis base or halide, account for the most numerous family of these complexes. Important features related to structure, reactivity, properties and applications of diruthenium complexes have been reported [206-209]. The most common dimetal oxidation states are Ru_2(II,II) and Ru_2(II,III), the last being the thermodynamically most stable. The metal ions in the Ru_2(II,III), or $[Ru_2]^{5+}$, mixed-valence core are directly connected through a strong Ru-Ru bond of bond order 2.5. Diruthenium(II,III)-tetracarboxylatos show unique behavior and typical magnetic properties with high effective magnetic moments associated to the presence of three unpaired electrons.

The metal-metal multiply bonded Ru_2(II,II) cores are stabilized by the coordination of four equatorial carboxylate ligands to form $[Ru_2(O_2CR)_4]^+$ complexes which show the paddlewheel typical structure (Fig. 7). The nature of the axial L ligand has significant influence on the type of species formed in the solid state that can vary from dinuclear complexes to multinuclear extended polymeric chains in which the dinuclear units are linked by the bridging axial ligands [206, 207]. The presence of chloride favors the formation of axial bridges as illustrated by the crystal structure, *e.g.,* of the complex $[Ru_2(O_2CCH_3)_4Cl]$, tetrakis(acetato)chloridodiru-thenium(II,III), that shows a polymeric structure in which the ruthenium centers are linked by the halide bridges into an infinite *zig-zag* chain [207].

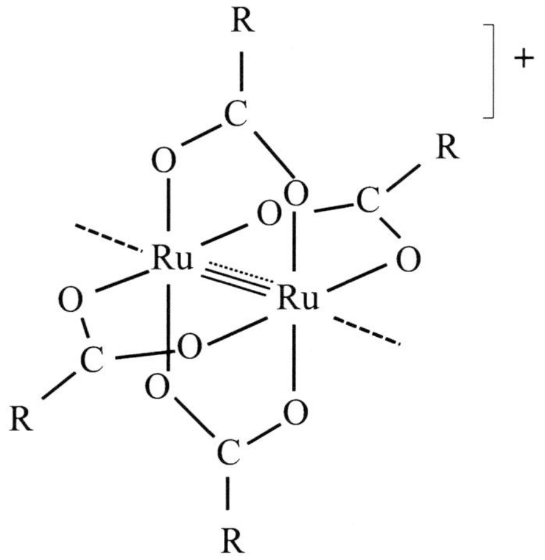

Fig. (7). Generic structure of the $[Ru_2(O_2CR)_4]^+$ metal-metal bonded complex.

The reactivity and chemical behavior of the $[Ru_2(O_2CR)_4Cl]$ compounds in solution has been scarcely explored. Nevertheless, it has been reported that these complexes can undergo ligand substitution reactions with the exchange of the relatively labile chloride ligand with the solvent (S) to give the correspondent axially substituted species, *e.g.*, the neutral $[Ru_2(O_2CR)_4Cl(S)]$ and the cationic $[Ru_2(O_2CR)_4(S)_2]^+$ complexes. The predominant species in solution will depend mainly on the nature of the solvent (if it is coordinating or not). The presence of excess of chloride in solution may favor the formation of the $[Ru_2(O_2CR)_4Cl_2]^-$ anionic complex. The redox potential of the Ru_2(II,III) dimetal cores has been reported for only few compounds [207], but the observed values are in the range accessible physiologically. Thus, these compounds might be possibly activated by reduction process to give the correspondent Ru_2(II,II) reduced cores in the biological environment.

In contrast to both of the other two classes of complexes, *e.g.*, the Ru(III) and Ru(II) mononuclear complexes and the Ru(II) organometallic compounds, the diruthenium(II,III) metal-metal bonded complexes have received much less attention with regard to the antitumor/anticancer properties. The first studies reported at the literature around the 1990s [102] revealed the slight antineoplastic activity against P388 leukemia cells for the complexes $[Ru_2(O_2CCH_3)_4Cl]$ and $[Ru_2(O_2CCH_3CH_2)_4Cl]$; however, no further biological studies were reported perhaps due to the poor solubility of these compounds in water. Another article, published in 2002, described the cytotoxicity against HeLa and CoLo 320DM human cancer cell lines for the complexes: (a) $[Ru_2(O_2CR)_4L_2]PF_6$, L = imidazole, 1-methylimidazole or water, R = CH_3, L = ethanol, R = Fc (ferrocenyl) or Fc-CH=CH-, and (b) $M_3[Ru_2(O_2CR)_4(H_2O)_2]$, M = Na^+, R = m-$C_6H_4SO_3^-$, M = K^+, R = p-$C_6H_4SO_3^-$. The IC_{50} values varied from 120 to 950 μmol L^{-1}, and the antineoplastic activity was shown to be higher for the most water soluble *m*-phenylsulfonate derivatives, while the poorly water soluble imidazole derivatives were found to be non-cytotoxic [210]. A study on the interaction of diruthenium-tetracarboxylatos with the 9-ethylguanine biomolecule was reported, however, no significant clues about the elucidation of the biological activity for this type of compounds could be suggested [211, 212].

Therefore, the most recent studies on diruthenium(II,III) metal-metal multiply bonded complexes with the aim of exploiting their anticancer properties are totally centered in our research group. We have used the strategy of combining the Ru_2(II,III) cores with organic pharmaceuticals of clinical use to develop a novel class of diruthenium(II,III)-(pharmaceuticals) metallodrugs which has been pioneered shown to be promising candidates to target glioma.

Diruthenium(II,III)-(Pharmaceuticals) Metallodrugs

An interesting approach to the design of novel metallodrugs is the coordination of metal centers to biologically active ligands *(e.g.*, drugs capable of exerting their own effects). This strategy can be exploited in several ways to promote, *e.g.*, synergistic effects from metal and ligands favoring alternative mechanisms of action, improvement in solubility, enhancement of the biological activity, reduction of undesirable side-effects, modulation of redox-activity, and enhancement of cellular uptake, among others effects.

Following this approach, a novel class of potential anticancer metallodrugs has been designed by combining the diruthenium(II,III) core with carboxylic organic pharmaceuticals. The leading compound of this class, a diruthenium-ibuprofen complex [61], is currently undergoing preclinical studies targeting glioma models, as presented further on this chapter.

The main pharmaceuticals selected for the design of this novel series of metallodrugs belong to the group of the Non-Steroidal Anti-Inflammatory Drugs (NSAIDs) which comprises a variety of carboxylic acids such as those shown in Fig. (**8**). Another interesting carboxylic ligand is the γ-linolenic acid (GLA), Fig. (**8**), which has also been combined with the diruthenium(II,III) center, as presented further.

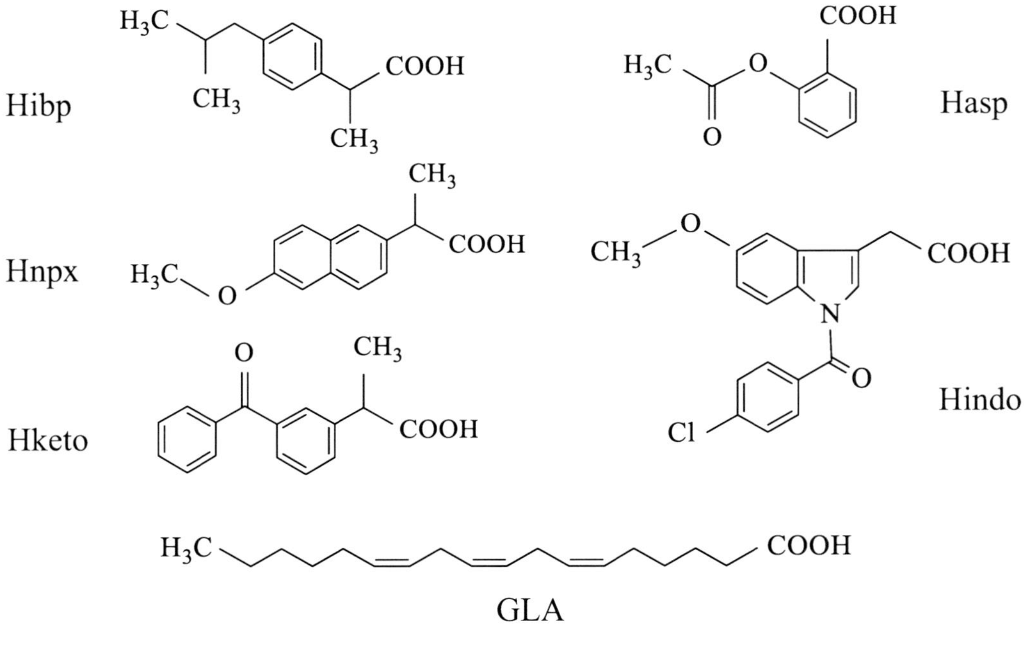

Fig. (8). Structures of the ibuprofen (Hibp), naproxen (Hnpx), ketoprofen (Hketo), aspirin (Hasp) and indomethacin (Hind) NSAIDs, and the γ-linolenic acid (GLA).

NSAIDs are worldwide used to treat inflammation (as anti-inflammatory), as well as pain (as analgesic) and fever (as antipyretic), which are caused by diverse physiological and/or pathological conditions. The mechanism of the anti-inflammatory action is associated primarily to the biosynthesis of prostaglandins

(PGs) involving the inhibition of both isoforms (COX-1 and COX-2) of the cyclooxygenase (COX) enzyme in the pathway of the metabolism of the arachidonic acid. The inhibition of COX-2 (that is induced by extracellular stimuli) is related to the inflammation process, while the inhibition of the COX-1 (a constitutive enzyme) has been associated to side-effects, mainly the gastrointestinal irritation or ulceration caused by the NSAIDs [213].

The wide range of applications together with the fact that some of NSAIDs are readily available in the market without need of medical prescription has accounted for a high consumption of these drugs all over the world. The indiscriminate use of these drugs by population is a matter of serious concern because, despite the pharmacological/medicinal benefits, the prolonged use of NSAIDs may cause severe damage to the gastrointestinal tract. The most popular anti-pyretic and analgesic NSAID drug also prescribed for coronary artery disease and stroke [214], the Aspirin®, is well-known to induce gastrointestinal side-effects as gastric lesions, ulcerations and erosions [214]. A large number of patient-consumers of NSAIDs suffer from severe gastrointestinal problems, the treatments show high cost, and the side-diseases may even cause the patient death [215].

In addition to the well-established classical clinical uses, NSAIDs may also show anticancer related properties, as has been revealed in clinical trials more recently. The long-term use of NSAIDs has been associated to a significant reduction of risk of a variety of malignances, *e.g.,* colorectal, gastric, breast, prostate, lung and skin cancers [216-231]. The long-term use of aspirin significantly reduced the risk of gastric and colon cancers [228]. NSAIDs were found to exert anti-carcinogenic effects in animal experimental models [232-235]. Gastric tumors chemically induced in mice were reduced not only by aspirin, but also by other NSAIDs such as ibuprofen, indomethacin and sulindac [232, 233]. NSAIDs were also capable of inhibiting the growth of transplanted tumors and carcinogen-induced skin tumors in animals [234, 235]. The protective effect of NSAIDs on neoplasia, however, seems to depend on the continuous use of the drugs. The anticancer effects of NSAIDs were shown to be reversible, the tumor recurrence increased shortly after drug use was discontinued. The regular intake of ibuprofen was shown to be chemopreventive for breast cancer [236] and to decrease the growth of non-small cell lung cancer *in vitro* [237]. Aspirin and other NSAIDs were capable of inhibiting cell proliferation and inducing apoptosis in several cancer cell lines what was considered to be relevant to antitumor activity and to prevention of carcinogenesis [225, 238, 239]. Although the mechanism of action associated to the anticancer related pharmacological effects of NSAIDs still remains unclear, it may involve the drug properties of inhibiting the COX enzymes [240]. In particular, the anticancer effect of NSAIDs might be mainly related to the inhibition of COX-2 which is over expressed in several types of cancer and has been associated with tumorigenesis [217]. NSAIDs-induced apoptosis mechanisms may also be involved [241-244]. Moreover, it has been suggested that both COX-dependent and COX-independent mechanisms might play a role in NSAID induced apoptosis [225, 228, 245, 246]. However, despite all the promising anticancer properties of the NSAIDs, the high doses required to produce anti-carcinogenic effects and to induce apoptosis have been considered as a key limitation for their use aiming the treatment of cancer.

A number of NSAIDs contain carboxylic acid (RCOOH) functional groups that can be deprotonated (*d*-) to give the correspondent *d*-NSAIDs in the form of the derived $RCOO^-$ carboxylate anions, which are potential ligands capable of coordinating metal ions. Metal-NSAID complexes having the $[M_2(O_2CR)_4]$ paddlewheel framework, in which each oxygen atom of the $RCOO^-$ bridging anion coordinates individually to two metal (M) ions of the same metal, were shown to exhibit interesting biological properties. The approach of coordinating NSAIDs to metal ions may promote the enhancement of the biological activity and/or the decrease of undesirable side-effects, in relation to those of the correspondent non-coordinated organic drugs. Classical examples are the copper(II) complexes of NSAIDs. The benefits, *e.g.*, the anti-inflammatory activity and principally the ability to reduce gastrointestinal ulcerogenic effects, shown by these complexes, accounted for the entrance of a copper-indomethacin metallodrug into veterinary clinic to treat inflammation in dogs and horses [247, 248].

The ability of carboxylic-drug ligands to bridge two metal ions can also be exploited to stabilize multiply bonded dimetallic cores. In our first work, in 1996, the ibuprofen (Hibp) NSAID, in its both isomeric forms, the *(R,S)*-racemic and the *(S)(+)*-enantiomer, was shown to interact with the $[Mo_2Cl_8]^{4-}$ unit, stabilizing the $[Mo]^{4+}$ quadruple metal-metal bonded core to give the complex of the formula

$[Mo_2(ibp)_4]$. The reaction with *(S)(+)*-ibuprofen gave a non-crystalline solid, while the racemic mixture led to the preferential crystallization of $[Mo_2(R\text{-ibp})_2(S\text{-ibp})_2]$. The stereochemistry of the crystal showed that the chiral ibuprofenate (ibp) ligands coordinate to the dimolybdenum core "in a sequence that forms a centrosymmetric non-chiral complex" [249].

The possibility of stabilizing multiple metal-metal bonds by NSAID-derived carboxylate ligands prompted us to study further the interactions of the ibuprofen and other analogous pharmaceuticals with the Ru_2(II,III) mixed-valence core. To the best of our knowledge, aside the researches from our group, only one article from 1989, briefly describing the reactivity of the diruthenium core with aspirinato was published [250], but lacking any mention to further perspectives for biological studies.

Our first report on diruthenium(II,III)-NSAID, named here DIRUNSAID, complexes was published in 2000, describing the synthesis and the characterization of the diruthenium-ibuprofen, Ruibp, metallodrug of the formula $[Ru_2(ibp)_4Cl]$, ibp = ibuprofenate. The anti-inflammatory and the ulcerogenic activities of Ruibp were compared with those of the analogue copper(II) complex, Cuibp, $[Cu_2(ibp)_4]$, and of the ibuprofen (Hibp) parent drug [251]. The oral administrations of Cuibp and Ruibp inhibited the development of carrageenan-induced edema in rats at the same level of Hibp, suggesting that the anti-inflammatory effects were not lost after the coordination of the drug to these metal ions. Interestingly, the metallodrugs were capable of reducing significantly (to about 50%) the gastric lesion indexes in relation to Hibp. The results for Cuibp were not totally unexpected since the analogues Cu-aspirin [252] and Cu-flurbiprofen [253] also showed protective anti-ulcer effect, even though Cu complexes of naproxen and ketoprofen were ulcerogenic [254, 255]. The findings for Ruibp, however, were quite surprisingly, since for the first time a complex of ruthenium with NSAID was found to exert anti-inflammatory, anti-ulcerogenic properties [251]. The combined anti-inflammatory/gastroprotective effects, although unusual, might be therapeutically desirable, since the available common anti-inflammatory pharmaceuticals show potential for gastrointestinal erosion.

Subsequently, taking into account the ability of Ru-based complexes to exert antitumor activity [reported at that time in some references as, *e.g.*, 76, 77, 86, 88,

102, 112, 256-258] and also the potential for cancer therapy demonstrated by NSAIDs, we started, from the late 1990s, to investigate the antitumor/anticancer properties of the DIRUNSAID metallodrugs, in particular against glioma models. Despite the biological potential of ruthenium compounds, there are still few reports into this direction, as for example, one study from 2004 reporting that the mononuclear complex $K_2[RuCl_4(dmgly)]\cdot 2H_2O$, dmgly = *N,N*-dimethylglycine, was toxic to C6 glioma cells *in vitro* but not to primary astrocytes [258].

Gliomas are primary brain tumors very difficult to treat by the available conventional procedures [259, 260]. One of the most malignant tumors is the glioblastoma multiforme (GBM), classified by the World Health Organization (WHO) as grade IV and associated to genetic alterations related to, *e.g.,* the control of cell growth, migration, apoptosis, and invasion [261]. The current treatment, consisting of surgical resection followed by radiotherapy and/or chemotherapy, has provided little improvements, in part because of the highly invasive nature and resistance of GBM to conventional methods [262]. The patient average survival is about only one year after surgery and the poor survival is mainly related to the post-surgical re-incidence of the tumor [262-264]. COX and PGs may be important to the tumor related processes since they are involved in cell growth, survival, migration/invasion and angiogenesis processes; COX-2 expression is up regulated in gliomas and may be associated to poor patient prognosis [265-269]; the COX-2 inhibitor effects on progression of tumor in patients with GBM are under studies in clinical trials [270, 271]. In summary, the current poor prognosis for glioma requires the search for novel drugs that may offer improvement to the treatment of patients, especially those with GBM. In fact, new treatment options are under testing in clinical trials and pilot studies, including the bevacizumab anti-angiogenic drug [272-276]; and other drugs are also in development to treat glioma [277-281]. Nevertheless, particularly due to the severe side-effects and poor median survival in first-line therapy [282], the treatment of patients diagnosed with glioma is still challenging for scientists and clinicians, requiring the urgent need for novel therapeutic drugs with different mechanisms of action.

In this context, we have studied the effects of the DIRUNSAID metallodrugs on glioma models. The first article, published in 1998, reported the synthesis and the characterization as well as the antiproliferative activity of four complexes, *i.e.*, [Ru_2(*d*-NSAID)$_4$Cl], *d*-NSAID = ibp or asp, and [Ru_2(*d*-NSAID)$_4$(H_2O)$_2$]PF_6, *d*-NSAID = npx or ind, compared with those of the NSAID parent drugs, in tumor-cell proliferation of C6 rat glioma cells *in vitro* [283]. The Ruibp and Runpx metallodrugs exhibited the most significant effects and showed increased antiproliferative activity in the C6 cell line compared to their correspondent Hibp and Hnpx drugs, respectively. The inhibitory effects were found to be time dependent and did not involve direct cytotoxicity as shown by cell viability assays. Moreover, since the C6 cell line does not express COX-2 *in vitro*, the observed effects for the DIRUNSAID metallodrugs, taking into account the NSAID component, may be associated to either COX-1 or non-COX related mechanisms. The substantial enhancement of the C6 rat glioma cell antiproliferative activity after the coordination of the NSAIDs to the Ru_2(II,III) core was assigned to a synergistic effect from the metal and the organic drug ligand. In the same report [283], we also showed that these DIRUNSAID metallodrugs were not active in other tested human tumors, such as the Hep2 larynx and the T24/83 bladder human tumors.

The promising activity of the complexes on inhibiting the C6 glioma cell proliferation encouraged further studies for which Ruibp was selected as the leading DIRUNSAID metallodrug. The intracellular effects of the metallodrug upon C6 rat glioma were investigated and important targets of action were identified. The effects of exposure to Ruibp were examined upon "C6 cell cycle distribution, mitochondrial membrane potential, reactive oxygen species generation and mRNA and protein expression of E2F1, cyclin D1, c-myc, pRb, p21, p27, p53, Ku70, Ku80, Bax, Bcl2, cyclooxygenase 1 and 2 (COX-1 and COX-2)" [284]. The main alterations in the mRNA and protein expression were observed for p21 and p27 cyclin-dependent kinase inhibitors that were increased. A decrease in anti-apoptotic Bcl2 expression as well as an increase in pro-apoptotic Bax expression accompanied a slight increase in apoptosis and a substantial decrease in the mitochondrial membrane potential. The exposure of the cells to Ruibp led to an increase in protein expression of COX-1 (responding to a significant loss of production of PGE_2) which is a well-known target for the NSAID, suggesting an intracellular action of the ibuprofen. The findings were in agreement with possible degradation of Ruibp within the cytoplasm thus releasing the organic drug to inhibit the COX-1 activity [284]. Ruibp was also shown to interact with the human serum albumin (HSA) leading to conformational changes in the secondary structure but without causing cleavage of the protein. If the effects against glioma cells are predominantly due to the ibuprofen alone, to some coordinated ibuprofen, or to ibuprofen plus some ruthenium species is not known yet. However, it is certain that the ruthenium plays a key role in the mode of action of Ruibp, and that synergistic effects from Ru and ibuprofen are important for the biological activity, since the coordination of the NSAID to the Ru_2(II,III) core leads to enhancement of the antiproliferative effects in relation to those found for Hibp [283].

The following step was to investigate the effects of Ruibp on the proliferation of human glioma cell lines *in vitro*. Five cell lines (U87MG, U138MG, A172, T98G and U251MG) were examined and the two ones (A172 and U87MG) expressing the wild type p53 were shown to be the most sensitive to the effects of the metallodrug. The acute and chronic toxicology of Ruibp in normal Wistar rats was investigated. Ruibp was tested for antitumor activity "by either chronic 14 days intra-peritoneal administration or chronic Alzet osmotic pump infusion, in the rat C6 orthotopic glioma model *in vivo*" [285]. The intra-peritoneal injection of the metallodrug led to the inhibition of tumor area with no significant toxic effects, but there was an increase in blood neutrophils and monocytes as well as a decrease in blood lymphocytes. The direct infusion of the metallodrug into the tumor *via* the Alzet osmotic pump caused similar inhibition of tumor area, but without modifying the differential blood leukocyte counts. The results of these studies proved the potential of Ruibp as an inhibitor of tumor growth *in vivo* [285]. The Hibp drug, separately, was found to suppress T98G human glioma cell proliferation, migration and to induce apoptosis *in vitro*, and to cause significant inhibition of T98G migration [261].

In addition to the NSAID class of pharmaceuticals, we have also studied the interaction of the γ-linolenic acid (GLA) with the Ru_2(II,III) core. The complex RuGLA of the formula [Ru_2(*d*-GLA)$_4$Cl], *d*-GLA = deprotonated carboxylate anion derived from the GLA, named here as DIRUGLA, was prepared, characterized and tested in glioma cells.

GLA, similarly to other polyunsaturated fatty acids, inhibits the glioma cell proliferation *in vitro*, and exerts antitumor effects in various types of tumor *in vivo*, in animal models and human clinical studies [286-295]. It was shown to promote DNA damage in the C6 rat glioma cells *in vitro* [296]. The mechanism of action involves modification in energy and lipid metabolism, ROS production and caspase activation, cytochrome-c release and apoptosis [297-300].

The activity of DIRUGLA was tested in C6 rat glioma cells by analyzing "cell number, viability, lipid droplet formation, apoptosis, cell cycle distribution, mitochondrial membrane potential and reactive oxygen species (ROS)" [301]. The C6 cell proliferation was inhibited by the metallodrug in a time and concentration dependent manner. The EC_{50} of RuGLA was found to decrease with increasing exposure time. RuGLA was shown to enter into the cells. A significant increase in sub-G_1 apoptotic cell population occurred in the cells treated with RuGLA. The presence of the compound led to a decrease on the mitochondrial membrane potential. An increase on ROS generation was observed for the cells that maintained a high mitochondrial membrane potential. The decreased mitochondrial membrane potential and the increased ROS generation were suggested to be involved in triggering apoptosis in the cells exposed to the metallodrug [301]. In the sequence, the anti-proliferative activity and the effects on tumor morphology of RuGLA were investigated and compared with those of GLA, both in the C6 rat glioma cells *in vitro* and in an orthotopic model in the Wistar rat *in vivo* [302]. RuGLA was shown to inhibit the C6 cell proliferation, and to cause marked changes in the cell morphology *in vitro* that suggested its incorporation into the cells. Endocytotic vesicles were impregnated with the metal, suggesting a receptor-mediated binding and uptake of RuGLA. The metallodrug was found to cause possible DNA damage during the *S*-phase of the cell cycle. It was also shown to inhibit C6 cell proliferation *in vivo* with changes in tumor morphology that confirmed the cellular uptake. The mode of action may be related to glioma cell interactions with the extracellular matrix. The drug may also have anti-angiogenic properties which need further investigation. RuGLA, that does not appear to act *via* cytotoxic mechanisms (as shown by "unaltered cell viability, lactate dehydrogenase leakage and apoptotic index") [302] can be a potential low-toxicity drug candidate for antiproliferative therapy of glioma.

Besides the studies focused on glioma, we have also investigated the effects of three DIRUNSAID metallodrugs in the HT-29 and Caco-2 human colon carcinoma cell lines, which express high and low levels of COX-2 respectively [303]. All the three tested complexes, *i.e.*, $[Ru_2(d\text{-NSAID})_4Cl]$, *d*-NSAID = ibp or keto, and $[Ru_2(d\text{-NSAID})_4(H_2O)_2]PF_6$, *d*-NSAID = npx, showed mild anti-proliferative activity in both types of colorectal cancer cells. Ruibp and Runpx showed slight higher activity in Caco-2 than in HT-29 cells, suggesting that COX-2 inhibition is not totally responsible for the effects of these metallodrugs. Both of complexes were able to affect to some extent the production/activity of MMP-2 and MMP-9 by HT-29 cells. The low dependence of the DIRUNSAID effects on the COX-2 expression levels is probably associated to the non-selective inhibition of COX-1 and COX-2 by the parent NSAIDs (ibuprofen, ketoprofen and naproxen). Since the analogous aspirin NSAID was found to influence cellular processes, such as apoptosis and angiogenesis, and suggested to act through COX-independent pathways, the results for the DIRUNSAID metallodrugs were considered to reinforce the questioning about the "rationale of focusing simply on COX-2 inhibition for an anti-cancer strategy" [303].

Simultaneously to the development of novel diruthenium(II,III)-(pharmaceuticals) metallodrugs, and the investigations on their anticancer/antitumor properties, we have also performed studies with the aim of elucidating relevant processes which may be involved in their mechanism of action. The biological activity of diruthenium(II,III) metallodrugs in the physiological environment is prone to involve, *e.g.,* ligand substitution reactions (such as chloride/water axial exchange), oxidation-reduction processes, and interactions with relevant bio-ligands, proteins, enzymes. In this context, we have recently started to perform studies on the reactivity of this class of metallodrugs. The prototype non-drug complex $[Ru_2(O_2CCH_3)_4Cl]$ was selected as a model for the first studies due to its higher solubility in water compared to the analogous DIRUNSAID complexes. The non-drug complex was examined for the reactivity in the form of the correspondent diaqua-Ru_2 species, $[Ru_2(O_2CCH_3)_4(H_2O)_2]^+$, which predominates in aqueous solution. The diaqua-substituted complex was firstly investigated for water/chloride exchange ligand reactions, and was shown to undergo stepwise substitution reactions in which the two axial water molecules are successively replaced by the chloride ligands. Both of the sequential axial substitution reactions are enthalpy driven as suggested from the determined thermodynamic parameters ($\Delta H°$, $\Delta S°$ and $\Delta V°$) [304]. Following these studies, the diaqua-Ru_2 species were examined for the reactions with low-molecular-weight biomolecules, *i.e.,* the amino acids (*aa*) glycine (gly), cysteine (cys), histidine (his) and tryptophan (trp). Kinetic studies, based on the determination of kinetic rate laws and rate constants, revealed that the diaqua-Ru_2 species reacts with the biomolecules by exchanging one axially-coordinated water molecule by the *aa* ligand to give the corresponding aqua-(*aa*)-Ru_2 substituted species. The value of the kinetic rate constant was shown to depend on the nature of the incoming *aa* ligand. The axial substitution of the first water ligand by the *aa* followed the relative order cys >> trp ~ gly. The most significant effects on the axial substitution kinetics were found for the amino acids cys and his, probably due to the presence of the coordinating thiol and imidazole groups, respectively. The $[Ru_2(O_2CR)_4]^+$ paddlewheel framework was shown to remain stable during the ligand substitution reactions and to be mostly preserved in the presence of the *aa* [304].

Taking into account the key role of redox processes in the mode of action of anticancer metal-based drugs, we have also started to exploit the behavior of the diruthenium(II,III) complexes in the presence of relevant bio-reducing agents. Kinetic studies for the reactions of the diaqua-complex $[Ru_2(O_2CCH_3)_4(H_2O)_2]^+$ with glutathione (GSH) and ascorbic acid were conducted [305]. In the presence of either GSH or ascorbic acid, the diaqua-Ru_2 complex was shown to undergo a first step reaction involving ligand substitution with the displacement of the axially-coordinated water molecule by the reducing agent. In both of cases, the first step reaction was followed by an intra-molecular electron transfer process leading to the reduction of the dimetallic center from $[Ru_2]^{5+}$ to $[Ru_2]^{4+}$. The kinetics of the substitution reaction with the GSH was found to be much faster than that with the ascorbic acid what was explained on the basis of the stronger donor character of the thiol group of glutathione. Moreover, in contrast to the reaction with ascorbic acid, for which the electron transfer process did not lead to further decomposition processes, the electron transfer by GSH was found to promote the cleavage of the paddlewheel structure. The activation parameters for the ligand substitution reactions were in agreement with a dissociative mechanism controlled by the release of the weakly bonded axial water ligand from the diaqua-Ru_2 species, and the activation volume suggested a dissociative interchange (I_d) mechanism. The dissociative nature of this reaction step may be associated to the labilization of the axially coordinated water by the Ru-Ru multiple bond. The reaction with ascorbic acid was affected by the presence of chloride in excess which favored a significant slowing down in the reaction as a result of the coordinated water/free chloride competing substitution since chloride is a stronger nucleophile than ascorbate [305].

Furthermore, we have started studies with the aim of investigating the interactions of the diruthenium(II,III)-(pharmaceuticals) metallodrugs with proteins. In a recent paper, we reported the interactions of the non-drug complex $[Ru_2(O_2CCH_3)_4Cl]$ with the model protein hen egg-white lysozyme (HEWL) [306]. Studies in solution gave evidence for the maintenance of the dimetal core, while two of the four acetate ligands are released by the interaction of the diruthenium complex with the protein. The crystal structure data agree with the results in solution, showing that the "HEWL binds two diruthenium moieties, at Asp101 and Asp119, respectively, with the concomitant release of two acetate ligands from each diruthenium original complex" [306].

The findings from our studies on the reactivity and interactions of bio-relevant molecules with the non-drug complex $[[Ru_2(O_2CCH_3)_4Cl]$, a model to elucidate the behavior of the $[Ru_2(O_2CR)_4]^+$ paddlewheel framework, gave the first key insights to the possible biological targets and mode of action of the Ru_2(II,III) metallodrugs. Researches with the main objectives of designing novel and/or modified diruthenium(II,III)-(pharmaceuticals) metallodrugs and expanding the studies on their interactions with relevant biomolecules, bio-targets and drug carriers, *etc.*, are undergoing in our laboratories. In addition, we are also performing studies to extend the research on biological/pharmacological properties of the metallodrugs, especially with the aim of exploiting their potential to target glioma cancer therapy.

CONCLUSION

Studies on Ru-based anticancer drugs are still in their beginning compared to the Pt drugs that play key role as chemotherapeutic drugs in the current cancer treatments.

Nevertheless, the fast evolution of scientific research focused on ruthenium in recent years is highly encouraging to the development of novel generations of Ru-based chemotherapeutic drugs. Significant progress has been achieved with the entrance of NAMI-A and KP1019 (and its analogue KP1339) into human clinical trials, and at the present other promising Ru-complexes are undergoing preclinical studies. The selected Ru-based drugs discussed in this chapter, nonetheless, represent only part of the rich field available to be exploited for the design of novel Ru-based metallodrugs. Difficulty in finding structure/(mechanism of action)/(anticancer activity) rationale correlations (accounted mainly for the structural diversity, variable oxidation states and distinctly different properties, *e.g.*, chemical, physico-chemical, biochemical, biological and pharmacological properties) of numerous classes of Ru compounds, still challenges the scientific community. Nevertheless, the current knowledge collected on this field offers important insights for further studies aiming to the development of novel Ru-anticancer drug candidates for clinical studies.

ACKNOWLEDGEMENTS

The author gratefully acknowledge the Brazilian research agencies Fundação de Amparo à Pesquisa do Estado de São Paulo (FAPESP) for financial support (in particular, grant 2011/06592-1), and Conselho Nacional de Desenvolvimento Cientifico e Tecnológico (CNPq) and Coordenação de Aperfeiçoamento de Pessoal de Nível Superior (CAPES) for fellowships, related to the development of the research on the diruthenium (II,III)-based metallodrugs presented here. The author also acknowledge all the collaborators involved in these studies, in particular, Prof. A. Colquhoun from the Department of Cell and Developmental Biology, University of São Paulo, for the effective collaboration on the biological studies of the diruthenium complexes in glioma models.

CONFLICT OF INTEREST

The author confirms that this chapter contents have no conflict of interest.

REFERENCES

[1] Orvig C, Abrams MJ. Medicinal inorganic chemistry: introduction. Chem Rev 1999; 99: 2201-3.

[2] Jones CJ, Thornback JR. Medicinal applications of coordination chemistry. RSC Publishing: Cambridge 2005.

[3] Gielen M, Tiekink ERT. Metallotherapeutic Drugs & Metal-based Diagnostic Agents - The use of metals in medicine. West Sussex: John Wiley & Sons Ltd 2005.

[4] Farrer NJ, Sadler PJ. Medicinal inorganic chemistry: state of the art, new trends, and a vision of the future. In Alessio E, Ed. Bioinorganic Medicinal Chemistry. Weinheim: Wiley-VCH Verlag & Co. KGaA 2011;1-48.

[5] Guo Z, Sadler P J. Metals in medicine. Angew Chem Int Ed 1999; 38: 1512-31.

[6] Dabrowiak JC. Metals in Medicine. West Sussex: John Wiley & Sons Ltd 2009.

[7] Hambley WT. Developing new metal-based therapeutics: challenges and opportunities. Dalton Trans 2007: 4929-37.

[8] Silva JJRF, Williams RPJ. The Biological Chemistry of the Elements - The inorganic chemistry of life. 2nd ed. Oxford: Oxford University Press 2001.

[9] Wilkins PC, Wilkins RG. Inorganic Chemistry in Biology. Oxford: Oxford Science Publications 1997.

[10] Bertini I, Gray HB, Lippard S, Valentine J, Eds. Bioinorganic Chemistry. California: University Science Books 1994.

[11] Barry NPE, Sadler PJ. Exploration of the medical periodic table: towards new targets. Chem Commun 2013; 49: 5106-31.

[12] van Rijt SH, Sadler PJ. Current applications and future potential for bioinorganic chemistry in the development of anticancer drugs. Drug Discov Today 2009; 14: 1089-97.

[13] Romero-Canelón I, Sadler PJ. Next-generation metal anticancer complexes: multitargeting *via* redox modulation. Inorg Chem 2013; 52: 12276-91.

[14] Meggers E. Exploring biologically relevant chemical space with metal complexes. Curr Opin Chem Biol 2007; 11: 287-92.

[15] Kelland LR. The resurgence of platinum-based cancer chemotherapy. Nat Rev Cancer 2007; 7: 573-84.

[16] van Zutphen S, Reedijk J. Targeting platinum anti-tumour drugs: Overview of strategies employed to reduce systemic toxicity. Coord Chem Rev 2005; 249: 2845-53.

[17] Reedijk J. Platinum anticancer coordination compounds: study of DNA binding inspires new drug design. Eur J Inorg Chem 2009; 10: 1303-12.

[18] Wheate NJ, Walker S, Craig GE, Oun R. The status of platinum anticancer drugs in the clinic and in clinical trials. Dalton Trans 2010; 39: 8113-27.

[19] Brabec V, Kasparkova J. ^{78}Pt platinum-based drugs. In: Gielen M, Tiekink ERT, Eds. Metallotherapeutic Drugs & Metal-based Diagnostic Agents - The use of metals in medicine. West Sussex: John Wiley & Sons Ltd 2005, pp. 489-506.

[20] Kostova I. Platinum-based anticancer agents, frontiers in anti-cancer drug discovery. In: Atta-ur-Rahman, Choudhary MI, Eds. Frontiers in Anti-Cancer Drug Discovery, Bussum: Bentham Science Publishers 2010, vol. 1, pp. 298-339.

[21] Dhar S, Lippard SJ. Current status and mechanism of action of platinum-based anticancer drugs. In: Alessio E, Ed. Bioinorganic Medicinal Chemistry. Weinheim: Wiley-VCH Verlag & Co KGaA 2011; 79-96.

[22] Lippert B. Cisplatin, Chemistry and Biochemistry of a Leading Anticancer Drug. Weinheim: Wiley-VCH 1999.

[23] Jung Y, Lippard SJ. Direct cellular responses to platinum-induced DNA damage. Chem Rev 2007; 107 1387-407.

[24] Stathopoulos GP. Cisplatin: process and future. JBUON 2013; 18: 564-69.
[25] Rosenberg B, Vancamp LV, Trosko JE, Mansour VH. Platinum compounds: a new class of potent antitumor agent. Nature 1969; 222: 385-86.
[26] Feldman D R, Bosl GJ, Sheinfeld J, Motzer RJ. Medical treatment of advanced testicular cancer. J Am Med Assoc 2008; 299: 672-84.
[27] Reedijk J. New clues for platinum antitumor chemistry: Kinetically controlled metal binding to DNA. Proc Natl Acad Sci USA 2003; 100: 3611-16.
[28] Ahmad S, Isab A, Ali S. Structural and mechanistic aspects of platinum anticancer agents. Trans Met Chem 2006; 31: 1003-16.
[29] Wong E, Giandomenico CM. Current status of platinum-based antitumor drugs. Chem Rev 1999; 99: 2451-66.
[30] Wang D, Lippard SJ. Cellular processing of platinum anticancer drugs. Nat Rev Drug Disc 2005; 4: 307-20.
[31] Brabec V, Kasparkova J. Modifications of DNA by platinum complexes - Relation to resistance of tumors to platinum antitumor drugs. Drug Res Updates 2005; 8: 131-46.
[32] Graf N, Lippard SJ. Redox activation of metal-based prodrugs as a strategy for drug delivery. Adv Drug Deliv Rev 2012; 64: 993-1004.
[33] Bhargava A, Vaishampayan UN. Satraplatin: leading the new generation of oral platinum agents. Expert Opin Investig Drugs 2009; 18: 1787-7.
[34] Nemirovski A, Vinograd I, Takrouri K, Mijovilovich A, Rompel A, Gibson D. New reduction pathways for ctc-$[PtCl_2(CH_3CO_2)_2(NH_3)(Am)]$ anticancer prodrugs. Chem Commun 2010; 46: 1842-44.
[35] Ronconi L, Sadler PJ. Using coordination chemistry to design new medicines. Coord Chem Rev 2007; 251: 1633-48
[36] Oberoi HS, Nukolova NV, Kabanov AV, Bronich TK. Nanocarriers for delivery of platinum anticancer drugs. Adv Drug Deliv Rev 2013; 65: 1667-85.
[37] Duncan R. Polymer conjugates as anticancer nanomedicines. Nat Rev Cancer 2006; 6: 688-701.
[38] Moghimi SM, Hunter AC, Murray JC. Nanomedicine: current status and future prospects. FASEB J 2005; 19: 311-30.
[39] Lovejoy KS, Lippard SJ. Non-traditional platinum compounds for improved accumulation, oral bioavailability, and tumor targeting. Dalton Trans 2009; 48: 10651-59.
[40] Borrelli A, Schiattarella A, Musella A, Mancini R, Capasso C, De Luca V, Carginale V, Sanseverino M, Tornesello AL, Gori E, Pica A, Di Santi A, Basile F, Iacobellis F, Colacurci N, Cobellis L, Mancini A. A molecular carrier to transport and deliver cisplatin into endometrial cancer cells. Chem Biol Drug Des 2012; 80: 9-16.
[41] Burger KNJ, Staffhorst RWHM, De Vijlder HC, Velinova MJ, Bomans PH, Frederik PM, De Kruijff B. Nanocapsules: lipid-coated aggregates of cisplatin with high cytotoxicity. Nat Med 2002; 8: 81-4.
[42] Stathopoulos GP, Boulikas T, Kourvetaris A, Stathopoulos J. Liposomal Oxaliplatin in the Treatment of Advanced Cancer: A Phase I Study. Anticancer Res 2006; 26: 1489-93.
[43] Boulikas T. Clinical overview on Lipoplatin™: a successful liposomal formulation of cisplatin. Expert Opin Investig Drugs 2009; 18: 1197-218.
[44] Feazell RP, Nakayama-Ratchford N, Dai H, Lippard SJ. Soluble single-walled carbon nanotubes as longboat delivery systems for platinum(IV) anticancer drug design. J Am Chem Soc 2007; 129: 8438-9.

[45] Mukhopadhyay S, Barnes CM, Haskel A, Short SM, Barnes KR, Lippard SJ. Conjugated platinum(IV)-peptide complexes for targeting angiogenic tumor vasculature. Bioconjugate Chem 2008; 19: 39-49.

[46] Dhar S, Gu FX, Langer R, Farokhzad OC, Lippard SJ. Targeted delivery of cisplatin to prostate cancer cells by aptamer functionalized Pt(IV) prodrug-PLGA-PEG nanoparticles Proc. Natl Acad Sci USA 2008; 105: 17356-61.

[47] Dhar S, Daniel WL, Giljohann DA, Mirkin CA, Lippard SJ. Polyvalent oligonucleotide gold nanoparticle conjugates as delivery vehicles for platinum(IV) warheads. J Am Chem Soc 2009; 131: 14652-53.

[48] Stathopoulos GP, Boulikas T, Lipoplatin formulation review article. J Drug Deliv 2012; 2012 (ID 581363): 1-10.

[49] Boulikas T. Low toxicity and anticancer activity of a novel liposomal cisplatin (Lipoplatin) in mouse xenografts. Oncol Rep 2004; 12: 3-12.

[50] Ang WH, Dyson PJ. Classical and non-classical ruthenium-based anticancer drugs: towards targeted chemotherapy. Eur J Inorg Chem 2006; 20: 4003-18.

[51] Cepeda V, Fuertes MA, Castilla J, Alonso C, Quevedo C, Pérez JM. Biochemical mechanisms of cisplatin cytotoxicity. Anti Canc Agents Med Chem 2007; 7: 3-18.

[52] Dwyer FP, Gyarfas EC, Rogers WP, Koch JH: Biological activity of complex ions. Nature 1952; 170: 190-1.

[53] Dwyer FP, Mayhew E, Roe EMF, Shulman A. Inhibition of Landschütz ascites tumour growth by metal chelates derived from 3,4,7,8-tetramethyl-1,10-phenanthroline. Br J Cancer 1965; 19:195-9.

[54] http://apps.webofknowledge.com, accessed on January and April, 2014.

[55] Lentzen O, Moucheron C, Mesmaeker A K. $_{44}$Ru Perspectives of ruthenium complexes in cancer theraphy. In: Gielen M, Tiekink ERT, Eds. Metallotherapeutic Drugs & Metal-based Diagnostic Agents - The use of metals in medicine. West Sussex: John Wiley & Sons Ltd 2005; 359-78.

[56] Bratsos I, Gianferrara T, Alessio E, Hartinger CG, Jakupec MA, Keppler BK. Ruthenium and other non-platinum anticancer compounds. In: Alessio E, Ed. Bioinorganic Medicinal Chemistry. Weinheim: Wiley-VCH Verlag & Co KGaA 2011; 151-74.

[57] Jakupec MA, Galanski M, Arion VB, Hartinger CG, Keppler BK. Antitumor metal compounds: more than theme and variations. Dalton Trans 2008; 2: 183-94.

[58] Kostova I. Ruthenium complexes as anticancer agents. Curr Med Chem 2006; 13: 1085-107.

[59] Bergamo A, Sava G. Ruthenium complexes can target determinants of tumor malignancy. Dalton Trans 2007; 13: 1267-72.

[60] Levina A, Mitra A, Lay PA. Recent developments in ruthenium anticancer drugs. Metallomics 2009; 1: 458-70.

[61] de Oliveira Silva D. Perspectives for novel mixed diruthenium-organic drugs as metallopharmaceuticals in cancer therapy. Anti Canc Agents Med Chem 2010; 10: 312-23.

[62] Fink G S. Arene ruthenium complexes as anticancer agents. Dalton Trans 2010; 39: 1673-88.

[63] Ang WH, Casini A, Sava, G, Dyson PJ. Organometallic ruthenium-based antitumor compounds with novel modes of action. J Organomet Chem 2011; 696: 989-98.

[64] Sava G, Bergamo A, Dyson PJ. Ruthenium anticancer compounds: myths and realities of the emerging metal-based drugs. Dalton Trans 2011; 40: 9069-75.

[65] Gasser G, Ott I, Metzler-Nolte N. Organometallic anticancer compounds. J Med Chem 2011; 54: 3-25.

[66] Sava G, Bergamo A, Dyson PJ. Metal-based antitumour drugs in the post-genomic era: what comes next? Dalton Trans 2011; 40: 9069-75.

[67] Bergamo A, Gaiddon C, Schellens JHM, Beijnen JH, Sava G. Approaching tumour therapy beyond platinum drugs. Status of the art and perspectives of ruthenium drug candidates. J Inorg Biochem 2012; 106: 90-9.

[68] Hartinger CG, Metzler-Nolte N, Dyson PJ. Challenges and opportunities in the development of organometallic anticancer drugs. Organometallics 2012; 31: 5677-85.

[69] Komeda S, Casini A. Next-generation anticancer metallodrugs. Curr Top Med Chem 2012; 12: 219-35.

[70] Fink GS. Water-soluble arene ruthenium complexes: From serendipity to catalysis and drug design. J Organom Chem 2014; 751: 2-19.

[71] Nazarov AA, Hartinger CG, Dyson PJ. Opening the lid on piano-stool complexes: An account of ruthenium(II)-arene complexes with medicinal applications. J Organom Chem 2014; 751: 251-60.

[72] Reisner E, Arion VB, Keppler BK, Pombeiro AJL. Electron-transfer activated metal-based anticancer drugs. Inorg Chim Acta 2008; 361: 1569-83.

[73] Gianferrara T, Bratsos I, Alessio E. A categorization of metal anticancer compounds based on their mode of action. Dalton Trans 2009; 37: 7588-98.

[74] Reedijk, J. Metal-ligand exchange kinetics in platinum and ruthenium complexes. Platinum Metals Rev. 2008, 52, 2-11.

[75] Jungwirth U, Kowol CR, Keppler BK, Hartinger CG, Berger W, Heffeter P. Anticancer activity of metal complexes: involvement of redox processes. Antioxid Redox Signal 2011; 15: 1085-127.

[76] Sadler PJ. Inorganic chemistry and drug design. Adv Inorg Chem 1991; 36: 1-48.

[77] Clarke MJ. Ruthenium metallopharmaceutics. Coord Chem Rev 2003; 236: 209-33.

[78] Bartel C, Egger AE, Jakupec MA, Heffeter P, Galanski M, Berger W, Keppler BK. Influence of ascorbic acid on the activity of the investigational anticancer drug KP1019. J Biol Inorg Chem 2011; 16:1205-15

[79] Huheey JE, Keiter EA, Keiter RL. Inorganic Chemistry: Principles of Structure and Reactivity; 4th Ed. New York: Happer Collins College Publishers 1993.

[80] Varmus H. The new era in cancer research. Science 2006; 312: 1162-5.

[81] Dyson PJ, Sava G. Metal-based antitumor drugs in the post genomic era. Dalton Trans 2006; 16: 1929-33.

[82] Casini A. Exploring the mechanisms of metal-based pharmacological agents *via* an integrated approach. J Inorg Biochem 2012; 109: 97-106.

[83] Carter DC, Ho JX. Structure of serum albumin. Adv Protein Chem 1994; 45: 153-203.

[84] Sun H, Li H, Sadler PJ. Transferrin as a metal ion mediator. Chem Rev 1999; 99: 2817-42.

[85] Timerbaev AR, Hartinger CG, Aleksenko SS, Keppler BK. Interactions of antitumor metallodrugs with serum proteins: advances in characterization using modern analytical methodology. Chem Rev 2006; 106: 2224-48.

[86] Clarke MJ. Ruthenium complexes: potential roles in anticancer pharmaceutics. In: Keppler BK, Ed. Metal Complexes in Cancer Chemotherapy. New York: VCH 1993; 129-56.

[87] Clarke MJ, Zhu F, Frasca, DR. Non-platinum chemotherapeutic metallopharmaceuticals. Chem Rev 1999; 99: 2511-33.

[88] Mestroni G, Alessio E, Sava G, Pacor S, Coluccia M. The development of tumor-inhibiting ruthenium-dimethylsulfoxide complexes. In: Keppler BK, Ed. Metal Complexes in Cancer Chemotherapy. New York: VCH 1993; 157-85.

[89] De Oliveira Silva D, Toma HE. Propriedades e importância dos sulfóxidos de rutênio. Química Nova 1993; 16: 40-8.

[90] Bratsos I, Bergamo A, Sava G, Gianferrara T, Zangrando E, Alessio E. Influence of the anionic ligands on the anticancer activity of Ru(II)-dmso complexes: Kinetics of aquation and *in vitro* cytotoxicity of new dicarboxylate compounds in comparison with their chloride precursors. J Inorg Biochem 2008; 102: 606-17.

[91] Alessio E, Mestroni G. Nardin G, Attia WM, Calligaris M, Sava G, Zorzet S. *Cis*- and *trans*-dihalotetrakis(dimethylsulfoxide)ruthenium(II) complexes ($RuX_2(DMSO)_4$ X; = CI, Br): Synthesis, Structure, and Antitumor Activity. Inorg Chem 1988; 27: 4099-106.

[92] Sava G, Pacor S, Zorzet S, Alessio E, Mestroni G. Antitumor properties of Dimethylsulphoxide ruthenium(II) complexes in the Lewis lung carcinoma system. Pharmacol Res 1989; 21: 617-28.

[93] Coluccia M, Sava G, Loseto F, Nassi A, Boccarelli A, Giordano D, Alessio E, Mestroni G. Anti-leukaemic action of $RuCl_2(DMSO)_4$ isomers and prevention of brain involvement on P388 leukaemia and on P338/DDP subline. Eur J Cancer 1993; 29A: 1873-9.

[94] Cabrera E, Cerecetto H, Gonzalez M, Gambino D, Noblia P, Otero L, Parajon-Costa B, Anzellotti A, Sanchez-Delgado R, Azqueta A, de Cerain AL, Monge A. Ruthenium (II) nitrofurylsemicarbazone complexes: new DNA binding agents. Eur J Med Chem 2004; 39: 377-82.

[95] Wu A, Kennedy DC, Patrick BO, James BR. Ruthenium(II) sulfoxide-maltolato and -nitroimidazole complexes: synthesis and MTT assay. Inorg Chem 2003; 42: 7579-86.

[96] Toma HE, De Oliveira Silva D. Chromatographic, spectroscopic and electrochemical characterization of geometrical isomers of the diclorobis(2,6-dimethylpyrazine bis(dimethylsulphoxide)ruthenium(II) complex. Polyhedron 1991; 10: 1699-704.

[97] Toma HE, De Oliveira Silva D. Elution behavior of N-heterocyclic derivatives of mixed ruthenium(II)-sulfoxide complexes in reversed-phase high performance liquid chromatography. Chromatographia 1991; 32: 546-8.

[98] De Oliveira Silva D, Toma HE. Linkage isomerization and electrochemical behavior of two geometrical isomers of dichlorobis(dimethylsulfoxide)bis(t-butylpyridine)ruthenium(II). Can J Chem 1994; 72: 1705-8.

[99] De Oliveira Silva D, Saika JJ, Toma HE. Photochemical behavior of the dichlorobis(dimethylsulfoxide)bis(t-butylpyridine)ruthenium(II) complex. J Photochem Photobiol A: Chemistry 1998; 112: 209-12.

[100] Brindell M, Kulis E, Elmroth SKC, Urbanska K, Stochel G. Light-induced anticancer activity of $[RuCl_2(DMSO)_4]$ complexes. J Med Chem 2005; 48: 7298-304.

[101] Mura P, Camalli M, Casini A, Gabbiani C, Messori L. Trans-cis-cis-$[RuCl_2(DMSO)_2(2\text{-amino-5-methyl-thiazole})_2]$, (PMRu52), a novel ruthenium(II) compound acting as a strong inhibitor of cathepsin B. J Inorg Biochem 2010; 104: 111-7.

[102] Keppler BK, Lipponer K, Stenzel B, Kratz F. New tumor-inhibiting ruthenium complexes. In: Keppler BK, Ed. Metal Complexes in Cancer Chemotherapy. New York: VCH 1993; 187-220.

[103] Berger MR, Garzon FT, Keppler BK, Schmäehl D. Efficacy of new ruthenium complexes against chemically induced autochthonous colorectal carcinoma in rats. Anticancer Res 1989; 9: 761-5.

[104] Bratsos I, Jednera S, Gianferrara T, Alessio E. Ruthenium anticancer compounds: challenges and expectations. Chimia 2007; 61: 692-7.

[105] Schluga P, Hartinger CG, Egger A, Reisner E, Galanski M, Jakupec M, Keppler BK. Redox behavior of tumor-inhibiting ruthenium(III) complexes and effects of physiological reductants on their binding to GMP. Dalton Trans 2006; 1796-802.

[106] Ravera M, Baracco S, Cassino C, Zanello P, Osella D. Appraisal of the redox behaviour of the antimetastatic ruthenium(III) complex [ImH][$RuCl_4$(DMSO)(Im)], NAMI-A. Dalton Trans 2004; 2347-51.

[107] Brindell M, Piotrowska DA, Shoukry A, Stochel G, van Eldik R. Kinetics and mechanism of the reduction of (ImH)[*trans*-$RuCl_4$(dmso)(Im)] by ascorbic acid in acidic aqueous solution. J Biol Inorg Chem 2007; 12: 809-18.

[108] Brindell M, Stawoska I, Supel J, Skoczowski A, Stochel G, van Eldik R. The reduction of (ImH)[trans-$Ru^{III}Cl_4$(dmso)(Im)] under physiological conditions: preferential reaction of the reduced complex with human serum albumin. J Biol Inorg Chem 2008; 13: 909-18.

[109] Cocchietto M, Zorzet S, Sorc A, Sava G. Primary tumor, lung and kidney retention and antimetastasis effect of NAMI-A following different routes of administration. Invest New Drugs 2003; 21: 55-62.

[110] Sava G, Capozzi I, Clerici K, Gagliardi G, Alessio E, Mestroni G. Pharmacological control of lung metastases of solid tumors by a novel ruthenium complex. Clin Exp Metastasis 1998; 16: 371-9.

[111] Sava G, Bergamo A, Zorzet S, Gava B, Casarsa C, Cocchietto M, Furlani A, Scarcia V, Serli B, Iengo E, Alessio E, Mestroni, G. Influence of chemical stability on the activity of the antimetastasis ruthenium compound NAMI-A. Eur J Cancer 2002; 38: 427-35.

[112] Bergamo A, Gagliardi R, Scarcia V, Furlani A, Alessio E, Mestroni G, Sava G. *In vitro* cell cycle arrest, *in vivo* action on solid metastasizing tumors, and host toxicity of the antimetastatic drug NAMI-A and cisplatin. J Pharmacol Exp Ther 1999; 289: 559-64.

[113] Sava G, Zorzet S, Turrin C, Vita F, Soranzo MR, Zabucchi G, Cocchietto M, Bergamo A, DiGiovine S, Pezzoni G, Sartor L, Garbisa S. Dual action of NAMI-A in inhibition of solid tumor metastasis: selective targeting of metastatic cells and binding to collagen. Clin Cancer Res 2003; 9: 1898-1905.

[114] Alessio E, Mestroni G, Bergamo A, Sava G. Ruthenium antimetastatic agents. Curr Top Med Chem 2004; 4: 1525-35.

[115] Rademaker-Lakhai JM, van den Bongard D, Pluim D, Beijnen JH, Schellens JHM. A phase I and pharmacological study with imidazolium-trans-DMSO-imidazole-tetrachlororuthenate, a novel ruthenium anticancer agent. Clin Cancer Res 2004; 10: 3717-27.

[116] Casarsa C, Mischis MT, Sava G. TGFβ_1 regulation and collagen-release-independent connective tissue re-modelling by the ruthenium complex NAMI-A in solid tumours. J Inorg Biochem 2004; 98: 1648-54.

[117] Sava G, Frausin F, Cocchietto M, Vita F, Podda E, Spessotto P, Furlani A, Scarcia V, Zabucchi G. Actin-dependent tumour cell adhesion after short-term exposure to the antimetastasis ruthenium complex NAMI-A. Eur J Cancer 2004; 40: 1383-96.

[118] Frausin F, Scarcia V, Cocchietto M, Furlani A, Serli B, Alessio E, Sava G. Free exchange across cells, and echistatin-sensitive membrane target for the metastasis inhibitor NAMI-A

(imidazolium *trans*-imidazoledimethylsulfoxidetetrachlororuthenate) on KB tumor cells. J Pharm Exp Ther 2005; 313: 227-33.

[119] Gava B, Zorzet S, Spessotto P, Cocchietto M, Sava G. Inhibition of B16 melanoma metastases with the ruthenium complex imidazolium *trans*-imidazoledimethylsulfoxide tetrachlororuthenate and down-regulation of tumor cell invasion. J Pharm Exp Ther 2006; 317: 284-91.

[120] Frausin F, Cocchietto M, Bergamo A, Searcia V, Furlani A, Sava G. Tumor cell uptake of the metastasis inhibitor ruthenium complex NAMI-A and its *in vitro* effects on KB cells. Cancer Chemother Pharmacol 2002; 50: 405-11.

[121] Ravera M, Baracco S, Cassino C, Colangelo D, Bagni G, Sava G, Osella D. Electrochemical measurements confirm the preferential bonding of the antimetastatic complex [ImH][$RuCl_4$(DMSO)(Im)] (NAMI-A) with proteins and the weak interaction with nucleobases. J Inorg Biochem 2004; 98: 984-90.

[122] Pluim D, van Waardenburg RCAM, Beijnen JH, Schellens JHM. Cytotoxicity of the organic ruthenium anticancer drug NAMI-A is correlated with DNA binding in four different human tumor cell lines. Cancer Chemother Pharmacol 2004; 54: 71-8.

[123] Grössl M, Reisner E, Hartinger CG, Eichinger R, Semenova O, Timerbaev AR, Jakupec MA, Arion VB, Keppler BK. Structure-activity relationships for NAMI-A-type complexes (HL)[trans-$RuCl_4$L(S-dmso)ruthenate(III)] (L = imidazole, indazole, 1,2,4-triazole, 4-amino-1,2,4-triazole, and 1-Methyl-1,2,4-triazole): aquation, redox properties, protein binding, and antiproliferative activity. J Med Chem 2007; 50: 2185-93.

[124] Bergamo A, Messori L, Piccioli F, Cocchietto M, Sava G. Biological role of adduct formation of the ruthenium(III) complex NAMI-A with serum albumin and serum transferrin. Invest New Drugs 2003; 21: 401-11.

[125] Pacor S, Zorzet S, Cocchietto M, Bacac M, Vadori M, Turrin C, Gava B, Castellarin A, Sava G. Intratumoral NAMI-A treatment triggers metastasis reduction, which correlates to CD44 regulation and tumor infiltrating lymphocyte recruitment. Pharmacol Exp Ther 2004; 310: 737-74.

[126] Vacca A, Bruno M, Boccarelli A, Coluccia M, Ribatti D, Bergamo A, Garbisa S, Sartor L, Sava G. Inhibition of endothelial cell functions and of angiogenesis by the metastasis inhibitor NAMI-A. Br J Cancer 2002; 86: 993-8.

[127] Zorzet S, Bergamo A, Cocchietto M, Sorc A, Gava B, Alessio E, Iengo E, Sava G. Lack of *in vitro* cytotoxicity, associated to increased G2-M cell fraction and inhibition of matrigel invasion, may predict *in vivo*-selective antimetastasis activity of ruthenium complexes. J. Pharmacol Exp Ther 2000; 295: 927-33.

[128] Levina A; Lay PA. Influence of an anti-metastatic ruthenium(III) prodrug on extracellular protein-protein interactions: studies by bio-layer interferometry. Inorg Chem Front 2014; 1: 44-8.

[129] Messori L, Merlino A. Ruthenium metalation of proteins: the X-ray structure of the complex formed between NAMI-A and hen egg white lysozyme. Dalton Trans 2014; 43: 6128-31.

[130] Vadori M, Pacor S, Vita F, Zorzet S, Cocchietto M, Sava G. Features and full reversibility of the renal toxicity of the ruthenium-based drug NAMI-A in mice. J Inorg Biochem 2013; 118: 21-7.

[131] Bergamo A, Masi A, Jakupec MA, Keppler BK, Sava G. Inhibitory effects of the ruthenium complex KP1019 in models of mammary cancer cell migration and invasion. Metal-Based Drugs 2009; 681270.

[132] Seelig MH, Berger MR, Keppler BK. Antineoplastic activity of three ruthenium derivatives against chemically induced colorectal carcinoma in rats. J Cancer Res Clin Oncol 1992; 118: 195-200.

[133] Frühauf S, Zeller WJ. New platinum, titanium, and ruthenium complexes with different patterns of DNA damage in rat ovarian tumor cells. Cancer Res 1991; 51: 2943-8.

[134] Kapitza S, Jakupec MA, Uhl M, Keppler BK, Marian B. The heterocyclic ruthenium(III) complex KP1019 (FFC14A) causes DNA damage and oxidative stress in colorectal tumor cells. Cancer Lett 2005; 226: 115-21.

[135] Kapitza S, Pongratz M, Jakupec MA, Heffeter P, Berger W, Lackinger L, Keppler BK, Marian B. Heterocyclic complexes of ruthenium(III) induce apoptosis in colorectal carcinoma cells. J Cancer Res Clin Oncol 2005; 131: 101-10.

[136] Hartinger CG, Jakupec MA, Zorbas-Seifried S, Groessl M, Egger A, Berger W, Zorbas H, Dyson PJ, Keppler BK. KP1019, A new redox-active anticancer agent - preclinical development and results of a clinical phase I study in tumor pat. Chem Biodivers 2008; 5: 2140-55.

[137] Pieper T, Borsky K, Keppler BK. Non-platinum antitumor compounds. Top Biol Inorg Chem 1999; 1: 171-99.

[138] Hartinger CG, Zorbas-Seifried S, Jakupec MA, Kynast B, Zorbas H, Keppler BK. From bench to bedside-preclinical and early clinical development of the anticancer agent indazolium trans-[tetrachlorobis(1H-indazole)ruthenate(III)] (KP1019 or FFC14A). J Inorg Biochem 2006; 100: 891-904.

[139] Hartinger CG, Keppler BK. CE in anticancer metallodrug research - an update. Electrophoresis 2007; 28: 3436-46.

[140] Dömötör O, Hartinger CG, Bytzek AK, Kiss T, Keppler BK, Enyedy EA. Characterization of the binding sites of the anticancer ruthenium(III) complexes KP1019 and KP1339 on human serum albumin *via* competition studies. J Biol Inorg Chem 2013; 18: 9-17.

[141] Pongratz A, Schluga P, Jakupec MA, Arion VB, Hartinger CG, Allmaier G, Keppler BK. Transferrin binding and transferrin-mediated cellular uptake of the ruthenium coordination compound KP1019, studied by means of AAS, ESI-MS and CD spectroscopy. J Anal At Spectrom 2004; 19: 46-51.

[142] Heffeter P, Böck K, Atil B, Hoda MAR, Körner W, Bartel C, Jungwirth U, Keppler. BK, Micksche M, Berger W, Koellensperger G. Intracellular protein binding patterns of the anticancer ruthenium drugs KP1019 and KP1339. J Biol Inorg Chem 2010; 15: 737-48

[143] Hummer AA, Heffeter P, Berger W, Filipits M, Batchelor D, Büchel GE, Jakupec MA, Keppler B K, Rompel A. X-ray absorption near edge structure spectroscopy to resolve the *in vivo* chemistry of the redox-active indazolium trans-[tetrachlorobis(1H-indazole) ruthenate(III)] (KP1019). J Med Chem 2013; 56: 1182-96.

[144] Hummer AA, Rompel A. X-Ray absorption spectroscopy: a tool to investigate the local structure of metal-based anticancer compounds *in vivo*. In: Christov CZ, Ed. Biomolecular spectroscopy: advances from integrating experiments and theory. Book series: Advances in protein chemistry and structural biology. San Diego: Elsevier 2013; 93: 257-305.

[145] Hummer AA, Rompel A. The use of X-ray absorption and synchrotron based micro-X-ray fluorescence spectroscopy to investigate anti-cancer metal compounds *in vivo* and *in vitro*. Metallomics, 2013; 5: 597-614.
[146] Heffeter P, Atil B, Kryeziu K, Groza D, Koellensperger G, Körner W, Jungwirth U, Mohr T, Keppler BK, Berger W. The ruthenium compound KP1339 potentiates the anticancer activity of sorafenib *in vitro* and *in vivo*. Eur J Cancer 2013; 49: 3366-75.
[147] Heffeter P, Riabtseva A, Senkiv Y, Kowol CR, Körner W, Jungwith U, Mitina N, Keppler BK, Konstantinova T, Yanchuk I, Stoika R, Zaichenko A, Berger W. Nanoformulation improves activity of the (pre)clinical anticancer ruthenium complex KP1019. J Biom Nanotechnol 2014; 10: 877-84.
[148] Dale LD, Tocher JH; Dyson TM, Edwards DI, Tocher DA. Studies on DNA damage and induction of SOS repair by novel multifunctional bioreducible compounds.2. A metronidazole adduct of a ruthenium-arene compound. Anti-Cancer Drug Design 1992; 7: 3-14.
[149] Dougan SJ, Sadler PJ. The design of organometallic ruthenium arene anticancer agents. Chimia, 2007; 61: 704-15.
[150] Dyson PJ. Systematic design of a targeted organometallic antitumor drug in pre-clinical development. Chimia 2007; 61: 698-703.
[151] Yan YK, Melchart M, Habtemariam A, Sadler PJ. Organometallic chemistry, biology and medicine: ruthenium arene anticancer complexes. Chem Commun 2005; 38: 4764-76.
[152] John RO, Arion VB, Jakupec MA, Keppler BK. Ruthenium(II)-arene complex with heterocyclic ligands as prospective antitumor agent. Metal Ions in Biology and Medicine 2006; 9: 40-5.
[153] Huxham LA, Cheu ELS, Patrick BO, James BR. The synthesis, structural characterization, and *in vitro* anti-cancer activity of chloro(p-cymene) complexes of ruthenium(II) containing a disulfoxide ligand. Inorg Chim Acta 2003; 352: 238-46.
[154] Fetzer L, Boff B, Ali M, Xiangjun M, Collin J, Sirlin C, Gaiddon C, Pfeffer M. Library of second-generation cycloruthenated compounds and evaluation of their biological properties as potential anticancer drugs: Passing the nanomolar barrier. Dalton Trans 2011; 40: 8869-78.
[155] Zheng W, Luo Q, Lin Y, Zhao Y, Wang X, Du Z, Hao X, Yu Y, Lü S, Ji L, Li X, Yang L, Wang F. Complexation with organometallic ruthenium pharmacophores enhances the ability of 4-anilinoquinazolines inducing apoptosis. Chem Commun 2013; 49: 10224-6.
[156] Yellol GS, Donaire A, Yellol JG, Vasylyeva V, Janiak C. Ruiz J. On the antitumor properties of novel cyclometalated benzimidazole Ru(II), Ir(III) and Rh(III) complexes. Chem Commun 2013; 49: 11533-5.
[157] Kilpin KJ, Crot S, Riedel T, Kitchen JA, Dyson PJ. Ruthenium(II) and osmium(II) 1,2,3-triazolylidene organometallics: a preliminary investigation into the biological activity of 'click' carbene complexes. Dalton Trans 2014; 43: 1443-8.
[158] Oehninger L, Stefanopoulou M, Alborzinia H, Schur J, Ludewig S, Namikawa K, Muñoz-Castro A, Köster RW, Baumann K, Wölfl S, Sheldrick WS, Ott I. Evaluation of arene ruthenium(II) N-heterocyclic carbene complexes as organometallics interacting with thiol and selenol containing biomolecules. Dalton Trans 2013; 42: 1657-66.
[159] Schäfer S, Ott I, Gust R, Sheldrick WS. Influence of the polypyridyl (pp) ligand size on the DNA binding properties, cytotoxicity and cellular uptake of organoruthenium(II)

complexes of the type $[(\eta^6\text{-}C_6Me_6)Ru(L)(pp)]^{n+}$ [L = Cl, n = 1; L = $(NH_2)_2CS$, n = 2]. Eur J Inorg Chem 2007; 3034-46.

[160] Morris RE, Aird RE, Murdoch PDS, Chen H, Cummings J, Hughes ND, Parsons S, Parkin A, Boyd G, Jodrell DI, Sadler PJ. Inhibition of cancer cell growth by ruthenium(II) arene complexes. J Med Chem 2001; 44: 3616-21.

[161] Scolaro C, Bergamo A, Brescacin L, Delfino R, Cocchietto M, Laurenczy G, Geldbach TJ, Sava G, Dyson PJ. *In vitro* and *in vivo* evaluation of ruthenium(II)–arene PTA complexes. J Med Chem 2005; 48: 4161-71.

[162] Wang F, Habtemariam A, Van-der-Geer E, Fernández R, Melchart M, Deeth RJ, Aird R, Guichard S, Fabbiani FP, Lozano-Casal P, Oswald IDH, Jodrell DI, Parsons S, Sadler PJ. Controlling ligand substitution reactions of organometallic complexes: Tuning cancer cell cytotoxicity. Proc Natl Acad Sci USA 2005; 102: 18269-74.

[163] Habtemariam A, Melchart M, Fernandez R, Parsons S, Oswald IDH, Parkin A, Fabbiani FP, Davidson JE, Dawson A, Aird RE, Jodrell DI, Sadler PJ. Structure–activity relationships for cytotoxic ruthenium(II) arene complexes containing N,N-, N,O-, and O,O-chelating ligands. J Med Chem 2006; 49: 6858-68.

[164] Peacock AFA, Habtemariam A, Fernández R, Walland V, Fabbiani F, Parsons S, Aird RE, Jodrell DI, Sadler PJ. Tuning the reactivity of osmium(II) and ruthenium(II) arene complexes under physiological conditions. J Am Chem Soc 2006; 128: 1739-48.

[165] Bruijnincx PC, Sadler PJ. Controlling platinum, ruthenium, and osmium reactivity for anticancer drug design. Adv Inorg Chem 2009; 1-62.

[166] Babak MV, Meier SM, Legin AA, Razavi MSA, Roller A, Jakupec MA, Keppler BK, Hartinger CG. Am(m)ines make the difference: organoruthenium am(m)ine complexes and their chemistry in anticancer drug development, Chem Eur J 2013; 19: 4308-18.

[167] Fernandez R, Melchart M, Habtemariam A, Parsons S, Sadler PJ. Use of chelating ligands to tune the reactive site of half-sandwich ruthenium(II)-arene anticancer complexes. Chem Eur J 2004; 10: 5173-9.

[168] Aird RE, Cummings J, Ritchie AA, Muir M, Morris RE, Chen H, Sadler PJ, Jodrell DI. *In vitro* and *in vivo* activity and cross resistance profiles of novel ruthenium (II) organometallic arene complexes in human ovarian cancer. Br J Cancer 2002; 86: 1652-7.

[169] Hayward RL, Schornagel QC, Tente R, Macpherson JS, Aird RE, Guichard S, Habtemariam A, Sadler PJ, Jodrell DI. Investigation of the role of Bax, p21/Waf1 and p53 as determinants of cellular responses in HCT116 colorectal cancer cells exposed to the novel cytotoxic ruthenium(II) organometallic agent, RM175. Cancer Chemother Pharmacol 2005; 55: 577-83.

[170] Bergamo A, Masi A, Peacock AFA, Habtemariam A, Sadler PJ, Sava G. *In vivo* tumour and metastasis reduction and *in vitro* effects on invasion assays of the ruthenium RM175 and osmium AFAP51 organometallics in the mammary cancer model. J Inorg Biochem 2010; 104: 79-86.

[171] Novakova O, Chen H, Vrana O, Rodger A, Sadler PJ, Brabec V. DNA interactions of monofunctional organometallic ruthenium(II) antitumor complexes in cell-free media Biochemistry 2003; 42: 11544-54.

[172] Chen H, Parkinson JA, Parsons S, Coxall RA, Gould RO, Sadler PJ, Organometallic ruthenium(II) diamine anticancer complexes: arene-nucleobase stacking and stereospecific hydrogen-bonding in guanine adducts. J Am Chem Soc 2002; 124: 3064-82.

[173] Chen H, Parkinson JA, Morris RE, Sadler PJ. Highly selective binding of organometallic ruthenium ethylenediamine complexes to nucleic acids: novel recognition mechanisms. J Am Chem Soc 2003; 125: 173-86.
[174] Casini A, Gabbiani C, Michelucci E, Pieraccini G, Monet G, Dyson PJ, Messori L, Exploring metallodrug-protein interactions by mass spectrometry: comparisons between platinum coordination complexes and an organometallic ruthenium compound. J Biol Inorg. Chem 2009; 14: 761-70.
[175] Casini A, Hartinger CG, Nazarov AA, Dyson PJ. Organometallic antitumour agents with alternative modes of action top. Organomet Chem 2010; 32: 57-80.
[176] Loughrey BT, Williams ML, Healy PC, Innocenti A, Vullo D, Supuran CT, Parsons PG, Poulsen SA. Novel organometallic cationic ruthenium(II) pentamethylcyclopentadienyl benzenesulfonamide complexes targeted to inhibit carbonic anhydrase. J Biol Inorg Chem 2009; 14: 935-45.
[177] Wu K, Hu W, Luo Q, Li X, Xiong S, Sadler PJ, Wang F. Competitive binding sites of a ruthenium arene anticancer complex on oligonucleotides studied by mass spectrometry: ladder-sequencing *versus* top-down. J Am Soc Mass Spectrom 2013; 24: 410-20.
[178] Wang F, Xu J, Habtemariam A, Bella J, Sadler PJ. Competition between glutathione and guanine for a ruthenium(II) arene anticancer complex: detection of a sulfenato intermediate. J Am Chem Soc, 2005; 127: 17734-43.
[179] Wang F, Weidt S, Xu J, Mackay CL, Langridge-Smith PRR, Sadler PJ. Identification of clusters from reactions of ruthenium arene anticancer complex with glutathione using nanoscale liquid chromatography Fourier transform ion cyclotron mass spectrometry combined with ^{18}O-labeling. J Am Soc Mass Spectrom 2008; 19: 544-9.
[180] Blunden BM, Lu H, Stenzel MH. Enhanced delivery of the RAPTA-C macromolecular chemotherapeutic by conjugation to degradable polymeric micelles biomacromolecules 2013; 14: 4177-88.
[181] Bergamo A, Masi A, Dyson PJ, Sava G. Modulation of the metastatic progression of breast cancer with an organometallic ruthenium compound. Int J Oncol 2008; 33: 1281-9.
[182] Casini A, Gabbiani C, Sorrentino F, Rigobello MP, Bindoli A, Geldbach TJ, Marrone A, Re N, Hartinger CG, Dyson PJ, Messori L. Emerging protein targets for anticancer metallodrugs: inhibition of thioredoxin reductase and cathepsin B by antitumor ruthenium(II)−arene compounds. J Med Chem 2008; 51: 6773-81.
[183] Wu B, Ong MS, Groessl M, Adhireksan Z, Hartinger CG, Dyson PJ, Davey CA. A ruthenium antimetastasis agent forms specific histone protein adducts in the nucleosome core. Chem Eur J 2011; 17: 3562-6.
[184] Guidi F, Modesti A, Landini I, Nobili S, Mini E, Bini L, Puglia M, Casini A, Dyson PJ, Gabbiani C, Messori L. The molecular mechanisms of antimetastatic ruthenium compounds explored through DIGE proteomics. J Inorg Biochem 2013; 118: 94-9.
[185] Ang WH, De Luca A, Chapuis-Bernasconi C, Juillerat-Jeanneret L, Lo Bello M, Dyson PJ. Organometallic ruthenium inhibitors of glutathione-*S*-transferase P1-1 as anticancer drugs. Chem Med Chem 2007; 2: 1799-806.
[186] Ang WH, Parker LJ, De Luca A, Juillerat-Jeanneret L, Morton CJ, Lo Bello M, Parker MW, Dyson P J. Rational design of an organometallic glutathione transferase inhibitor. Angew Chem Int Ed 2009; 48: 3854-7.

[187] Vock CA, Ang WH, Scolaro C, Phillips AD, Lagopoulos L, Juillerat-Jeanneret L., Sava G, Scopelliti R, Dyson PJ. Development of ruthenium antitumor drugs that overcome multidrug resistance mechanisms. J Med Chem 2007; 50: 2166-75.

[188] Auzias M, Therrien B, Fink GS, Šÿtěpnička P, Ang WH, Dyson PJ. Ferrocenoyl pyridine arene ruthenium complexes with anticancer properties: synthesis, structure, Electrochemistry, and Cytotoxicity. Inorg Chem 2008; 47: 578-83.

[189] Meier SM, Hanif M, Adhireksan Z, Pichler V, Novak M, Jirkovsky E, Jakupec MA, VB, Davey CA, Keppler BK, Hartinger CG. Novel metal(II) arene 2-pyridinecarbothioamides: a rationale to orally active organometallic anticancer agents. Chem Sci 2013; 4: 1837-46.

[190] Berger I, Hanif M, Nazarov AA, Hartinger CG, John RO, Kuznetsov ML, Groessl M, Schmitt F, Zava O, Biba F, Arion VB, Galanski M, Jakupec MA, Juillerat-Jeanneret L, Dyson P J, Keppler BK. *In vitro* anticancer activity and biologically relevant metabolization of organometallic ruthenium complexes with carbohydrate-based ligands. Chem Eur J 2008; 14: 9046-57.

[191] Hanif M. Nazarov AA, Hartinger CG, Kandioller W, Jakupec MA, Arion VB, Dyson P J, Keppler BK. Osmium(II)-*versus* ruthenium(II)-arene carbohydrate-based anticancer compounds: similarities and differences. Dalton Trans 2010; 39: 7345-52.

[192] Hanif M, Nazarov AA, Hartinger CG. Synthesis of $[Ru^{II}(\eta^6\text{-}p\text{-cymene})(PPh_3)(L)Cl]PF_6$ complexes with carbohydrate-derived phosphites, imidazole or indazole co-ligands. Inorg Chim Acta 2012; 380: 211-5.

[193] Hartinger CG, Nazarov AA, Ashraf SM, Dyson PJ, Keppler BK. Carbohydrate-metal complexes and their potential as anticancer agents. Curr Med Chem 2008; 15: 2574-91.

[194] Kurzwernhart A, Kandioller W, Bartel C, Baechler S, Trondl R, Muehlgassner G, Jakupec M A, Arion VB, Marko D, Keppler BK, Hartinger CG. Targeting the DNA-topoisomerase complex in a double-strike approach with a topoisomerase inhibiting moiety and covalent DNA binder. Chem Commun 2012; 48: 4839-41.

[195] Turel I, Kljun J, Perdih F, Morozova E, Bakulev V, Kasyanenko N, Byl JAW, Osheroff N. First ruthenium organometallic complex of antibacterial agent ofloxacin. Crystal structure and interactions with DNA. Inorg Chem 2010; 49: 10750-2.

[196] Turel I, Kljun J. Interactions of metal ions with DNA, its constituents and derivatives, which may be relevant for anticancer research. Curr Top Med Chem 2011; 11: 2661-87.

[197] Kljun J, Bytzek AK, Kandioller W, Bartel C, Jakupec MA, Hartinger CG, Keppler BK, Turel I. Physicochemical studies and anticancer potency of ruthenium η-p-cymene complexes containing antibacterial quinolones. organometallics 2011; 30: 2506-12.

[198] Zhang L, Carroll P, Meggers E. Ruthenium complexes as protein kinase inhibitors. Org Lett 2004; 6: 521-3.

[199] Bregman H, Williams DS, Atilla GE, Carroll PJ, Meggers E. An organometallic inhibitor for glycogen synthase kinase 3. J Am Chem Soc 2004; 126: 13594-5.

[200] Debreczeni JE, Bullock AN, Atilla GE, Williams DS, Bregman H, Knapp S, Meggers E. Ruthenium half-sandwich complexes bound to protein kinase Pim-1. Angew Chem Int Ed 2006; 45: 1580-5.

[201] Smalley KS, Contractor R, Haass NK, Kulp AN, Atilla-Gokcuman GE, Williams DE, Bregman H, Flaherty KT, Soengas MS, Meggers E, Herlyn M. An organometallic protein kinase inhibitor pharmacologically activates p53 and induces apoptosis in human melanoma cells. Cancer Res 2007; 67: 209-17.

[202] Mendoza-Ferri MG, Hartinger CG, Eichinger RE, Stolyarova N, Jakupec MA, Nazarov AA, Severin K, Keppler BK. Influence of the spacer length on the *in vitro* anticancer activity of dinuclear ruthenium-arene compounds. Organometallics 2008; 27: 2405-7.

[203] Novakova O, Nazarov AA, Hartinger CG, Keppler BK, Brabec V. DNA interactions of dinuclear Ru-II arene antitumor complexes in cell-free media. Biochem Pharmacol 2009; 77: 364-74.

[204] Morais TS, Silva TJL, Marques F, Robalo MP, Avecilla F, Madeira PJA, Mendes PJG, Santos, I, Garcia MH. Synthesis of organometallic ruthenium(II) complexes with strong activity against several human cancer cell lines. J Inorg Biochem 2012; 114: 65-74.

[205] Côrte-Real L, Matos AP, Alho I, Morais TS, Tomaz AI, Garcia MH, Santos I, Bicho MP, Marques F. Cellular uptake mechanisms of an antitumor ruthenium compound: the endosomal/lysosomal system as a target for anticancer metal-based drugs. Microsc Microanal 2013;19: 1122-30.

[206] Cotton F A, Murillo CA, Walton RA. Multiple bonds between metal atoms, 3rd ed. New York: Springer Science and Busines Media Inc 2005.

[207] Aquino MAS. Diruthenium and diosmium tetracarboxylates: synthesis, physical properties and applications. Coord Chem Rev 1988; 170: 141-202.

[208] Aquino MAS. Recent developments in the synthesis and properties of diruthenium tetracarboxylates. Coord Chem Rev 2004; 248: 1025-45.

[209] Ribeiro G, Vichi FM, de Oliveira Silva D. Synthesis, characterization and adsorption properties of porous mixed valent diruthenium(II,III)-terephthalate and diruthenium(II,III)-adipate polymers. J Mol Struc 2008; 890: 209-14.

[210] Van Rensburg CEJ, Kreft E, Swarts JC, Dalrymple SR, Macdonald DM, Cooke MW, Aquino MAS. Cytotoxicity of a series of water-soluble mixed valent diruthenium tetracarboxylates. Anticancer Res 2002; 22: 889-92.

[211] Dunbar KR, Matonic JH, Saharan VP, Crawford CA, Christou G. Structural evidence for a new metal-binding mode for guanine bases: implications for the binding of dinuclear antitumor agents to DNA. J Am Chem Soc 1994; 116: 2201-2.

[212] Crawford CA, Day EF, Saharan VP, Folting K, Huffman JC, Dunbar KR, Christou G. N-7,O-6 bridging 9-ethylguanine (9-EtGH) groups in dinuclear metal-metal bonded complexes with bond orders of one, two or four. J Chem Soc Chem Commun 1996; 1113-4.

[213] Foye WO, Lemke TL, Williams DA. Principles of Medicinal Chemistry, 4rd ed. New York: Lippincott Williams & Wilkins 1995.

[214] Vane JR, Flower RJ, Botting RM. History of aspirin and its mechanism of action. Stroke 1990; 21: 12-23.

[215] Griffin MR, Sheiman JM. Prospects for changing the burden of nonsteroidal anti-inflammatory drug toxicity. Am J Med 2001; 110: S33-7.

[216] Herendeen JM, Lindley C. Use of NSAIDs for the chemioprevention of colorectal cancer. Ann Pharmacother 2003; 37: 1664-74.

[217] Pereg D, Lishner M. Non-steroidal anti-inflammatory drugs for the prevention and treatment of cancer. J Int Med 2005; 258: 115-23.

[218] Thun MJ, Henley SJ, Patrono C. Nonsteroidal Anti-inflammatory Drugs as Anticancer Agents: Mechanistic, Pharmacologic, and Clinical Issues. J Nat Cancer Inst 2002; 94: 252-66.

[219] Gupta RA, DuBois RN. Aspirin, NSAIDS, and colon cancer prevention: mechanisms? Gastroenterology 1998; 114: 1095-8.
[220] Rao CV, Reddy BS. NSAIDs and chemoprevention. Curr. Cancer Drug Targets 2004; 4: 29-42.
[221] Giovannucci E, Egan KM, Hunter DJ, Stampfer MJ, Colditz GA, Willett WC, Speizer FE. Aspirin and the risk of colorectal cancer in women. N Engl J Med 1995; 333: 609-14.
[222] Farrow DC, Vaughan TL, Hansten PD, Stanford JL, Risch HA, Gammon MD, Chow WH, Dubrow R, Ahsan H, Mayne ST, Schoenberg JB, West AB, Rotterdam H, Fraumeni Jr JF, Blot W J. Use of aspirin and other nonsteroidal anti-inflammatory drugs and risk of esophageal and gastric cancer. Cancer Epidemiol Biomarkers Prev 1998; 7: 97-102.
[223] Akre K, Ekstrom AM, Signorello LB, Hansson LE, Nyren O. Aspirin and risk for gastric cancer: a population-based case-control study in Sweden. Br J Cancer 2001; 84: 965-8.
[224] Baron JA, Sandler RS. Nonsteroidal anti-inflammatory drugs and cancer prevention. Annu Rev Med 2000; 51: 511-23.
[225] Dai Y, Wang WH. Non-steroidal anti-inflammatory drugs in prevention of gastric cancer. World. J Gastroenterol 2006; 12: 2884-9.
[226] Zaridze D, Borisova E, Maximovitch D, Chkhikvadze V. Aspirin protects against gastric cancer: results of a case-control study from Moscow Russia. Int J Cancer 1999; 82: 473-6.
[227] Greenberg ER, Baron JA, Freeman DH Jr, Mandel JS, Haile R. Reduced risk of large-bowel adenomas among aspirin users. The Polyp Prevention Study Group. J Natl Cancer Inst 1993; 85: 912-6.
[228] Dube C, Rostom A, Lewin G, Tsertsvadze A, Barrowman N, Code C, Sampson M, Moher D. The use of aspirin for primary prevention of colorectal cancer: a systematic review prepared for the U.S. Preventive Services Task Force. Ann Intern Med 2007; 146: 365-75.
[229] Gridley G, McLaughlin JK, Ekbom A, Klareskog L, Adami HO, Hacker DG, Hoover R, Fraumeni JFJr. Incidence of cancer among patients with rheumatoid arthritis. J Natl Cancer Inst 1993; 85: 307-11.
[230] Wang WH, Huang JQ, Zheng GF, Lam SK, Karlberg J, Wong BC. Non-steroidal anti-inflammatory drug use and the risk of gastric cancer: a systematic review and meta-analysis. J Natl Cancer Inst 2003; 95: 1784-91.
[231] Schreinemachers DM, Everson RB. Aspirin use and lung, colon, and breast cancer incidence in a prospective study. Epidemiology 1994; 5: 138-46.
[232] Tanaka T, Kojima T, Yoshimi N, Sugie S, Mori H. Inhibitory effect of the non-steroidal anti-inflammatory drug, indomethacin on the naturally occurring carcinogen, 1-hydroxyanthraquinone in male ACI/N rats. Carcinogenesis 1991; 12: 1949-52.
[233] Hu PJ, Yu J, Zeng ZR, Leung WK, Lin HL, Tang BD, Bai AH, Sung JJ. Chemoprevention of gastric cancer by celecoxib in rats. Gut 2004; 53: 195-200.
[234] Sawaoka H, Kawano S, Tsuji S, Tsujii M, Gunawan ES, Takei Y, Nagano K, Hori M. Cyclooxygenase-2 inhibitors suppress the growth of gastric cancer xenografts *via* induction of apoptosis in nude mice. Am J Physiol 1998; 274: 1061-7.
[235] Beazer-Barclay Y, Levy DB, Moser AR, Dove WF, Hamilton SR, Vogelstein B, Kinzler KW. Sulindac suppresses tumorigenesis in the Min mouse. Carcinogenesis 1996; 17: 1757-60.
[236] Harris RE, Kasbari S, Farrar WB. Prospective study of nonsteroidal anti-inflammatory drugs and breast cancer. Oncol. Rep 1999; 6: 71-3.

[237] Hida T, Leyton J, Makheja AN, Ben-Av P, Hla T, Martinez A, Mulshine J, Malkani S, Chung P, Moody TW. Non-small cell lung cancer cycloxygenase activity and proliferation are inhibited by non-steroidal antiinflammatory drugs. Anticancer Res 1998; 18: 775-82.

[238] Chan TA. Nonsteroidal anti-inflammatory drugs, apoptosis, and colon-cancer chemoprevention. Lancet Oncol 2002; 3: 166-74.

[239] Chan TA, Morin PJ, Vogelstein B, Kinzler KW. Mechanisms underlying nonsteroidal antiinflammatory drug-mediated apoptosis. Proc Natl Acad Sci USA 1998; 95: 681-6.

[240] Fitzgerald GA. COX-2 and beyond: approaches to prostaglandin inhibition in human disease. Nat Rev Drug Discov 2003; 2: 879-91.

[241] Jana NR. NSAIDs and apoptosis. Cell Mol Life Sci 2008; 65: 1295-301.

[242] Green DR, Kroemer G. The pathophysiology of mitochondrial cell death. Science 2004; 305: 626-9.

[243] Green DR. Apoptotic pathways: ten minutes to dead. Cell 2005; 121: 671-4.

[244] Green DR, Kroemer G. Pharmacological manipulation of cell death: clinical applications in sight? J Clin Invest 2005; 115: 2610-7.

[245] Shiff SJ, Koutsos MI, Qiao L, Rigas B. Nonsteroidal Antiinflammatory Drugs Inhibit the Proliferation of Colon Adenocarcinoma Cells: Effects on Cell Cycle and Apoptosis. Expl Cell Res 1996; 222: 179-88.

[246] Smith ML, Hawcroft G, Hull MA. The effect of non-steroidal anti-inflammatory drugs on human colorectal cancer cells: evidence of different mechanisms of action. Eur J Cancer 2000; 36: 664-74.

[247] Sorenson JRJ. In: Sorenson JRJ, Ed. Biology of copper complexes. New York: Humana Press 1987.

[248] Weder JE, Dillon CT, Hambley TW, Kennedy BJ, Lay PA, Biffin JR, Regtop HLN, Davies M. Copper complexes of non-steroidal anti-inflammatory drugs: an opportunity yet to be realized. Coord Chem Rev 2002; 232: 95-126.

[249] Cotton FA, de Oliveira Silva D. Preparation and crystal structure of a dimolybdenum(II) complex with the drug ibuprofen. Inorg Chim Acta 1996; 249: 57-61.

[250] Carvill A, Higgins P, McCann M, Ryan H, Shiels A. Synthesis, spectroscopic, electrochemical, and magnetic properties of dimolybdenum(II,II), diruthenium-(II,III) and -(II,II) complexes containing bridging aspirinate (2-acetoxybenzoate) ligands. J Chem Soc Dalton Trans 1989; 2435-41.

[251] Andrade A, Namora SF, Woisky RG, Wiezel G, Najjar R, Sertié JAA, de Oliveira Silva D. Synthesis and characterization of a diruthenium-ibuprofenato complex Comparing its anti-inflammatory activity with that of a copper(II)-ibuprofenato complex. J Inorg Biochem 2000; 81: 23-7.

[252] Willians DA, Walz DR, Foye WO. Synthesis and biological evaluation of tetrakis(acetylsalicylato)-μ-dicopper(II). J Pharm Sci 1976; 65: 126-8.

[253] Oga S, Taniguchi SF, Najjar R, Souza AR. Synthesis, characterization, and biological screening of a copper flurbiprofen complex with antiinflammatory effects. J Inorg Biochem 1991; 41: 45-51.

[254] Dendrinou-Samara C, Tsotsou G, Ekateriniadou LV, Korsaris AH, Raptopoulou CP, Terzis A, Kyriakidis DA, Kessissoglou DP. Anti-inflammatory drugs interacting with Zn(II), Cd(II) and Pt(II) metal ions. J Inorg Biochem 1998; 71: 171-9.

[255] Boyle E, Freeman PC, Goudie AC, Magan FR, Thompson M. Role of copper in preventing gastrointestinal damage by acidic anti-inflammatory drugs. J Pharm Pharmacol 1976; 28: 865-8.

[256] Grguric-Sipka SR, Vilaplana RA, Pérez JM, Fuertes MA, Alonso C, Alvarez Y, Sabo TJ, Vílchez-González F. Synthesis, characterization, interaction with DNA and cytotoxicity of the new potential antitumour drug cis-K[Ru(eddp)Cl_2]. J Inorg Biochem 2003: 97: 215-20.

[257] Bergamo A, Stocco G, Gava B, Cocchietto M, Alessio E, Serli B, Iengo E, Sava G. Distinct effects of dinuclear ruthenium(III) complexes on cell proliferation and on cell cycle regulation in human and murine tumor cell lines. J Pharmacol Expl Ther 2003; 305: 725-32.

[258] Djinovíc V, Momcilovíc M, Grguric-Sipka S, Trajkovic V, Stojkovic MM, Miljkovic D, Sabo T. Novel ruthenium complex K_2[Ru(dmgly)Cl_4]$\cdot 2H_2O$ is toxic to C6 astrocytoma cell line, but not to primary rat astrocytes. J Inorg Biochem 2004; 98: 2168-73.

[259] Armstrong TS. ONS Clinical Lectureship: Head's Up on Management of Patients with Malignant Glioma. Oncology Nursing Forum 2009; 36: E232-40.

[260] Bredel M. Translating biological insights into clinical endpoints in neuro-oncology. Lancet Oncol 2009; 10: 928-9.

[261] Gomes RN, Colquhoun A. E series prostaglandins alter the proliferative, apoptotic and migratory properties of T98G human glioma cells *in vitro*. Lipids in Health and Disease 2012; 11: 171.

[262] Lefranc F, Brotchi J, Kiss R. Possible future issues in the treatment of glioblastomas: Special emphasis on cell migration and the resistance of migrating glioblastoma cells to apoptosis. J Clin Oncol 2005; 23: 2411-22.

[263] Giese A, Bjerkvig R, Berens ME, Westphal M. Cost of migration: invasion of malignant gliomas and implications for treatment. J Clin Oncol 2003; 21: 1624-36.

[264] Maher EA, Furnari FB, Bachoo RM, Rowitch DH, Louis DN, Cavenee WK, DePinho RA. Malignant glioma: genetics and biology of a grave matter. Genes Dev 2001; 15: 1311-33.

[265] Zha S, Yegnasubramanian V, Nelson WG, Isaacs WB, De Marzo AM. Cyclooxygenases in cancer: progress and perspective. Cancer Lett 2004; 213: 1-20.

[266] Shono T, Tofilon PJ, Bruner JM, Owolabi O, Lang FF. Cyclooxygenase-2 expression in human gliomas: Prognostic significance and molecular correlations. Cancer Res 2001; 61: 4375-81.

[267] Kürzel F, Hagel C, Zapf S, Meissner H, Westphal M, Geise A. Cyclo-oxygenase inhibitors and thromboxane synthase inhibitors differentially regulate migration arrest, growth inhibition and apoptosis in human glioma cells. Acta Neurochir 2002; 144: 71-87.

[268] Nathoo N, Barnett GH, Golubic M. The eicosanoid cascade: possible role in gliomas and meningiomas. J Clin Pathol 2004; 57: 6-13.

[269] Wang M, Yoshida D, Liu S, Teramoto A. Prognostic significance of the immunohistochemical index of survivin in glioma: a comparative study with the MIB-1 index. J Neuro Oncology 2005; 72: 231-8.

[270] Drappatz J, Wen P. Non-cytotoxic drugs as potential treatments for gliomas. Curr Opi Neur 2004; 17: 663-73.

[271] Tuettenberg J, Grobholz R, Korn T, Wenz F, Rever R, Vajkoczy P. Continuous low-dose chemotherapy plus inhibition of cyclooxygenase-2 as an antiangiogenic therapy of glioblastoma multiforme. J Cancer Res Clin Oncol 2005; 131: 31-40.

[272] Friedman HS, Prados MD, Wen PY, Mikkelsen T, Schiff D, Abrey LE, Yung WK, Paleologos N, Nicholas MK, Jensen R, Vredenburgh J, Huang J, Zheng M, Cloughesy T. Bevacizumab Alone and in Combination With Irinotecan in Recurrent Glioblastoma. J Clin Oncol 2009; 27: 4733-40.

[273] Stupp R, Hegi ME, Mason WP, van den Bent MJ, Taphoorn MJB, Janzer RC, Ludwin SK, Allgeier A, Fisher B, Belanger K, Hau P, Brandes AA, Gijtenbeek J, Marosi C, Vecht CJ, Mokhtari K, Wesseling P, Villa S, Eisenhauer E, Gorlia T, Weller M, Lacombe D, Cairncross JG, Mirimanoff RO. Effects of radiotherapy with concomitant and adjuvant temozolomide *versus* radiotherapy alone on survival in glioblastoma in a randomised phase III study: 5-year analysis of the EORTC-NCIC trial. Lancet Oncol 2009; 10: 459-66.

[274] Wheeler CJ, Black KL, Liu G, Mazer M, Zhang XX, Pepkowitz S, Goldfinger D, Ng H, Irvin D, Yu JS. Vaccination Elicits Correlated Immune and Clinical Responses in Glioblastoma Multiforme Patients. Cancer Res 2008; 68: 5955-64.

[275] Fine HA. Toward a Glioblastoma Vaccine: Promise and Potential Pitfalls. J Clin Oncol 2004; 22: 4240-3.

[276] Steiner HH, Bonsanto MM, Beckhove P, Brysch M, Geletneky K, Ahmadi R, Schuele-Freyer R, Kremer P, Ranaie G, Matejic D, Bauer H, Kiessling M, Kunze S, Schirrmacher V, Herold-Mende C. Antitumor Vaccination of Patients With Glioblastoma Multiforme: A Pilot Study to Assess Feasibility, Safety, and Clinical Benefit. J Clin Oncol 2004; 22: 4272-81.

[277] Ferguson S, Lesniak MS. Convection enhanced drug delivery of novel therapeutic agents to malignant brain tumors. Curr Drug Deliv 2007; 4: 169-80.

[278] Wen PY, Kesari S, Drappatz J. Malignant gliomas: strategies to increase the effectiveness of targeted molecular treatment. Expert Rev Anticancer Ther 2006; 6: 733-54.

[279] Jiang H, Alonso MM, Gomez-Manzano C, Piao Y, Fueyo J. Oncolytic viruses and DNA-repair machinery: overcoming chemoresistance of gliomas. Expert Rev Anticancer Ther 2006; 6: 1585-92.

[280] Kim L, Glantz M. Chemotherapeutic options for primary brain tumors. Curr Treat Options Oncol 2006; 7: 467-78.

[281] Tuettenberg J, Friedel C, Vajkoczy P. Angiogenesis in malignant glioma-a target for antitumor therapy? Crit Rev Oncol Hematol 2006; 59: 181-93.

[282] Niewald M, Berdel C, Fleckenstein J, Licht N, Ketter R, Rube C. Toxicity after radiochemotherapy for glioblastoma using temozolomide - a retrospective evaluation. Radiat Oncol 2011; 6: 141.

[283] Ribeiro G, Benadiba M, Colquhoun A, de Oliveira Silva, D. Diruthenium (II,III) complexes of ibuprofen, aspirin, naproxen and indomethacin nonsteroidal anti-inflammatory drugs: synthesis, characterization and their effects on tumor-cell proliferation. Polyhedron, 2008; 27: 1131-7.

[284] Benadiba M, Santos RRP, de Oliveira Silva D, Colquhoun A. Inhibition of C6 rat glioma proliferation by [$Ru_2Cl(Ibp)_4$] depends on changes in p21, p27, Bax/Bcl2 ratio and mitochondrial membrane potential. J Inorg Biochem 2010; 104: 928-35

[285] Benadiba M, Costa IM, Rodrigo LSR, Santos FOS, de Oliveira Silva D, Colquhoun A. Growth inhibitory effects of [$Ru_2Cl(Ibp)_4$] in human glioma cells in vitro and in the rat C6 orthotopic glioma in vivo J Biol Inorg Chem 2014; DOI 10.1007/s00775-014-1143-4.

[286] Begin ME, Ells G, Das UN, Horrobin DF. Differential killing of human carcinoma cells supplemented with n-3 and n-6 polyunsaturated fatty acids. J Natl Cancer Inst 1986; 77: 1053-62.
[287] Das UN. Essential fatty acids, lipid peroxidation and apoptosis. Prostaglandins Leukot. Essent Fatty Acids 1999; 61: 157-63.
[288] Naidu MR, Das UN, Kishan A. Intratumoral gamma-linoleic acid therapy of human gliomas. Prostaglandins Leukot Essent Fatty Acids 1992; 45: 181-4.
[289] Das UN, Prasad VV, Reddy DR. Local application of gamma-linolenic acid in the treatment of human gliomas. Cancer Lett 1995; 94: 147-55.
[290] Leaver HA, Wharton SB, Bell HS, Leaver-Yap IM, Whittle IR. Highly unsaturated fatty acid induced tumor regression in glioma pharmacodynamics and bioavailability of gamma linolenic acid in an implantation glioma model: effects on tumor biomass, apoptosis and neuronal tissue histology. Prostaglandins Leukot Essent Fatty Acids 2002; 67: 283-92.
[291] Bakshi A, Mukherjee D, Bakshi A, Banerji AK, Das UN. Gammalinolenic acid therapy of human gliomas. Nutrition 2003; 19: 305-9.
[292] Leaver HA, Williams JR, Smith C, Whittle IR. Intracellular oxidation by human glioma cell populations: effect of arachidonic acid. Prostaglandins Leukot Essent. Fatty Acids 2004; 70: 449-53.
[293] Das UN. From bench to the clinic: gamma-linolenic acid therapy of human gliomas. Prostaglandins Leukot. Essent Fatty Acids 2004; 70: 539-52.
[294] Vartak S, Robbins ME, Spector AA. Polyunsaturated fatty acids increase the sensitivity of 36B10 rat astrocytoma cells to radiation induced cell kill. Lipids 1997; 32: 283-92.
[295] Vartak S, McCaw R, Davis CS, Robbins ME, Spector AA. Gammalinolenic acid (GLA) is cytotoxic to 36B10 malignant rat astrocytoma cells but not to 'normal' rat astrocytes. Br J Cancer 1998; 77: 1612-20.
[296] Benadiba M, Miyake JA, Colquhoun A. Gamma-linolenic acid alters Ku80, E2F1, and bax expression and induces micronucleus formation in C6 glioma cells *in vitro*. IUBMB Life 2009; 61: 244-51.
[297] Colquhoun A, Schumacher RI. Gamma-linolenic acid and eicosapentaenoic acid induce modifications in mitochondrial metabolism, reactive oxygen species generation, lipid peroxidation and apoptosis in Walker 256 rat carcinosarcoma cells. Biochim Biophys Acta 2001; 1533: 207-19.
[298] Colquhoun A, Schumacher RI. Modifications in mitochondrial metabolism and ultrastructure and their relationship to tumor growth inhibition by gamma-linolenic acid. Mol Cell Biochem 2001; 218: 13-20.
[299] Colquhoun A. Gamma-linolenic acid alters the composition of mitochondrial membrane subfractions, decreases outer mitochondrial membrane binding of hexokinase and alters carnitine palmitoyl transferase I properties in the Walker 256 rat tumor. Biochim Biophys Acta 2002; 1583: 74-84.
[300] Ramos KL, Colquhoun A. Protective role of glucose-6-phosphate dehydrogenase activity in the metabolic response of C6 rat glioma cells to polyunsaturated fatty acid exposure. Glia 2003; 43: 149-66.
[301] Ribeiro G, Benadiba M, de Oliveira Silva D, Colquhoun A. The novel ruthenium-g-linolenic complex $[Ru_2(aGLA)_4Cl]$ inhibits C6 rat glioma cell proliferation and induces changes in mitochondrial membrane potential, increased reactive oxygen species generation and apoptosis *in vitro*. Cell Biochem Funct 2010; 28: 15-23.

[302] Miyake JA, Benadiba M, Ribeiro G, de Oliveira Silva D, Colquhoun A. Novel ruthenium - gamma-linolenic acid complex inhibits C6 rat glioma cell proliferation *in vitro* and in the orthotopic c6 model *in vivo* after osmotic pump infusion. Anticancer Res 2014; 34: 1901-11.

[303] Santos RLSR, Bergamo A, Sava G, de Oliveira Silva D. Synthesis and characterization of a diruthenium(II,III)-ketoprofen compound and study of the *in vitro* effects on CRC cells in comparison to the naproxen and ibuprofen derivatives. Polyhedron 2012; 42: 175-81.

[304] Santos RLSR, van Eldik R, de Oliveira Silva d. Thermodynamics of axial substitution and kinetics of reactions with amino acids for the paddlewheel complex tetrakis(acetato)chloridodiruthenium(II,III). Inorg Chem 2012; 51: 6615-25.

[305] Santos RLSR, van Eldik R, de Oliveira Silva D. Kinetic and mechanistic studies on reactions of diruthenium(II,III) with biologically relevant reducing agents. Dalton Trans 2013; 42: 16796-805.

[306] Messori M, Marzo T, Sanches RNF, Hanif-Ur Rehman, de Oliveira Silva D, Merlino A. Unusual structural features in the lysozyme derivative of the tetrakis(acetato)chloride-diruthenium(II,III) complex. Angew Chem Int Ed 2014; DOI: 10.1002/anie.201403337 and 10.1002/ange.201403337.

CHAPTER 4

Molecularly-Targeted Therapeutic Strategies for Breast Cancer Focusing on HER2-Targeted Therapy, mTOR Inhibitor and Antiangiogenic Therapy

Teruhiko Fujii[*,1,2], Keisuke Miwa[1], Tomoyuki Ushijima[1], Mototsugu Matsunaga[1], Masaru Fukahori[1], Kotaro Yuge[1], Uhi Toh[3], Nobutaka Iwakuma[3], Ryuji Takahashi[3], Hiroki Takahashi[3], Miki Takenaka[3], Mai Mishima[3], Yoshito Akagi[3], Masayoshi Kage[2,4], Shino Nakagawa[5] and Maki Tanaka[6]

[1]Multidisciplinary Cancer Treatment Center, Kurume University, Kurume, Japan; [2]Center for Innovative Cancer Therapy, Kurume University, Kurume, Japan; [3]Department of Surgery, Kurume University, Kurume, Japan; [4]Department of Pathology, Kurume University, Kurume, Japan; [5]National Hospital Organization Kyushu Medical Cancer, Breast Care Center, Clinical Research Institute, Fukuoka, Japan; and [6]Kurume General Hospital, Kurume, Japan

Abstract: The development of chemotherapy or endocrine therapy has improved survival in patients of breast cancer. At the same time, molecularly-targeted therapy is also an important strategy. Molecularly-targeted therapeutic strategies is an effective for breast cancer, and clinical studies have shown its potential molecular targets which include human epidermal growth factor receptor (HER), mammalian target of rapamycin (mTOR), and vascular endothelial growth factor (VEGF). However, therapy for recurrence or metastatic patients is still palliative, and the possibility of inducing complete cure for breast cancer remains remote. For this reason, many new drugs and therapeutic strategies have been investigated. Here, we reviewed the up-to-date basic and clinical developments in molecularly-targeted therapy for breast cancer, focusing on HER, mTOR, and VEGF.

Keywords: Breast cancer, human epidermal growth factor receptor (HER), mammalian target of rapamycin (mTOR), molecularly-targeted therapy, vascular endothelial growth factor (VEGF).

***Corresponding Author Teruhiko Fujii:** Multidisciplinary Cancer Treatment Center, Kurume University, 67 Asahi-machi Kurume, 830-0011, Japan; Tel: +81-942-31-7748; Fax: +81-942-31-7749; E-mail: tfujii@med.kurume-u.ac.jp

Atta-ur-Rahman / M. Iqbal Choudhary (Eds.)

INTRODUCTION

The development of endocrine therapy or chemotherapy has improved survival in breast cancer patients, and molecularly-targeted cancer therapeutics is also effective approach. Molecularly-targeted therapy using drugs such as trastuzumab is an important strategy for breast cancer, and clinical studies have suggested that human epidermal growth factor receptor (HER), mammalian target of rapamycin (mTOR), and vascular endothelial growth factor (VEGF) are potential targets. Here, we reviewed up-to-date basic research and clinical developments in molecularly-targeted therapy for breast cancer.

HER2-TARGETED THERAPY

HER Family Signaling

The HER family, include human epidermal growth factor receptor 1 (HER1) (ErbB1 and epidermal growth factor receptor: EGFR), HER2 (ErbB2), HER3 (ErbB3), and HER4 (ErbB4), is an important target for anticancer treatments. They also play important roles in the progression of breast cancer. HER1 and HER2 overexpression is observed in 15-30% of breast cancers, and is associated with poor prognosis [1, 2]. HER3 overexpression is reported in 18% of breast cancers, HER3 overexpression is also associated with poor prognosis and it is suggested a route for resistance to drugs targeting HER1 or HER2 [2, 3]. In contrast, HER4 overexpression, seen in 12% of breast cancers, is correlated with differentiation and inhibition of cell growth; thus, it is suggested correlated with favorable prognosis in breast cancer [2, 3].

HERs have an extracellular domain (comprising domains I, II, III, and IV), a transmembrane segment and an intracellular kinase domain [4]. The extracellular domain of HER1, HER3, and HER4 receives extracellular signals from ligands, such as epidermal growth factor (EGF), transforming growth factor-α (TGF-α), amphiregulin, epiregulin, and heregulin; however, no direct ligand has been identified for HER2 [5, 6] (Fig. **1**). Because HER1, HER3, and HER4 is present in a closed conformation in which the dimerization domain cannot bind with anther HER without a ligand [5], the conformational change in the receptor is dependent

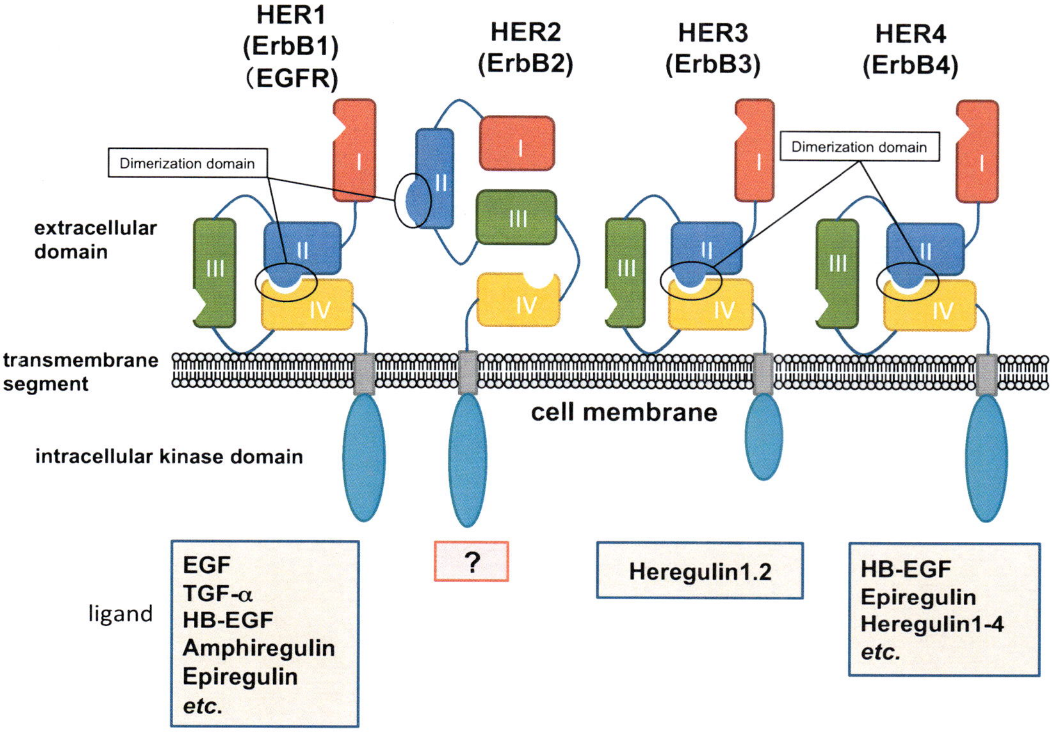

Fig. (1). HERs have an extracellular domain (comprising domains I, II, III, and IV), a transmembrane segment and an intracellular kinase domain [4]. The extracellular domain of HER1, HER3, and HER4 receives extracellular signals from ligands, such as EGF, TGF-α, amphiregulin, epiregulin, and heregulin; however, no direct ligand has been identified for HER2 [5, 6].

upon ligand binding. Domains I and III are concerned in folding the ligand to expose the dimerization domain in the active conformation and this process is needed for dimerization and activity of HER1, HER3, and HER4 [5, 7-9]. On the other hand, the HER2 permanently presents in an open conformation, thus the HER2 is always available for dimerization [5, 6]. The homodimer is formed by the two molecules of the same receptor and the heterodimers is formed by two different HERs (Fig. **2**). HER dimers have different signaling effect and potencies of heterodimers are stronger than homodimers [10]. Notably, HER3 only forms heterodimers and cannot form homodimers because it cannot bind adenosine triphosphate (ATP) and thus lacks intrinsic kinase activity. In particular, the HER2 and HER3 heterodimer has the strongest potential, it is suggested that this heterodimer is important in breast cancer proliferation and progression. Ligand

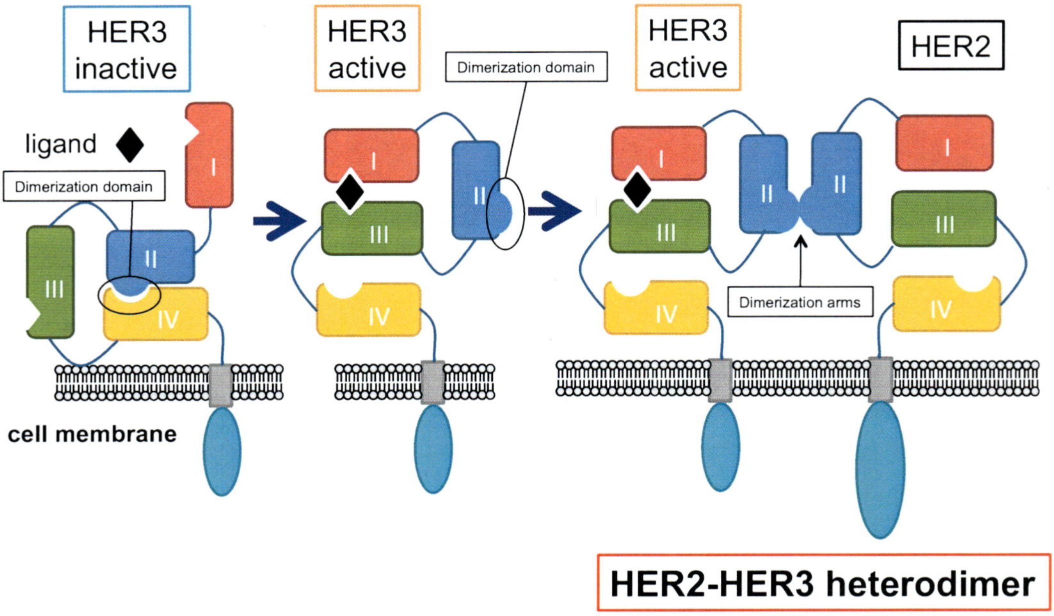

Fig. (2). Because HER1, HER3, and HER4 is present in a closed conformation in which the dimerization domain cannot bind with anther HER without a ligand [5], the conformational change in the receptor is dependent upon ligand binding. Domains I and III are concerned in folding the ligand to expose the dimerization domain in the active conformation and this process is needed for dimerization and activity of HER1, HER3, and HER4 [5, 7-9]. On the other hand, the HER2 permanently presents in an open conformation, thus the HER2 is always available for dimerization [5, 6]. Fig. (**2**) shows the heterodimeriztion developed by HER2 and HER3.

binding allows to form dimerization and the tyrosine kinase is autophosphorylated, thereby activating mitogen-activated protein kinase (MAPK) signaling and phosphoinositide 3-kinase (PI3K)/protein kinase B (Akt) signaling. Interestingly, HER2 homodimers predominantly activate the MAPK pathway but not the PI3K/Akt pathway [11]. In contrast, a significant role for the HER2-HER3 heterodimer interaction in promoting breast cancer tumorigenesis involves the PI3K/Akt pathway [12]. These dimerizations produce the cell growth, angiogenesis, migration and adhesion [1, 13-16].

Therapies Targeting the HER Family

Trastuzumab

Trastuzumab is a humanized monoclonal antibody that binds directly to domain IV of HER2 [17], suppressing HER2 signaling activity and marking tumor cells for further immunological response *via* antibody-dependent cellular cytotoxicity (ADCC) [18]. Trastuzumab is key drugs in the treatment strategy for HER2-positive breast cancer in metastatic setting, adjuvant, and neoadjuvant settings.

Effects of Trastuzumab in Metastatic Breast Cancer (MBC) Setting

The systemic therapy of metastatic breast cancer (MBC) or recurrence disease improves survival, however, it cannot cure. Thus, treatments should be smallest toxicity [19]. The efficacy and safety of trastuzumab monotherapy have been investigated in several phase II clinical studies for MBC as first-/second line treatment. In 1999, Baselga *et al.,* reported a phase II study which assessed the effect and toxicity of weekly trastuzumab monotherapy in HER2-positive MBC [20]. Most of the patients in that study had previously treated. Toxicity was minimal, and overall response rate (ORR) was 11.6%. From this study, trastuzumab has an acceptable tolerability and effective in pretreated patients with HER2-positive MBC [20]. Cobleigh *et al.,* also conducted a phase II study in 1999 [21]. In that trial, effect and tolerability of weekly trastuzumab monotherapy were evaluated in pretreated HER2-overexpressing MBC. Response rate (RR) was 15% and the median duration of survival was 13 months. The most common toxicity was cardiac dysfunction that observed in 4.7%. A study of first-line weekly trastuzumab monotherapy for HER2-overexpressing MBC was conducted in 2002 [22]. In 111 evaluable patients with HER2 (3+) overexpression by immunohistochemistry (IHC), RR was 35% and the clinical benefit rate (CBR) was 48%. Trastuzumab monotherapy as a first-line treatment was effective and has as acceptable tolerability for MBC. Furthermore, a study of first-line trastuzumab triweekly monotherapy (administered once every 3 weeks) for HER2-overexpressing MBC were reported in 2005 [23]. The ORR was 19%, CBR was 33%, and time to progression (TTP) was 3.4 months. Treating higher doses and administered once every 3 weeks did not change the effect and toxicity of trastuzumab and triweekly trastuzumab was found likely to represent a convenient alternative to weekly treatment in HER2-overexpressing MBC. Thus, because the RR of trastuzumab as monotherapy is 11-35% and it is well tolerated, trastuzumab monotherapy as first/second-line is effective for HER2-positive MBC (Table **1**). However, trastuzumab monotherapy should be indicated only for patients with no acute progression and for those with asymptomatic single bone metastasis or asymptomatic localization to the soft tissues. If patients have associated symptomatic visceral metastasis, they should receive a combination of chemotherapy and trastuzumab treatment.

Several of the phase II and III studies have demonstrated additive or synergistic efficacy in combination therapy of trastuzumab with chemotherapeutic agents. Slamon *et al.*, reported a phase III study of receiving chemotherapy with or without trastuzumab. Patients who had not pretreated with an anthracycline were administered with doxorubicin plus cyclophosphamide (AC) or epirubicin plus cyclophosphamide (EC) alone or in combination with trastuzumab. Patients who had pretreated with anthracycline were administered with paclitaxel monotherapy or in combination with trastuzumab [24]. The combination therapy of chemotherapy with trastuzumab resulted in an increased TTP (7.4 *vs* 4.6 months; $P < 0.001$), a higher ORR (50% *vs* 32%, $P < 0.001$), and longer overall survival (OS) (25.1 *vs* 20.3 months; $P = 0.01$). Combination of anthracycline and trastuzumab improved the TTP (7.8 *vs* 6.1 months; $P < 0.001$) and ORR (56% *vs* 42%, $P = 0.02$). Combination of paclitaxel and trastuzumab also improved the TTP (median, 6.9 *vs* 3.0 months; $P < 0.001$) and ORR (41% *vs* 17%, $P < 0.001$). However, trastuzumab was demonstrated with severe cardiotoxicity in 27% patients of anthracycline plus trastuzumab group compared with 13% of the paclitaxel plus trastuzumab group. From these data, the National Comprehensive Cancer Network (NCCN) guidelines point out that the 27% of cardiotoxicity in the combination of trastuzumab and anthracycline is too high; thus, this combination therapy should not use without a clinical study [19]. M77001 is comparing the effect and toxicity of trastuzumab plus docetaxel with docetaxel monotherapy in HER2-overexpressing MBC as a first-line treatment. Trastuzumab plus docetaxel was statistically superior to docetaxel monotherapy. ORR was 61% *vs* 34% ($P = 0.0002$), TTP was 11.7 *vs* 6.1 months ($P = 0.0001$), and OS was 31.2 *vs* 22.7 months ($P = 0.0325$), respectively [25]. Neutropenia was more commonly seen with trastuzumab plus docetaxel than with docetaxel alone, and symptomatic heart failure was seen in 1% of the combination group. These two trials indicate that combination treatment of taxane with trastuzumab is an effective treatment for MBC with few adverse events.

Trastuzumab with a taxane was also tested with or without carboplatin. Basic studies in HER2-positive breast cancer cell lines associated synergistic effects between trastuzumab plus carboplatin, trastuzumab plus docetaxel, and combination of trastuzumab plus docetaxel plus carboplatin [26-29]. Based on these data, the combination therapy of caboplatin with taxane and trastuzumab may be considered rational. The phase II clinical trials of the combination of trastuzumab with carboplatin or with carboplatin plus taxane for pretreated and refractory HER2-positive MBC showed significant clinical activity [30]. Robert *et al.*, conducted a phase III clinical study to evaluate the effect and toxicity of combination therapy of trastuzumab with paclitaxel with or without carboplatin as first-line treatment for HER2-positive MBC [31]. ORR was 52% for trastuzumab and paclitaxel with carboplatin (TPC) *vs* 36% for trastuzumab and paclitaxel (TP) (P = 0.04). Progression-free survival (PFS) was 10.7 months for TPC and 7.1 months for TP (hazard ratio [HR] 0.66, P = 0.03). Both regimens had an acceptable tolerability. The BCIRG 007 study was a phase III study comparing the efficacy of trastuzumab plus carboplatin (area under the serum concentration-time curve 6) and docetaxel (75 mg/m^2) (TCH) with trastuzumab plus docetaxel (100 mg/m^2) (TH) in HER2-positive MBC patients [32]. There was no statistical difference between TCH and TH in TTP (10.4 and 11.1months, HR 0.914, P = 0.57), RR (72% for both groups), or OS (37.4 and 37.1 months, HR 1.015, P = 0.99). The trial do not show improved efficacy with TCH group as compared with TH group. It was concluded that because the dose of docetaxel was higher in the TH group than that in the TCH group (100 *vs* 75 mg/m^2), the increased dose of docetaxel in the TH group should have abrogated the effect of carboplatin in the TCH group [32]. As both groups in this trial were effective, both TH and TCH combination therapy are acceptable options for HER2-positive MBC.

Table 1. Efficacy Outcomes from Clinical Trials of Trasuzumab Monotherapy in MBC Setting

Investigator	Phase	Setting	Regimen	N	Results	Refs.
Baselga *et al.*	II	Pretreated	T	46	ORR: 11.6%	[20]
Cobleigh *et al.*	II	Pretreated	T	222	RR: 15%, OS: 13M	[21]
Vogel *et al.*	II	First-line	T	114	RR HER2 IHC (3+): 35%, IHC(2+): 0% HER2 FISH (+): 34%, (-): 7%	[22]
Baselga *et al.*	II	First-line	T	105	ORR: 19%, CBR: 33%, TTP: 3.4M	[23]

T: trastuzumab; ORR: overall response rate; RR: response rate; OS: overall survival; IHC: immunohistochemistry; FISH: fluorescence *in situ* hybridization; CBR: clinical benefit rate; TTP: time-to-progression.

Furthermore, trastuzumab was evaluated in combination with vinorelbine. Vinorelbine is a chemotherapeutic vinca alkaloid agent that has been reported the synergistic effect with trastuzumab in basic studies [28]. The Trastuzumab and Vinorelbine or Taxane (TRAVIOTA) trial was evaluated the efficacy and safety of trastuzumab with vinorelbine or taxane combination treatment [33]. There was no statistical difference between trastuzumab with vinorelbine and trastuzumab with taxane in RR (51% *vs* 40%, P = 0.37) and TTP (8.5 *vs* 6.0 months, P = 0.09), and these two regimens had comparable rates of response and safety. The Herceptin plus Navelbine or Taxotere (HERNATA) trial was a phase III trial evaluating the efficacy and safety of first-line docetaxel plus trastuzumab or vinorelbine plus trastuzumab for HER2-positive advanced breast cancer (ABC) or MBC [34]. The TTP for docetaxel plus trastuzumab *vs* that for vinorelbine plus trastuzumab was 12.4 *vs* 15.3 months (HR = 0.94, P = 0.67), OS was 35.7 *vs* 38.8 months (HR 1.01, P = 0.98), and ORR was 59.3% in each arm; however, many patients in the docetaxel group could not continue treatment cause by adverse events (P < 0.001). It was concluded that the efficacy was not different between these two regimens, although the vinorelbine combination with trastuzumab had statistically fewer toxicities and should be acceptable first-line options for HER2-positive ABC or MBC.

Capecitabine is an orally-administered, enzymatically activated to fluorouracil (5-FU) in the tumor [35] and its combination with trastuzumab has also been investigated for MBC. Capecitabine has been reported the synergistic interaction with trastuzumab in basic studies [36]. Schaller *et al.,* reported the effect and tolerability of trastuzumab and capecitabine in a phase II trial of previously treated MBC [37]. In that study, ORR, PFS and OS were found to be 45%, 6.7 months, and 28 months, respectively. The Japan Breast Cancer Research Network (JBCRN) 00 trial was a phase II trial of combination of trastuzumab with capecitabine for HER2-positive MBC [38]. The RR was 65.0% in patients administered with first-line combination treatment of trastuzumab and capecitabine. TTP and OS were longer in first-line combination treatment of trastuzumab and capecitabine than in second- or third-line treatment (TTP, 280 *vs* 130 days, P < 0.05; OS, 780 *vs* 480 days, P < 0.05). In these two trials, treatment-related adverse events were hand-foot syndrome (HFS), nausea, diarrhea, motor dysfunction, stomatitis, fatigue, and vomiting. Most were mild adverse events, and much of the toxicity was manageable. As seen from the results presented above, clinical studies have reported that the combination of trastuzumab with paclitaxel alone or along with carboplatin, docetaxel, vinorelbine, and capecitabine is beneficial; thus, the NCCN guidelines have listed trastuzumab plus these agents as first-line regimens for HER2 overexpressed systemic disease [19].

Trastuzumab has also been tried in combination with gemcitabine or eribulin for MBC. Yardley *et al.,* evaluated the efficacy and safety of the trastuzumab and gemcitabine combination in HER2-positive MBC as first-/second-line therapy [39]. Gemcitabine is a cytidine analog that inhibits deoxyribonucleic acid (DNA) synthesis [40]. In that study, the ORR, PFS, and OS were 30%, 4 months, and 21 months. It was concluded that the combination therapy of trastuzumab with gemcitabine is clinically active, however, it seems less efficacy than trastuzumab in combination with vinorelbine or taxane [40]. As the role of trastuzumab and gemcitabine combination in patients pretreated with a trastuzumab for HER2-positive MBC was not clear by that trial, further studies of combination of gemcitabine and trastuzumab are needed to establish this combination therapy for MBC. Recently, the results of a phase II study designed to evaluate the toxicity and clinical activity of eribulin in first-line combination therapy with trastuzumab for HER2-overexpressing MBC were reported at the 36th San Antonio Breast Cancer Symposium (SABCS, 2013) [41]. Eribulin is a microtubule inhibitor used for the therapy of patients with MBC who have pretreated at least two chemotherapeutic agents. That study enrolled 52 patients, and the primary endpoint of ORR and secondary endpoint of PFS were 67% and 11.5 months, respectively. Eribulin in combination with trastuzumab appeared to have activity with acceptable toxicity. It is suggested that eribulin will be a good partner with trastuzumab for the treatment of MBC, but further exploration of this combination is warranted. Efficacy outcomes of trasuzumab with chemotherapy in MBC are summarized in Table **2**.

Effects of Trastuzumab in Adjuvant Setting

Several large clinical trials have been performed to evaluate the effect of trastuzumab in the adjuvant setting, and these trials have shown encouraging results. The similar study design of the National Surgical Adjuvant Breast and Bowel Project (NSABP) B-31 and the North Central Cancer Treatment Group (NCCTG) trial N9831 led to the combined analysis of the two studies [42]. These studies included treatment with the agents of AC followed by paclitaxel and 1 year with or without trastuzumab treatment with surgically removed HER2-overexpressing breast cancer. The primary endpoint was disease-free survival (DFS), which was significantly improved in the trastuzumab arm as compared with the control arm (85.3% *vs* 67.1%, HR 0.48, $P < 0.0001$). OS was also improved in the trastuzumab arm as compared with the control arm (91.4% *vs* 86.6%, HR 0.67, $P < 0.015$). The incidence of cardiotoxicity in the trastuzumab arm was 4.1% in trial B-31 and 2.9% in trial N9831. It was suggested that combination therapy of trastuzumab with paclitaxel after AC increases outcomes among postoperative HER2-overexpressing breast cancer. The Herceptin Adjuvant (HERA) trial is multicenter, randomized, phase III study evaluating the effect of trastuzumab for 1 and 2 years in the adjuvant setting with HER2-overexpressing early-stage breast cancer [43]. The 4-year DFS significantly improved in trastuzumab group as compared with that in the observation group (78.6% *vs* 72.2%, HR 0.76, $P < 0.0001$). However, OS did not improve (89.3% *vs* 87.7%, HR 0.85, $P = 0.11$). Higher incidences of severe and fatal toxicity were reported in patients on trastuzumab than in the observation group. Treatment with trastuzumab in adjuvant setting was demonstrated with significant activity at the 4-year median follow-up. Trastuzumab was an active in the adjuvant therapy of HER2-overexpressing breast cancer, although combined therapy with anthracycline-containing chemothrapy was associated with cardiotoxicity. The Breast Cancer International Research Group (BCIRG) 006 trial evaluated the effect and toxicity of a new non-anthracycline regimen with trastuzumab [44]. In that trial, early-stage breast cancer patients were assigned to treat AC followed by docetaxel (AC-T), the same treatment with trastuzumab (AC-T plus trastuzumab), or docetaxel and carboplatin with trastuzumab (TCH). The primary endpoint was DFS. DFS rates at 5 years were 75% in AC-T group, 84% in AC-T plus trastuzumab group (HR 0.64, $P < 0.001$; compared with AC-T), and 81% in TCH group (HR 0.75, $P = 0.04$; compared with AC-T). OS rates were 87%, 92% (HR 0.63, $P < 0.001$; compared with AC-T), and 91% (HR 0.77, $P = 0.04$; compared

Table 2. Efficacy Outcomes from Clinical Trials of Trasuzumab+Chemothrapy in MBC Setting

Investigator (Trial)	Phase	Setting	Regimen	N	Results	Refs.
Slamon *et al.*	III	First-line	T+PTX (triweekly) or T+A(E)C *vs* PTX (triweekly) or A(E)C	235 234	TTP: 7.4 *vs* 4.6M (P<0.001) ORR: 50 *vs* 32% (P<0.001) OS: 25.1 *vs* 20.3% (P = 0.01)	[24]
Marty *et al.* (M77001)	II	First-line	T+DTX *vs* DTX	92 94	ORR: 61 *vs* 34% (P = 0.0002) TTP: 11.7 *vs* 6.1M (P = 0.0001) OS: 31.2 *vs* 22.7M (P = 0.0325)	[25]
Robert *et al.*	III	First-line	T+PTX+carboplatin *vs* T+PTX	98 98	ORR: 52 *vs* 36% (P = 0.04) PFS: 10.7 *vs* 7.1M (HR 0.66, P = 0.03) OS: 35.7 *vs* 32.2M (HR 0.90, P = 0.76)	[31]
Valero *et al.* (BCIRG 007)	III	First-line	T+DTX(75)+carboplatin *vs* T+DTX(100)	131 131	RR: 72 *vs* 72% (P = 0.97) TTP: 10.4 *vs* 11.1M (HR 0.914, P = 0.57) OS: 37.4 *vs* 37.1M (HR 1.015, P = 0.99)	[32]
Burstein *et al.* (TRAVIOTA)	III	First-line	T+vinorelbine *vs* T+Taxane	41 40	RR: 51 *vs* 40% (P = 0.37) TTP: 8.5 *vs* 6.0M (P = 0.09)	[33]
Anderson *et al.* (HERNATA)	III	First-line	T+DTX *vs* T+vinorelbine	143 141	ORR: 59.3 *vs* 59.3% (P = 1.00) TTP: 12.4 *vs* 15.3M (HR 0.94, P = 0.67) OS: 35.7 *vs* 38.8M (HR 1.01, P = 0.98)	[34]
Schaller *et al.*	II	Pretreated	T+capecitabine	27	ORR: 45%, PFS: 6.7M, OS: 28M	[37]
Yamamoto *et al.* (JBCRN 00)	II	Pretreated	T+capecitabine	56	RR first line: 65.0%, senond or third line: 41.7% TTP first line: 280day, senond or third line: 130day OS first line: 780day, senond or third line: 480day	[38]
Yardley *et al.*	II	First or second-line	T+gemcitabine	41	ORR: 30%, PFS: 4M, OS: 21M	[39]
Wilks *et al.*	II	First-line	T+eribulin	52	ORR: 67%, PFS: 11.5M	[41]

T: trastuzumab; PTX: paclitaxel; AC: doxorubicin + cyclophosphamide; E: epirubicin; TTP: time-to-progression.; RR: response rate; OS: overall survival; ORR: overall response rate; PFS: progression-free survival; DTX: docetaxel.

with AC-T), respectively. No statistical differences in efficacy were found between the two trastuzumab groups, whereas both were superior to AC-T. As the risk-benefit ratio improved the non-anthracycline TCH regimen over AC-T plus trastuzumab, given its same efficacy and lower incidence of cardiac dysfunction, TCH will be considered the regimen of choice for patients with heart disease. The Finland Herceptin (FinHer) trial is a phase III study for axillary node positive or node negative with high risk breast cancer [45]. In that trial, patients received vinorelbine or docetaxel, followed by fluorouracil, epirubicin, and cyclophosphamide (FEC). HER2-overexpressed breast cancer patients were further treat or not to treat with trastuzumab, and the primary endpoint was DFS. The 3-year DFS was better in the trastuzumab treated arm than in trastuzumab control arm (89.3% *vs* 77.6%, HR 0.42, P = 0.01); however, there was no significant difference in OS between the two arms (96.3% *vs* 89.7%, HR 0.41, P = 0.07). The trial led to the conclusion that trastuzumab treated with vinorelbine or docetaxel is active in HER2-overexpressing breast cancer [45]. These clinical data have suggested that adjuvant trastuzumab therapy brings a significant benefit to early-stage breast cancer patients. Efficacy outcomes from clinical studies of trasuzumab in adjuvant setting are summarized in Table **3**. From these data, the NCCN guidelines and the St. Gallen consensus guidelines recommend that adjuvant trastuzumab treatment should be considered for node positive and node negative with high-risk early-stage HER2-overexpressing breast cancer [19, 46].

Table 3. Efficacy Outcomes from Clinical Trials of Trasuzumab in Adjuvant Setting

Investigator (Trial)	Phase	Regimen	N	Results	Refs.
Romond *et al.* (NSABP B-31 + NCCTG N9831)	III	surg→AC→PTX+T *vs* surg→AC→PTX	1672 1679	DFS: 85.3 *vs* 67.1% (HR 0.48, *P*<0.0001) OS: 91.4 *vs* 86.6% (HR 0.67, *P*<0.015)	[42]
Gianni *et al.* (HERA)	III	surg, chemo±rad→T (12M) *vs* surg, chemo±rad→observation	1703 1698	DFS: 78.6 *vs* 72.2% (HR 0.76, *P*<0.0001) OS: 89.3 *vs* 87.7% (HR 0.85, *P* = 0.11)	[43]
Slamon *et al.* (BCIRG 006)	III	surg→AC→DTX+T→T *vs* surg→DTX+carboplatin+T→T *vs* surg→AC→DTX	1073 1075 1073	DFS: 84 (HR 0.64, *P*<0.001) *vs* 81 (HR 0.75, *P* = 0.04) *vs* 75% OS: 92 (HR 0.63, *P*<0.001) *vs* 91% (HR 0.77, *P* = 0.04) *vs* 87%	[44]
Joensuu *et al.* (FinHer)	III	surg→DTX or V+T→FEC *vs* surg→DTX or V→FEC	116 116	DFS: 89.3 *vs* 77.6% (HR 0.42, *P* = 0.01) OS: 96.3 *vs* 89.7 % (HR 0.41 *P* = 0.07)	[45]

surg: surgery; AC: doxorubicin + cyclophosphamide; PTX: paclitaxel; chemo: chemotherapy; rad: radiation; FEC: fluorouracil + epirubicin + cyclophosphamide; DFS: disease-free survival; OS: overall survival; HR: hazard ratio; OS: overall survival; T: trastuzumab; DTX: docetaxel; V: vinorelbine.

The effect of adjuvant trastuzumab treatment for HER2-overexpressing small size breast cancer (less than 10 mm) is not clear. Gonzalez-Angulo *et al.,* demonstrated that HER2-overexpressing small size breast cancer patients had high-risk of recurrence than HER2-negative small size breast cancer patients. These results support that patients with HER2-overexpressing T1abN0M0 breast cancer have a high-risk of recurrence and should be considered for trastuzumab adjuvant treatment [47]. McArthur *et al.,* evaluated retrospectively the efficacy of adjuvant trastuzumab in patients with small tumor, node negative, HER2-overexpressing breast cancer. They suggested that patients even with small size HER2-overexpressing breast cancers may receive benefit from adjuvant trastuzumab treatment [48]. The NCCN guidelines designate the treatment of trastuzumab with chemotherapy as a category 1 recommendation in HER2-overexpressing breast cancer of more than 1 cm, and the NCCN guidelines also include a recommendation for trastuzumab adjuvant therapy in patients with node negative breast cancer that are 0.6 to 1.0 cm [19].

In the four initial clinical trials mentioned above [42-44], comparing 1 year duration of trastuzumab treated as adjuvant therapy *vs* observation showed a benefit for patients with HER2-overexpressing early-stage breast cancer. From those data, the US Food and Drug Administration (FDA) and the European Medicines Agency (EMA) approved the treatment of 1 year of trastuzumab in adjuvant therapy. However, the optimum duration of trastuzumab treatment is unclear. Recently, two sets of evidence regarding the duration of trastuzumab for adjuvant therapy have been reported. Goldhirsch *et al.,* compared 1 years of trastuzumab adjuvant therapy with 2 year therapy in the HERA trial [49]. Although there was no statistical difference in DFS between the 2-year treatment arm and the 1-year treatment arm (76% *vs* 75.8%, HR 0.99, P = 0.86), severe toxicities and cardiac dysfunction were observed more frequently in the 2-year arm than in the 1-year arm (grade 3-4 adverse events, 20.4% *vs* 16.3%; cardiac dysfunction, 7.2% *vs* 4.1%). Thus, 1 year of trastuzumab adjuvant treatment is more useful than 2 years of treatment for HER2-overexpressing early-stage breast cancer patients [49]. Another trial to examine duration of trastuzumab for adjuvant therapy is the Protocol for Herceptin as Adjuvant therapy with Reduced Exposure (PHARE) trial, which is an open-label, randomized phase III non-inferiority study of 6 months *vs* the 1 year of trastuzumab adjuvant therapy for HER2-positive early-stage breast cancer patients [50]. After 3-5 years follow-up, this trial could not show that 6 months of trastuzumab adjuvant therapy was non-inferior to 1 year of trastuzumab. From these two sets of data, 1 year of trastuzumab adjuvant therapy should be the optimum duration for HER2-positive early-stage breast cancer. As no clinical trials have been conducted to examine monotherapy with trastuzumab as an adjuvant treatment without concurrent or preceding chemotherapy, the efficacy of trastuzumab monotherapy for adjuvant therapy is not clear. The RESPECT (N-SAS BC07) trial is a multi-institutional prospective randomized controlled trial, which is being conducted to investigate the benefit of trastuzumab monotherapy compared with a combination therapy of trastuzumab and chemotherapy in women over 70 years old with HER2-overexpressing breast cancer [51]. This trial is ongoing, and the result may suggest the efficacy of trastuzumab monotherapy for adjuvant therapy.

Effects of Trastuzumab in Neoadjuvant Setting

Although neoadjuvant therapy with breast cancer increases incidences of operability on locally advanced tumor and rates of breast-conserving surgery, clinical studies of neoadjuvant therapy have not demonstrate an increase in DFS or OS compared with same treatment performed after breast operation [52]. Because patients with a pathological complete response (pCR) after trastuzumab neoadjuvant therapy in combination with chemotherapy followed by trastuzumab have a clinical activity [53], pCR has been used as a surrogate marker for efficacy in patients treated with neoadjuvant therapy in clinical trials. The widely used definition of pCR is no residual invasive cancer in the breast and axillary lymph nodes. In this part, we review the literature for HER2-targeted therapy in neoadjuvant clinical studies. A total of 7 clinical studies have conducted the combination of trastuzumab with neoadjuvant chemotherapeutic agents.

The MDACC study was a randomized with patients assigned to receive anthracycline and taxanes with or without trastuzumab in neoadjuvant setting [54]. The pCR rate in the combination group was 65% and chemotherapy alone group was 26%. There were no recurrences in the patients randomized to chemotherapy with trastuzumab, and the DFS at 1 and 3 years was 100% ($P = 0.04$) [55]. ABCSG-24 was a phase III trial and 90 patients were randomized to administer epirubicin plus docetaxel or epirubicin plus docetaxel plus capecitabine with or without trastuzumab in HER2-overexpressing breast cancer [56]. pCR rate was improved in the trastuzumab-added arm (40% *vs* 26.7%). The Neoadjuvant Herceptin (NOAH) trial evaluated the combination of trastuzumab with anthracycline and taxane with HER2-positive ABC in a neoadjuvant treatment [57]. The primary endpoint was 3-year event-free survival (EFS), which was significantly increased in the investigational arm (71% with trastuzumab *vs* 56% without trastuzumab, P = 0.013). The secondary endpoint was pCR which was also increased in the investigational arm (38% *vs* 19%, P = 0.001). Addition of trastuzumab was well tolerated, with no severe short-term cardiac failure. The Germany Breast Group/Gynecologic Oncology Study Group trial (the GeparQuattro trial) was a 3-arm phase III trial that evaluated how combination of trastuzumab with chemotherapy affected pCR rate of HER2-overexpressing breast cancer. Patients were administered with EC followed by docetaxel with or without trastuzumab and capecitabine preoperatively [58]. The pCR rate was 31.7% for treated with neoadjuvant trastuzumab plus chemotherapy and 15.7% for treated with chemotherapy alone. Pierga *et al.,* conducted a randomized phase II trial in which HER2-overexpressing breast cancer patients were randomized to administer EC followed by docetaxel with or without trastuzumab in neoadjuvant setting [59]. The pCR rate was improved in the chemotherapy with trastuzumab group (25.5% *vs* 19%), and the chemotherapy with trastuzumab was well tolerated. The Korean Cancer Study Group reported BR 07-01 study, which was investigated to assess the effect and toxicity of preoperative paclitaxel, gemcitabine, and trastuzumab in combination for HER2-overexpressing breast cancer [60]. The pCR rate was 58.5%, and adverse events were mild with few incidences of febrile neutropenia. The phase III American College of Surgeons' Oncology Group (ACOSOG) Z1041 study, reported at the 2013 Annual Meeting of the American Society of Clinical Oncology (ASCO), compared the pCR rate in Arm 1 (FEC followed by paclitaxel with trastuzumab) or Arm 2 (paclitaxel plus trastuzumab followed by FEC plus trastuzumab) in neoadjuvant setting [61]. The pCR rate was not found to differ between the two regimens (Arm 1 *vs* Arm 2 = 50.7% *vs* 48.6%) and it was concluded that high pCR rate was seen in combination of trastuzumab with anthracyclines and taxanes. Efficacy outcomes from clinical trials of trasuzumab in neoadjuvant setting are summarized in Table **4**. Overall, these studies showed an improvement in pCR rate with combination of trastuzumab with chemotherapy (pCR rate, 25.5-65%), compared to chemotherapy alone (pCR, 15.7-26.7%). However, no difference was seen

Table 4. Efficacy Outcomes from Clinical Trials of Trasuzumab in Neoadjuvant Setting

Investigator (Trial)	Phase	Regimen	N	Results	Refs.
Buzdar *et al.* (MDACC Neoadjuvant Trial)	III	T+PTX→T+FEC →surg *vs* PTX →FEC→surg	23 19	pCR: 65 *vs* 26 % (*P* = 0.016) DFS: 100 *vs* 85.3% (*P* = 0.041)	[54, 55]
Steger *et al.* (ABCSG-24)	III	T+E+DTX±C→surg *vs* E+DTX±C→surg	42 47	pCR: 40 *vs* 26.7%	[56]
Gianni *et al.* (NOAH)	III	T+A+PTX→T+PTX→T+CMF→surg→T *vs* A+PTX→PTX→CMF→surg	117 118	pCR: 38 *vs* 19% (*P* = 0.001) ORR: 87 *vs* 74% (*P* = 0.009) EFS: 71 *vs* 56% (HR 0.59, *P* = 0.013) OS: 87 *vs* 79% (HR 0.62, *P* = 0.114)	[57]
Untch *et al.* (GeparQuattro study)	III	T+(EC→DTX→C or EC→DTX+C or EC→ DTX) →surg→T *vs* EC→DTX→C or EC→DTX+C or EC→DTX →surg	445 1050	pCR: 31.7 *vs* 15.7% (*P* = 0.001)	[58]
Pierga *et al.*	II	EC→DTX+T→surg *vs* EC→DTX→surg	62 58	pCR: 25.5 *vs* 19%	[59]
Im *et al.* (BR 07-01)	II	T+PTX+gemcitabine→surg	53	pCR: 58.5%	[60]
Buzdar *et al.* (ACOSOG Z1041)	III	FEC→T+PTX→surg *vs* T+PTX→T+FEC→surg	138 142	pCR: 50.7 *vs* 48.6%	[61]

T: trastuzumab; PTX: paclitaxel; FEC: fluorouracil + epirubicin + cyclophosphamide; surg: surgery; E: epirubicin; DTX: docetaxel; C: capecitabine; A: anthracycline; CMF: cyclophosphamide + methotrexate + fluorouracil; EC: epirubicin + cyclophosphamide; pCR: pathological complete response; DFS: disease-free survival; ORR: overall response rate; EFS: event-free survival; HR: hazard ratio; OS: overall survival.

between trastuzumab plus chemotherapy and chemotherapy alone in terms of breast conserving surgery [62]. In the toxicity profile, the addition of trastuzumab did not improve the incidence of cardiac or non-cardiac adverse events. Concurrent treatment of trastuzumab and anthracyclines has been performed in several randomized studies, such as MDACC, NOAH, and GeparQuattro trials, with no increase in cardiac dysfunction. Since the influence of the cardiac dysfunction after long-term progress observation is unknown in neoadjuvant setting, concurrent treatment of anthracyclines and trastuzumab should be prudent. Furthermore, since there is no high-level evidence with respect to trastuzumab without chemotherapy in neoadjuvant settings, treatment with trastuzumab alone should not be performed unless as a clinical trial.

Recently, Schwartzberg *et al.,* reported a phase I/II trial of neoadjuvant carboplatin, eribulin, and trastuzumab (ECH) for operable HER2-overexpressing breast cancer at the ASCO 2013 Annual Meeting [63]. That study was designed to determine the maximum tolerated dose (MTD) of eribulin in addition with carboplatin and trastuzumab (phase I) and to determine the effect and toxicity of the ECH regimen (phase II) given as neoadjuvant therapy with stage IIA to IIIB breast cancer patients. Phase I had a planned enrollment of 12 patients, and phase II planned 44 additional patients. The primary endpoint is efficacy as measured by clinical response prior to surgery. This trial is currently ongoing [64].

Trastuzumab-DM1 (T-DM1)

Trastuzumab-DM1 (T-DM1) is an antibody-drug conjugate (ADC) which combines the trastuzumab and the potent antimicrotubule drug fungal toxin DM1 (derivative of maytansine1) using a highly stable linker [65, 66]. DM1 has *in vitro* cytotoxicity 10-200 times that of taxanes or vinca alkaloids [65, 67]. After T-DM1 binds to HER2, HER2 are internalized with T-DM1 by endocytosis, and intracellular release of DM1, then DM1 suppresses the cancer cells. Thus, T-DM1 selectively kills HER2-positive breast cancer cells, decreasing toxicity to non-tumoral tissues. Preclinical studies showed T-DM1 to strongly inhibit proliferation of HER2-overexpressing breast cancer cell lines, evoking ADCC similar to that of trastuzumab. Xenograft tumors in Severe Combined Immunodeficient (SCID) mice were significantly inhibited by T-DM1. T-DM1 was active even with cross-resistance to trastuzumab and tyrosine kinase inhibitor such as lapatinib [68].

Effects of T-DM1 in MBC Setting

In a phase I trial, T-DM1 was demonstrated with reversible mild toxicity and substantial clinical efficacy (RR was 44%) in a heavily previous treated patients [69]. In a phase II study, T-DM1 monotherapy was shown to have an acceptable tolerability with no dose-limiting cardiac dysfunction, with an ORR of 25.9%, and a PFS of 4.6 months [70]. Another phase II trial was investigated to determine whether T-DM1 was active in HER2-overexpressing MBC patients who had pretreated standard anti-HER2 therapies [71]. ORR was 34.5%, CBR was 48.2%, and PFS was 6.9 months with mild adverse events. These data suggest that T-DM1 monotherapy is active and has promising efficacy in heavily pretreated HER2-overexpressing MBC patients. The TDM4450g study was a phase II study to evaluate T-DM1 against trastuzumab with docetaxel (HT) as first-line treatment for HER2-overexpressing MBC [72]. Primary endpoints were PFS and safety. Although the ORR and OS were similar for T-DM1 and trastuzumab plus docetaxel (ORR: 64.2% *vs* 58.0%; HR of death for T-DM1 relative to HT was 1.06, P = 0.889), PFS was statistical increased in T-DM1 group (14.2 *vs* 9.2 months, HR 0.594, P = 0.0353). T-DM1 had an acceptable tolerability *vs* HT, with a fewer severe toxicity (46.4% *vs* 90.9%). From these data, T-DM1 for HER2-overexpressing MBC patients as a first line therapy provided a significant activity in PFS, with an accepted tolerability. In the EMILIA study, HER2-overexpressing ABC patients who had been previously treated with taxanes and trastuzumab were assigned to receive either T-DM1 or lapatinib plus capecitabine [73]. The combination treatment of lapatinib with capecitabine is a standard option for patients who have experienced disease progression during previous treatment with trastuzumab, and this combination increases the TTP in patients pretreated with trastuzumab plus an anthracycline or plus a taxanes [74]. The primary endpoints of the EMILIA study were PFS, OS, and toxicity. PFS was 9.6 months with T-DM1 *vs* 6.4 months with lapatinib and capecitabine group (HR 0.65, P < 0.001), and OS was 30.9 months *vs* 25.1 months (HR 0.68, P < 0.001) [73]. Incidence of severe adverse events was higher with lapatinib plus capecitabine group than with T-DM1 (57% *vs* 41%). T-DM1 statistical improved PFS and OS with few adverse events than lapatinib with capecitabine in HER2-overexpressing MBC patients. On the basis of these results, the NCCN guidelines recommend T-DM1 as the preferred option for treatment of HER2-overexpressing MBC patients who have previously treated with trastuzumab-based regimen [19]. Efficacy outcomes of T-DM1 in MBC setting are summarized in Table **5**.

Effects of T-DM1 in Neoadjuvant or Adjuvant Setting

Moreover, T-DM1 is being tested in neoadjuvant or adjuvant settings. NCT01196052 is a phase II trial which will evaluate the toxicity and activity of T-DM1 after the completion of anthracycline-based neoadjuvant or adjuvant chemotherapy in early-stage HER2-overexpressing breast cancer patients. Accrual for this study is complete [75]. The KATHERINE study will assess the activity and toxicity of T-DM1 *vs* trastuzumab as adjuvant therapy with HER2-

Table 5. Efficacy Outcomes of T-DM1 in MBC Setting

Investigator (Trial)	Phase	Setting	Regimen	N	Results	Refs.
Krop *et al.*	I	Pretreated	T-DM1	24	MTD: 3.6mg/Kg, RR: 44%	[69]
Burris *et al.*	II	Pretreated	T-DM1	112	ORR: 25.9%, PFS: 4.6M	[70]
Krop *et al.*	II	Pretreated	T-DM1	110	ORR: 34.5%, CBR: 48.2%, PFS:6.9M	[71]
Hurvitz *et al.* (TDM4450g)	II	First-line	T-DM1 *vs* T+DTX	67 70	PFS 14.2 *vs* 9.2M (HR 0.594, *P* = 0.0353) ORR 64.2 *vs* 58.0%	[72]
Verma *et al.* (EMILIA)	III	Pretreated	T-DM1 *vs* lapatinib+ capecitabine	495 496	PFS 9.6 *vs* 6.4M (HR 0.65, *P*<0.001) OS 30.9 *vs* 25.1M (HR 0.68, *P*<0.001) ORR 43.6 *vs* 30.8% (*P*<0.001)	[73]

T-DM1: trastuzumab-DM1; DTX: docetaxel; MTD: maximum tolerated dose; RR: response rate; ORR: overall response rate; PFS: progression-free survival; CBR: clinical benefit rate; HR: hazard ratio.

overexpressing breast cancer patients who have residual tumor in the breast or axillary lymph nodes after operation. This study is actively in progress [76]. Comparison of T-DM1 *vs* trastuzumab with standard hormone therapy in neoadjuvant setting is also under the investigation [77].

Pertuzumab

Trastuzumab is clinically effective, as mentioned above, but a significant proportion of HER2-overexpressing breast cancer patients either do not respond or eventually become resistant to trastuzumab [22, 24]. Because mitogenic potencies of heterodimers are stronger than homodimers, it is suggested that the ligand-dependent activation of HER1, HER3, or HER4 might be important for trastuzumab resistance [78]. In preclinical studies, trastuzumab inhibited HER2 homodimer-mediated breast cancer cell growth but not heterodimer-mediated one, and this means that ligand-independent HER2 activation is inhibited by trastuzumab [11]. Pertuzumab is a humanized monoclonal antibody that mainly block dimerization of HER2 and HER3, thereby suppressing the intracellular signaling correlated with proliferation and progression [79-81]. Ghosh *et al.,* also reported that pertuzumab inhibited breast cancer cell growth induced by heregulin

[11]. This result suggested that pertuzumab can inhibit ligand-dependent HER2 dimerization and signaling [82].

Effects of Pertuzumab in MBC Setting

Although a phase I clinical study of pertuzumab monotherapy yielded promising results [83], phase II trials have reported pertuzumab monotherapy to have limited effects for HER2-positive MBC patients [84, 85]. Therefore, the combination of pertuzumab with trastuzumab as a dual blockade therapy was investigated. Pertuzumab and trastuzumab bind to different HER2 extracellular domain (trastuzumab binds to domain IV, and pertuzumab binds to the dimerization arm of domain II), and it has been suggested that a combination of the two antibodies might suppress proliferation more active than either antibody alone [80, 86]. Indeed, *in vivo* data from breast cancer xenograft models demonstrated that the combination of trastuzumab and pertuzumab therapy showed a synergistic antitumor activity, which was not achieved by either agent alone [82]. Overall, the different mechanisms of trastuzumab and pertuzumab combination therapy can act in a complementary fashion to supply a stronger blockade of HER2-mediated intracellular signaling than either antibody alone.

To explore the mechanisms of this synergistic effect, a small phase II trial was investigated by Portera *et al.* [87]. In that study, ORR was 18%, however, the trial was prematurely terminated because 54.5% of patients presented with cardiac dysfunction. The same combination of trastuzumab with pertuzumab was also tested in the phase II study with HER2-positive MBC patients [88]. The ORR was 24.2% and the CBR was 50%. The combination therapy was effective and had acceptable tolerability in pretreated with trastuzumab patients. In that large phase II trial, the incidence of cardiac dysfunction was minimal, and it is noteworthy that combination of pertuzumab with trastuzumab did not result in increased cardiac toxicities. To determine whether those therapeutic activities were effect of the combination of pertuzumab with trastuzumab or of pertuzumab monotherapy, a third separate cohort treated with pertuzumab monotherapy was recruited to the BO17929 study [89]. ORR was 3.4% and CBR was 10.3%, during pertuzumab alone. In combination therapy with trastuzumab and pertuzumab, the ORR was 17.6% and CBR was 41.2%. PFS was increase with combination therapy group than with pertuzumab alone group (17.4 *vs* 7.1 weeks). From these results, it was indicated that the combination therapy of pertuzumab with trastuzumab may be more active than either agent alone. According to the NCCN guidelines, for patients with breast cancer progression after trastuzumab treatment without pertuzumab, a line of treatment containing pertuzumab plus trastuzumab with or without a chemotherapy may be considered [19]. From these promising phase II results, a randomized registration phase III clinical study, Clinical Evaluation of Pertuzumab and Trastuzumab (CLEOPATRA) was conducted to evaluate the efficacy and safety of pertuzumab and trastuzumab combination therapy as first-line treatment [90]. In that study, HER2-overexpressing MBC patients were assigned to administer placebo plus trastuzumab plus docetaxel (placebo group) or pertuzumab plus trastuzumab plus docetaxel (pertuzumab group) [90]. The PFS was 12.4 months in the placebo group, as compared with 18.5 months in the pertuzumab group (HR 0.62, $P < 0.001$). OS demonstrated a strong tendency in improvement of pertuzumab group without increase in cardiac toxicity. A confirmatory OS analysis of the CLEOPATRA study was recently presented after a median follow-up of 30 months [91]. In that second interim analysis, the combination of pertuzumab plus trastuzumab plus docetaxel significantly improved OS for HER2-positive MBC patients as compared to trastuzumab and chemotherapy (median OS not reached in the pertuzumab group *vs* 37.6 months in the control group, HR 0.66; $P = 0.0008$). In the pertuzumab group, RR also showed improvement (80.2% *vs* 69.3%, $P = 0.001$), and the toxicities were generally mild. There was no increase in cardiac toxicities. From results of the CLEOPATRA study, the combination of pertuzumab plus trastuzumab plus docetaxel may become the standard first-line therapy for HER2-overexpressing MBC. In addition, clinical studies of pertuzumab plus trastuzumab plus other chemotherapeutic agents are ongoing to test the best partner to pertuzumab plus trastuzumab. One such study is the Pertuzumab Herceptin Evaluation with Xeloda (PHEREXA) phase II study, which assesses the activity and toxicity of a combination of trastuzumab plus capecitabine with or without pertuzumab in HER2-overexpressing MBC patients [92]. Another study is the VELVET trial phase II trial that will evaluate the activity and toxicity of pertuzumab combination with vinorelbine and trastuzumab as first-line therapy for MBC or locally advanced HER2-overexpressing breast cancer patients [93]. Recently, the results of a phase II trial of pertuzumab plus trastuzumab and paclitaxel combination therapy were reported at the 2013 ASCO Annual Meeting. 36 patients were evaluable at 6 months: 29/36 (81%) patients were progression-free (4 had complete response [CR], 14 had partial response [PR], and 11 had stable disease [SD]), and 7 patients showed progression) [94].

T-DM1 and pertuzumab bind to distinct epitopes on HER2 extracellular domain, and have different mechanisms, suggesting that this combination therapy may have stronger complete blockade of HER2-mediated intracellular signaling. A phase Ib/II study of pertuzumab with T-DM1 combination treatment for ABC or MBC has been investigated, in which, PR was observed in 9 of 23 patients [95]. In another phase Ib/II trial, patients received pertuzumab and T-DM1 as first-line therapy or in a relapsed setting (defined as progression on prior HER2-directed therapy for MBC) [96]. In that study, ORR was 41% in the first-line arm and 42% in the relapsed arm. Because those initially phase Ib/II study results reported well tolerated and promising effect in HER2-positive MBC patients, the randomized, 3-arm, phase III MARIANNE trial is currently underway to investigate the activity and toxicity of pertuzumab with T-DM1 or T-DM1 alone, *vs* the combination of trastuzumab with taxanes in HER2-overexpressing previously untreated MBC patients [97]. The recruitment target for this study is 1092 patients, and the primary endpoint is PFS and secondary endpoint is incidence of adverse events. The results of this clinical trial are expected to reveal whether T-DM1 plus pertuzumab should be the new treatment strategy for HER2-positive MBC. Efficacy outcomes of pretuzumab in MBC setting is summarized in Table **6**.

Effects of Pertuzumab in Neoadjuvant or Adjuvant Setting

The impact of this dual anti-HER2 inhibition in metastatic disease has been translated to the adjuvant or neoadjuvant setting. Although the increased pCR rates demonstrate with the combination of trastuzumab with standard chemotherapeutic agents, about 30-70% patients do not experience a pCR, and about 15% of patients recurrent after neoadjuvant treatment, associating required resistance or the presence of *de novo* [98]. Therefore, dual blockade with a combination of targeting treatments have been investigated. The Neoadjuvant Study of Pertuzumab and Herceptin in an Early Regimen Evaluation (NeoSphere) study assess the efficacy and safety of the following combination therapy arms: trastuzumab plus docetaxel, docetaxel plus trastuzumab plus pertuzumab, trastuzumab plus pertuzumab, and docetaxel plus pertuzumab [99]. The CR plus PR rates were 79.8%, 88.1%, 67.6%, and 71.4%, respectively, while pCR rates were 29%, 45.8%, 16.8%, and 24%, respectively. These results showed greater antitumor effect in the docetaxel plus trastuzumab plus pertuzumab arm. Furthermore, the trastuzumab plus pertuzumab arm was also well tolerated and improved efficacy, which is expected to establish the molecularly targeted therapy that does not involve cytotoxic agents for selected patients. Interestingly, hormone-receptor-negative arm showed a higher pCR rate than other arms, it was suggesting that hormone receptor status should be an intrinsic factor of the tumors [99]. Efficacy outcomes of NeoSphere study is summarized in Table **6**.

The APHINITY trial will evaluate the clinical activity and toxicity of pertuzumab in combination with chemotherapy plus trastuzumab as adjuvant setting in HER2-overexpressing breast cancer patients [100]. The recruitment target for this study is 4800 patients, and the primary endpoint is invasive DFS. The results are expected to assess the role of pertuzumab in adjuvant setting for early-stage breast cancer. For early-stage HER2-overexpressing breast cancer, ongoing adjuvant APHINITY study, may define the future standards of care in terms of dual HER2 blockade and the type of concomitant chemotherapy administered [101].

Tyrosine Kinase Inhibitors

Lapatinib

Lapatinib is reversible an orally-administered small molecule tyrosine kinase inhibitor (TKI) that selectively inhibits HER1 and HER2 [102]. Lapatinib suppressing the intracellular signaling of the MAPK-, PI3K/Akt-, and mammalian target of rapamycin (mTOR)-dependent pathway, thus lapatinib associated with cell cycles or apoptosis of breast cancer cells [103]. Phosphatase and tensin homolog (PTEN) has tumor-suppressor effect in PI3K/Akt signaling, and decrease of PTEN, or up-regulation of insulin-like growth factor 1 receptor (IGF-1R) signaling, might be important for trastuzumab resistance [104, 105]. Lapatinib inhibits the HER2 signaling by blocking the intracellular tyrosine

Table 6. Efficacy Outcomes from Clinical Trials of Pertuzumab.

Investigator (Trial)	Phase	Setting	Regimen	N	Results	Refs.
Portera *et al.*	II	MBC pretreated	T+P	11	ORR:18%	[87]
Baselga *et al.*	II	MBC Pretreated	T+P	66	ORR: 24.2%, CBR: 50%, PFS: 5.5M	[88]
Cortes *et al.* (BO17929)	II	MBC Pretreated	P monotherapy T+P (addition of T)	29	ORR: 3.4%, CBR: 10.3%, PFS: 7.1M ORR: 17.6%, CBR: 41.2%, PFS: 17.4M	[89]
Baselga *et al.* (CLEOPATRA)	III	MBC First-line	P+T+DTX *vs* placebo+T+DTX	402 406	ORR: 80.2 *vs* 69.3% ($P = 0.001$) PFS: 18.5 *vs* 12.4M (HR 0.62, $P<0.001$) OS: HR 0.64, $P = 0.005$ (the interim result is not statistically significant and is deemed exploratory)	[90, 91]
Miller *et al.*	Ib/II	MBC Pretreated	P+T-DM1	37	ORR: 39%	[95]
Dieras *et al.*	Ib/II	MBC First-line Pretreated	P+T-DM1	first-line: 22 pretreated: 45	ORR first line: 41% pretreated: 42%	[96]
Gianni *et al.* (NeoSphere)	II	Neoadjuvant	T+DTX→ surg+FEC+T *vs* T+P+DTX→ surg+FEC+T *vs* T+P→ surg+DTX+FEC+T *vs* P+DTX→ surg+FEC+T	107 107 107 96	pCR 29.0 *vs* 45.8 *vs*16.8 *vs* 24.0%	[99]

MBC: metastatic breast cancer; T: trastuzumab; P: pertuzumab; DTX: docetaxel; T-DM1: trastuzumab-DM1; surg: surgery; FEC: fluorouracil + epirubicin + cyclophosphamide; ORR: overall response rate; CBR: clinical benefit rate; PFS: progression-free survival; HR: hazard ratio; OS: overall survival; pCR: pathological complete response.

kinase activity of HER1 and HER2, and lapatinib is suggested to avoid the resistance of trastuzumab associated with the loss of PTEN [106] and the up-regulation of IGF-1R signaling [107]. Further, lapatinib can bind to the p95 truncated variant of HER2 (p95 HER2) and lapatinib suppresses cell growth in trastuzumab resistant cells expressing p95 HER2 [108]. These data supports that lapatinib is one of the promising therapeutic option for trastuzumab resistant breast cancer [109].

Effects of Lapatinib in MBC Setting

A phase II clinical study was investigated to assess the clinical activity and toxicity of single-agent lapatinib (1250 or 1500 mg once daily) in stage IIIB/IV HER2-overexpressing breast cancer patients who was trastuzumab-refractory [110]. ORR was 7.7% and 5.1%, and CBR was 14.1% and 9.0%. TTP was 15.3 weeks, and OS was 79 weeks. Another phase II study (EGF20009) also demonstrated that first-line lapatinib monotherapy had clinical activity and had acceptable tolerability in HER2-positive ABC or MBC [111]. These results suggest that first-line lapatinib monotherapy demonstrates clinical activity and has an acceptable tolerability in pretreated HER2-positive MBC.

Conventional chemotherapeutic drugs, such as capecitabine and taxanes, have also been tested with lapatinib. In phase III trial, HER2-overexpressing MBC patients who had pretreated with anthracycline, taxane, and trastuzumab were received combination treatment of lapatinib with capecitabine [74]. The median TTP was 8.4 months in the combination arm, and 4.4 months in the capecitabine monotherapy arm. The combination therapy was superior to capecitabine alone, and it was well tolerated. That trial led to approval of the use of lapatinib plus capecitabine in MBC patients. EGF30001 was a phase III study comparing lapatinib plus paclitaxel with placebo plus paclitaxel for HER2-positive MBC as first-line treatment. That trial also demonstrated that the lapatinib plus paclitaxel group was significantly superior to placebo plus paclitaxel [112]. In HER2-positive patients, ORR was 63.3% and 37.8%, and TTP was 36.4 and 25.1 weeks, respectively. The rate of diarrhea and rash was statistically higher in the paclitaxel plus lapatinib arm; however, the incidence of cardiotoxicity was low. These data suggested that patients receiving combination therapy with lapatinib exhibited better prognosis in comparison to those receiving chemotherapy alone in HER2-positive MBC.

Basic experiments have demonstrated that lapatinib is also effective in combination with trastuzumab, and the two agents are not cross-resistant [103, 113, 114]. EGF104900 was phase III trial comparing the efficacy of lapatinib monotherapy and in combination with trastuzumab with HER2-overexpressing patients who was progressed prior trastuzumab therapy [115]. Combination therapy of Lapatinib with trastuzumab was superior to lapatinib monotherapy for

PFS (11.1 *vs* 8.1months, HR 0.74, P = 0.011) and OS (14 *vs* 9.5 months, HR 0.74, P = 0.026). The most frequent toxicity was diarrhea, which was more commonly seen in the combination arm; however, the rate of cardiactoxicity was low. This study suggested that combination therapy of lapatinib with trastuzumab indicates a cytotoxic agent-free option that was well tolerated and reduced the risk of disease progression. Efficacy outcomes of lapatinib in MBC setting are summarized in Table **7**.

Effects of Lapatinib in Neoadjuvant or Adjuvant Setting

Dual HER2 inhibition is being examined in neoadjuvant and adjuvant settings. The Chemotherapy Herceptin and Lapatinib in Operable Breast Cancer (CHER-LOB) study was neoadjuvant phase II study of taxanes-anthracycline in combination with trastuzumab alone, lapatinib alone, or combination of trastuzumab with lapatinib in patients with HER2-overexpressing, stage II to IIIA operable breast cancer [116]. In each of the three groups, chemotherapy consisted of weekly paclitaxel followed by FEC for four courses. The patients randomly assigned to group A were treated with trastuzumab; those in group B, received lapatinib; and in group C, were treated with combination of trastuzumab and lapatinib. The pCR rates were 25% in group A, 26.3% in group B, and 46.7% in group C (P = 0.019). The Translational Breast Cancer Research Consortium (TBCRC) protocol 006 was phase II trial of neoadjuvant therapy without chemotherapy in HER2-positive operable breast cancer patients [117]. Patients received lapatinib and trastuzumab, and interestingly, estrogen receptor (ER)-positive patients also received hormonal therapy with letorozle. The overall pCR was 27%, including 21% for patients with ER-positive patients and 36% for ER-negative patients. It was concluded that selected HER2-overexpressing breast cancer patients may avoid cytotixic agents, and stronger blockade of HER receptors and ER is a promising strategy warranting further investigation. Two randomized neoadjuvant trials examined the combination of trastuzumab or lapatinib to taxane based chemotherapy. The Neoadjuvant Lapatinib and/or Trastuzumab Treatment Optimization (NeoALTTO) study was a phase III neoadjuvant trial which compared lapatinib alone, trastuzumab alone and in combination with paclitaxel for HER2-overexpressing breast cancer [118]. pCR

Table 7. Efficacy Outcomes from Clinical Trials of Lapatinib in MBC Setting.

Investigator (Trial)	Phase	Setting	Regimen	N	Results	Refs.
Blackwell *et al.*	II	MBC pretreated	L (1250mg, 1500mg)	78	RR: 7.7%, 5.1% CBR: 14.1%, 9.0% TTP: 15.3weeks OS: 79weeks	[110]
Gomez *et al.* (EGF20009)	II	MBC first-line	L	138	ORR: 24%, CBR: 31% PFS rate: 43% (6M)	[111]
Geyer *et al.* (EGF100151)	III	MBC pretreated	L+capecitabine *vs* capecitabine	163 161	TTP: 8.4 *vs* 4.4 M (HR 0.49, *P*<0.001) ORR: 22 *vs* 14%	[74]
Di Leo *et al.* (EGF30001)	III	MBC first-line	L+PTX *vs* PTX	49 37 (HER2 positive only)	TTP: 36.4 *vs* 25.1 weeks (HR 0.53, *P* = 0.005) ORR: 63.3 *vs* 37.8% (*P* = 0.023)	[112]
Blackwell *et al.* (EGF104900)	III	MBC pretreated	L+T *vs* L	148 148	PFS: 11.1 *vs* 8.1 M (HR 0.74, *P* = 0.011) OS: 14 *vs* 9.5M (HR 0.74, *P* = 0.026)	[115]
Guarneri *et al.* (CHER-LOB)	II	Noeadjuvant	T+(PTX→FEC)→surg *vs* L+(PTX→FEC)→surg *vs* (T+L)+(PTX→FEC)→ surg	36 39 46	pCR: 25 *vs* 26.3 *vs* 46.7% (*P* = 0.019)	[116]
Rimawi *et al.* (TBCRC 006)	II	Neoadjuvant	T+L+letrozole (ER positive) →surg+adjuvant	64	pCR: 27%	[117]
Baselga *et al.* NeoALTTO	III	Neoadjuvant	L+PTX→surg→FEC→L *vs* T+PTX→surg→FEC→T *vs* T+L+PTX→surg→FEC→ T+L	154 149 152	pCR: 24.7 *vs* 29.5 *vs* 51.3%	[118]
Carey *et al.* (CALGB 40601)	III	neoadjuvant	PTX+T→surg *vs* PTX+T+L→surg *vs* T+L→surg (closed)	120 118 67	pCR: 40 *vs* 51 *vs* 32%	[119]
Holmes *et al.* (US Oncology)	II	neoadjuvant	T→T(FEC→PTX)→surg *vs* L→L(FEC→PTX)→surg *vs* T+L→T+L(FEC→PTX) →surg	total 100	pCR: 54 *vs* 45 *vs* 74%	[120]

Table 7 contd.....

Investigator (Trial)	Phase	Setting	Regimen	N	Results	Refs.
Untch *et al.* (GeparQuinto GBG44)	III	neoadjuvant	T+(EC→DTX)→surg *vs* L+(EC→DTX)→surg	309 311	pCR: 30.3 *vs* 22.7%	[121]
Robidoux *et al.* (NSABP B-41)	III	neoadjuvant	AC→PTX+T→surg *vs* AC→PTX+L→surg *vs* AC→PTX+T+L→surg	177 171 106	pCR: 52.5 *vs* 53.2 *vs* 62.0%	[122]

MBC: metastatic breast cancer; L: lapatinib; PTX: paclitaxel; T: trastuzumab; FEC: fluorouracil + epirubicin + cyclophosphamide; surg: surgery; ER: estrogen receptor; EC: epirubicin + cyclophosphamide; DTX: docetaxel; AC: doxorubicin + cyclophosphamide; RR: response rate; CBR: clinical benefit rate; TTP: time-to-progression; HR: hazard ratio; ORR: overall response rate; PFS: progression-free survival; OS: overall survival; pCR: pathological complete response.

rates were 24.7% for lapatinib monotherapy, 29.5% for trastuzumab monotherapy, and 51.3% for the lapatinib plus trastuzumab. Clinical and translational results of the CALGB 40601 study were reported at the 2013 ASCO Annual Meeting. That study was a phase III neoadjuvant study of weekly treatment of paclitaxel and trastuzumab with or without lapatinib in HER2-overexpressing breast cancer patients [119]. In that trial, pCR rates were 51% in the paclitaxel plus trastuzumab plus lapatinib arm, 40% in the paclitaxel plus trastuzumab group, and 32% in the trastuzumab plus lapatinib group. The pCR rates in the paclitaxel plus trastuzumab group were not statistically different from that in the paclitaxel plus trastuzumab plus lapatinib group (P = 0.11). This data are qualitatively similar to those of the NeoALTTO trial. In contrast, three trials (US Oncology study, GeparQuinto study, and NSABP B-41) have investigated the combination of trastuzumab or lapatinib with anthracycline or taxane-based chemotherapy. The US Oncology study assessed the neoadjuvant administration of trastuzumab, lapatinib, or the combination of both, followed by FEC and then weekly paclitaxel with the continuation of the same anti-HER2 agents [120]. The pCR rates were 54% for trastuzumab, 45% for lapatinib, and 74% for the combination of lapatinib and trastuzumab. The GeparQuinto GBG 44 trial was a phase III study involving patients with untreated HER2-overexpressing operable or locally ABC [121]. Patients received neoadjuvant treatment with EC (four cycle) followed by docetaxel (four cycle) with either trastuzumab (ECH-TH group) or lapatinib (ECL-TL group) throughout all cycles before surgery. pCR rates were 30.3% in the ECH-TH group and 22.7% in the ECL-TL group (P = 0.04). NSABP B-41 was a phase III neoadjuvant clinical study with HER2-positive breast cancer patients. Patients received AC followed by weekly paclitaxel concurrently with trastuzumab, lapatinib, or a combination of trastuzumab plus lapatinib. pCR was noted in 52.5% in the trastuzumab arm, 53.2% in the lapatinib arm, and 62.0% in the combination arm. In that study, substitution of lapatinib for trastuzumab in combination with standard chemotherapeutic agents resulted in similar high percentages of pCR [122].

Combination of HER2-targeted therapy resulted in significantly higher pCR percentages than HER2-directed monotherapy. These data suggest that combination therapeutic strategy with trastuzumab and lapatinib is active for primary breast cancers; therefore, trials are being undertaken to further assess these findings in the adjuvant treatment. The Adjuvant Lapatinib and/or Trastuzumab Treatment Optimization (ALTTO) trial is a randomized phase III adjuvant trial comparing the efficacy of lapatinib monotherapy *vs* trastuzumab monotherapy *vs* trastuzumab followed by lapatinib *vs* lapatinib concomitantly with trastuzumab in HER2-overexpressing breast cancer patients [123]. The recruitment target for this study is 8381 patients, and the primary endpoint is DFS. The results are expected to confirm the role of lapatinib and trastuzumab in adjuvant setting for early-stage breast cancer. Efficacy outcomes of lapatinib in neoadjuvant setting are summarized in Table **7**.

Effects of Lapatinib in Brain Metastasis

Brain metastasis is often seen in patients with HER2-overexpressing MBC, and generally prognosis is poor. Since lapatinib is a small molecule TKI, it is suggested that lapatinib can cross the blood-brain barrier (BBB) to supply efficacious concentrations in the cerebrospinal fluid. In brain metastasis model with mice, lapatinib treatment inhibited the brain metastasis [124]. In clinical studies, lapatinib alone has observed antitumor effect for brain metastasis, and better response has been shown for the combination of capecitabine with lapatinib [125-127]. The LANDSCAPE trial was phase II, open label, multicenter study; eligible patients had HER2-overexpressing MBC with brain metastases not pretreated with whole brain radiotherapy, capecitabine, or lapatinib [128]. The objective central nervous system (CNS) response was 65.9%. These results support that lapatinib is an active anti-HER2 agent for brain metastasis from breast cancer.

Neratinib

Neratinib (HKI-272) is an orally-administered, small molecule TKI which inhibit the HER1, HER2, and HER4. Data from preclinical studies shows that neratinib reduces HER2 autophosphorylation with suppression of cell proliferation. Neratinib inhibit the intracellular signal transduction and cell cycle regulation such as the MAPK and PI3K/Akt pathways. Naratinib leads to cell arrest at the G1-S-phase of the cell cycle, and it inhibits the cancer cell growth [129].

Effects of Neratinib in MBC Setting

In a phase I study of neratinib in patients with advanced solid tumors, the dose-limiting toxicity (DLT) was diarrhea (grade 3); hence, the MTD was determined to be 320 mg [130]. PR was observed for 32%. In phase II study of neratinib monotherapy in patients with HER2-overexpressing ABC, the clinical activity and toxicity of neratinib were assessed in two cohorts: a prior trastuzumab treated arm and a no prior trastuzumab treated arm [131]. Neratinib 240 mg treatment orally once daily was chosen for this trial. PFS was 22.3 weeks in the prior trastuzumab treated arm and 39.6 weeks in the no prior trastuzumab treated arm, with an ORR of 24% and 56%. The common toxicities were diarrhea, nausea, vomiting, and fatigue; however, no neratinib-related, severe cardiac dysfunction was reported. Oral neratinib is an effective therapeutic agent and has an acceptable tolerability among both previously treated and no prior trastuzumab in HER2-overexpressing breast cancer patients. In another phase II study, the toxicity and clinical activity of neratinib monotherapy were compared with that of lapatinib plus capecitabine in HER2-overexpressing MBC and prior trastuzumab treatment [132]. Median PFS for neratinib was 4.5 *vs* 6.8 months for lapatinib plus capecitabine and OS was 19.7 *vs* 23.6 months. ORR (29% *vs* 41%; P = 0.067) and CBR (44% *vs* 64%; P = 0.003) were lower for the neratinib arm. Although the non-inferiority of neratinib was not seen when compared with lapatinib plus capecitabine, neratinib monotherapy showed relevant effective and well tolerated in HER2-

overexpressing MBC patients and may be an option for recurrent HER2-overexpressing MBC not suitable for lapatinib plus capecitabine combination therapy.

A phase I/II trial of the combination of neratinib with vinorelbine has been investigated [133]. Phase I of that study investigated the MTD of oral neratinib (160 or 240 mg/day) with vinorelbine (25 mg/m^2) in patients with solid tumors. Phase II was conducted to evaluate the safety, clinical activity, and pharmacokinetics of the combination in HER2-overexpressing MBC patients. Phase I established the MTD to be 240 mg of neratinib with 25 mg/m^2 of vinorelbine. The ORR in assessable phase II patients was 41% with no prior lapatinib and 8% with prior lapatinib. Neratinib plus vinorelbine treatment showed effective antitumor activity and had an acceptable toxicity in HER2-positive MBC patients. Further, a phase I/II trial of the combination of neratinib with paclitaxel has also been investigated [134]. Phase I of that study determined MTD to be oral neratinib 240 mg once daily plus weekly paclitaxel 80 mg/m^2 on days 1, 8, and 15 of each 28-day cycle. ORR was 73% and median PFS was 57.0 weeks. Neratinib and paclitaxel combination therapy was reported with higher adverse events than that of neratinib monotherapy, but was mild, and the combination therapy also showed clinical activity in HER2-overexpessing MBC patients. Efficacy outcomes of neratinib in MBC are summarized in Table **8**. From the results of that study, a phase III study is ongoing to assess the combination of neratinib with paclitaxel compared with trastuzumab plus paclitaxel in the first-line treatment. The recruitment target is 480 patients, and the primary endpoint is PFS [135].

Effects of Neratinib in Adjuvant Setting

Neratinib is also investigating as late adjuvant treatment in early-stage HER2-overexpressing breast cancer patients. Patients with surgically treated breast cancer who had administered standard adjuvant chemotherapy and finished 1 year of trastuzumab therapy were randomized to receive 1 year treatment of neratinib or placebo in a phase III study. The recruitment target for this study is 2842 patients, and the primary endpoint is DFS [136]. The results are expected to reveal the role of neratinib in HER2-positive breast cancer.

Table 8. Efficacy Outcomes from Clinical Trials of Neratinib and Afatinib in MBC Setting

Investigator	Phase	Regimen	N	Results	Refs.
Wong *et al.*	I	neratinib	25 (breast cancer)	MTD: 320mg PR: 32%	[130]
Burstein *et al.*	II	neratinib	66 (prior T) 70 (no prior T)	PFS prior T: 22.3 weeks, no prior T: 39.6 weeks ORR prior T: 24%, no prior T: 56%	[131]
Martin *et al.*	II	neratinib *vs* L+capecitabine	117 116	PFS: 4.5 *vs* 6.8M OS: 19.7 *vs* 23.6M ORR: 29 *vs* 41% ($P = 0.067$) CBR: 44 *vs* 64% ($P = 0.003$)	[132]
Awada *et al.*	I/II	neratinib+vinorelbine	12 (phase I) 79 (phase II)	MTD neratinib: 240mg, vinorelbine: 25mg/m^2 ORR prior L: 8%, no prior L: 41%,	[133]
Chow *et al.*	I/II	neratinib+PTX (weekly)	8 (phase I) 102 (phase II)	MTD neratinib: 240mg, PTX: 80mg/m^2 ORR: 73%, PFS: 57.0 weeks	[134]
Yap *et al.*	I	afatinib	53 (solid tumor)	MTD: 50mg daily PR: 3 patients (NSCLC) SD: 7 patients (NSCLC, esophagus carcinoma)	[140]
Lin *et al.*	II	afatinib	41	CBR: 46%, PFS: 15.1 weeks, OS: 61.0 weeks	[141]

L: lapatinib; PTX: paclitaxel; T: trastuzumab; MTD: maximum tolerated dose; PFS: progression-free survival; ORR: overall response rate; OS: overall survival; CBR: clinical benefit rate; PR: partial response; SD: stable disease; NSCLC: non-small-cell lung carcinoma.

Afatinib

Afatinib (BIBW 2992) is an oral, small molecule, anilinoquinazoline compound, and this drug is selective inhibitor of HER1, HER2, and HER4 tyrosine kinase. Further, afatinib suppresses HER1- and HER2-containing dimers [137, 138]. Afatinib has reported preclinical effect in various different tumor models. This TKI irreversibly binds HER1 and HER2, potently suppressing the kinase activity of wild-type and activated HER1 and HER2 mutants as well as inducing partial and complete tumor suppression in mouse models expressing HER1 and/or HER2 [137, 138]. Recently, at the 2013 ASCO Annual Meeting, Canonici *et al.*, reported the activity of afatinib monotherapy and combination therapy with trastuzumab in HER2-overexpressing breast cancer cell lines [139]. It was suggested that afatinib monotherapy has activity in HER2-overexpressing breast cancer, even in trastuzumab- and/or lapatinib-resistant breast cancer, and combination of afatinib with trastuzumab may be more effective than either agent alone in trastuzumab-sensitive breast cancer.

Effects of Afatinib in MBC Setting

A phase I trial of afatinib was investigated to determine toxicity, MTD, and preliminary antitumor efficacy [140]. That study enrolled 53 patients who were associated to different dose from 10 to 50 mg; MTD was determined to be 50 mg daily. Afatinib generally showed an acceptable tolerability, and the common toxicities were diarrhea, nausea, vomiting, rash, and fatigue. Three non-small-cell lung carcinoma (NSCLC) patients experienced confirmed PR, and 7 patients had disease stabilization lasting 6 months. A phase II study was conducted to explore afatinib activity in patients with HER2-overexpressing breast cancer after trastuzumab-refractory [141]. Forty-one patients were administered 50mg afatinib daily until disease progression. Four patients had PR, fifteen patients had SD as best response, and 46% achieved clinical activity. PFS was 15.1 weeks and OS was 61.0 weeks. The common toxicities were diarrhea and rush. To establish the role of afatinib in HER2-overexpressing, trastuzumab-refractory MBC patients, further investigation of afatinib in a larger clinical trial is warranted. Efficacy outcomes of afatinib in MBC are summarized in Table **8**.

At the 2012 ASCO Annual Meeting, three LUX-breast trials were presented. LUX-breast 1 is a phase III study comparing of afatinib and vinorelbine *vs* trastuzumab and vinorelbine in HER2-positive MBC patients pretreated with one regimen of trastuzumab [142]. The primary endpoint is PFS, and secondary endpoints is OS, objective response (OR), and toxicity. LUX-breast 2 is a phase II trial of afatinib in patients with HER2-positive MBC who is trastuzumab and/or lapatinib-refractory [143]. This trial is testing the activity and safety of afatinib monotherapy followed by afatinib beyond progression plus chemotherapeutic drugs in 120 patients with HER2-positive MBC, who failed on prior adjuvant and/or neoadjuvant lapatinib and/or trastuzumab. The primary endpoint is OR, and secondary endpoints are PFS, best overall response and duration of OR. LUX-breast 3 is a phase II trial of afatinib monotherapy or combination with vinorelbine *vs* investigator's choice of treatment in HER2-overexpressing breast cancer patients with brain metastasis progressing after trastuzumab or lapatinib treatments [144]. That study is to assess whether afatinib monotherapy or combination therapy with vinorelbine has clinical activity on brain metastases after failure of prior trastuzumab or lapatinib in patients with HER2-overexpressing breast cancer. Afatinib has very low molecular weight which suggests that it can pass through the BBB easily. Similar to lapatinib, afatinib could be effective in brain metastasis. We are expecting for confirmation from the LUX-breast 3 trial in brain metastasis patients treated with afatinib. Moreover, there are several other ongoing trials assessing the efficacy of afatinib in breast cancer, ether in single-agent or in combination with other HER2-targeted treatments, endocrine therapy, or chemotherapy [145].

mTOR INHIBITORS

mTOR is a serine-threonine protein kinase that plays a key role in the regulation of cell proliferation [146, 147]. mTOR have mTORC1 and mTORC2 complexes. The mTORC1 complex is existed of the mTOR catalytic subunit, regulatory associated protein of mTOR (raptor), proline-rich Akt substrate 40 kDa (PRAS40), and the protein mlST8/GβL [147, 148], and it is regulated by a number of intracellular signaling, such as the PI3K/Akt pathway. mTORC2 is existed of mTOR, rapamycin-insensitive companion of mTOR (rictor), mammalian stress-activated protein kinase interacting protein 1 (mSIN1), and mlST8/GβL [148]. PI3K activates the Akt by promoting translocation to the inner cellular membrane where it is phosphorylated and activated by phosphoinositide-dependent kinase (PDK) 1 and PDK 2 [149-151]. Akt prevents dimerization of tuberous sclerosis complex (TSC) 1 and 2, and also promotes phosphorylation of PRAS40 [152-154]. Inhibition of TSC dimerization and phosphorylation of PRAS40 allow mTORC1 to promote cell growth and proliferation *via* downstream transduction of proliferative signals through phosphorylation of the translational regulator eukaryotic initiation factor 4E-binding protein (4E-BP1) and the ribosomal protein S6 kinase, both of which are crucial to the regulation of protein synthesis [155]. In contrast, mTORC2 regulates and organizes the cellular actin cytoskeleton and regulation of Akt through phosphorylation [156]. For full activation, Akt requires phosphorylation by both mTORC and PI3K [146, 157]. The tumor suppressor PTEN is one of the most important negative regulators of the PI3K/Akt signaling pathway [158, 159]. Phosphatidylinositol-3,4,5-trisphosphate (PtdIns(3,4,5)P3) is a lipid second messenger and it controls the PI3K/Akt pathway, and PTEN suppresses the PI3K activity by PtdIns(3,4,5)P3 dephosphorylation [160]. Under normal conditions, PTEN acts as a negative regulator of this pathway, limiting the growth proliferation promoting effects mediated through activation of mTORC1. Mutations or gene amplifications in PI3K and mutations resulting in PTEN loss are reported in many cancers, making the mTOR signaling pathway a rational therapeutic target for cancer drugs [146, 157]. Rapamycin is a macrolide that was originally developed as an antifungal drug and was later recognized to have anticancer activities. The complex of rapamycin with FK506 binding protein (FKBP12) binds to mTORC1 and it inhibit mTORC1-mediated phosphorylation of the substrates S6 kinase 1 (S6K1) and 4E-BP1 [148]. In contrast, FKBP12-rapamycin cannot bind directly to mTORC2 [156, 161], suggesting that the effects of rapamycin on cellular signaling are due to inhibition of mTORC1 [148].

Effects of Temsirolimus in MBC Setting

Temsirolimus is an intravenous inhibitor of mTOR. In a phase I trial, temsirolimus was evaluated to determine toxicity and showed an acceptable tolerability. The most common adverse effects were rashes and stomatitis. PR was observed in 2 of 24 patients [162]. In a phase II study, weekly administered with 75 or 250mg of temsirolimus was associated with mild toxicity and ORR was 9.2% and TTP was 12 weeks in pretreated breast cancer patients [163]. Wolff *et al.,* reported phase III randomized study to compare the effects of placebo plus letrozole and temsirolimus plus letrozole in patients with aromatase inhibitor (AI) pretreated hormone-receptor positive MBC [164]. Grade 3-4 adversed events were more commonly in the temsirolimus plus letrozole arm than in the placebo plus letrozole arm. The combination of temsirolimus with letrozole did not increase the PFS, thus, temsirolimus plus letrozole is less effective than letrozole alone for patients with AI pretreated MBC. Efficacy outcomes from clinical trials of temsirolimus in MBC are summarized in Table **9**.

Table 9. Efficacy Outcomes from Clinical Trials of Temsirolimus and Everolimus in MBC Setting

Investigator (Trial)	Phase	Regimen	N	Results	Refs.
Raymond *et al.*	I	Temsirolimus	24	PR: 2 of 24 patients	[162]
Chan *et al.*	II	Temsirolimus	109	ORR: 9.2% TTP: 12 weeks	[163]
Wolff *et al.*	III	Letrozole+temsirolimus *vs* Letrozole+placebo	556 556	PFS: 8.9 *vs* 9.0M (HR 0.90, *P* = 0.25)	[164]
Ellard *et al.*	II	Everolimus	daily: 33 weekly: 16	RR daily: 12%, weekly: 0%	[165]
Morrow *et al.*	I/II	Everolimus+T	47	CBR: 34%, PFS: 4.1M	[168]
Andre *et al.*	I	Everolimus+PTX+T	31	recommended dose for everolimus: 10mg/day ORR: 44%, PFS: 34weeks	[169]
Jerusalem *et al.*	I	Everolimus+vinorelbine+T	47	recommended dose for everolimus 5mg/day and 30mg/week ORR: 19.1%, PFS: 30.7 weeks	[170]
O'Regan *et al.* (BOLERO-3)	III	Everolimus+vinorelbine+T *vs* Placebo+vinorelbine+T	284 286	PFS: 7.0 *vs* 5.78M (HR 0.78, *P* = 0.0067) ORR: 40.8 *vs* 37.2% (*P* = 0.2108) CBR: 59.2 *vs* 53.5% (*P* = 0.0945)	[171]

T: trastuzumab; PTX: paclitaxel; PR: partial response; CBR: clinical benefit rate; ORR: overall response rate; TTP: time-to-progression; PFS: progression-free survival; HR: hazard ratio; RR: response rate.

Effects of Everolimus in MBC Setting

Everolimus (RAD001) is an oral rapamycin analog that suppresses mTORC1 by the similar mechanism of rapamycin, but has different pharmacokinetics and solubility properties that increase its desirability for clinical use. A phase II trial resulted that RR with everolimus alone was 12 %, and the frequent severe toxicity were fatigue, pneumonitis, infection, and neutropenia [165]. Trastuzumab resistance has been involved with the action of the PI3K/Akt signaling and loss of PTEN is a powerful predictor for trastuzumab-resistance [104, 166]. In a basic study of PTEN loss and trastuzumab-resistant models, combination of everolimus with trastuzumab inhibited breast cancer growth [167]. That result suggested the favorite results for the combination of trastuzumab with everolimus for treating patients of trastuzumab-resistance conferred by PTEN deficiency. A phase I/II trial of trastuzumab in combination with everolimus assessed the toxicity and efficacy of this treatment in HER2-positive MBC patients that failed on trastuzumab treatment [168]. CBR was 34% and PFS was 4.1 months. Interestingly, PTEN-deficient patients showed decreased OS (P = 0.048). Further, everolimus has been investigated in addition of trastuzumab with chemotherapy. Combination treatment of everolimus with trastuzumab and paclitaxel in HER2-overexpressing MBC patients previously treated with trastuzumab has been evaluated [169]. The ORR of this combination group was 44%, and it had an acceptable tolerability. Combination of everolimus with trastuzumab and vinorelbine, everolimus showed an ORR of 19.1% and a PFS of 30.7 weeks [170]. Recently, at the 2013 ASCO Annual Meeting, results of the breast cancer trials of oral everolimus-3 (BOLERO-3) were reported [171]. This trial is a phase III to assess the activity of vinorelbine and trastuzumab with or without everolimus in HER2-overexpressing MBC patients resistant to trastuzumab and pre-ptreated with a taxane. PFS was 7.0 months in the everolimus arm as compared with 5.8 months in the placebo arm (HR 0.78, P = 0.0067). The most common toxicities included stomatitis, fatigue, neutropenia, and anemia. It was reported that addition of everolimus to vinorelbine and trastuzumab significantly prolonged PFS, and this combination therapy may be considered a novel and promising option in trastuzumab resistant HER2-overexpressing ABC. These clinical results suggest that combination therapy of everolimus with trastuzumab and chemotherapy has an acceptable tolerability and exhibits promising efficacy in heavily previously treated in HER2-positive MBC patients who failed on trastuzumab treatment. Efficacy outcomes from clinical trials of everolimus in MBC are summarized in Table **9**. Currently, the BOLERO-1 phase III study is investigating to evaluate the activity of addition of everolimus to trastuzumab and paclitaxel in HER2-overexpressing MBC as a first-line treatment [172]. The recruitment target for this study is 717 patients, and primary endpoint is PFS.

ANGIOGENESIS PATHWAY

Tumor Angiogenesis

The proper functioning of body tissues requires an adequate and ordered supply of blood *via* a system of arteries, veins, and capillaries. A blood supply is also essential for the malignant progression, invasion, and metastasis of solid tumors [173, 174]. In order to acquire sufficient blood flow, tumors stimulate blood vessel formation, in which angiogenesis plays a central role. Angiogenesis involves the production of new capillaries from pre-existing vessels [175], which then develop into the vessels that supply blood to the tumor. In the first avascular phase, tumor lesions remain dormant, and growth remains in a steady state where proliferation and apoptosis are balanced. Angiogenesis is required to progress beyond this stage [176], and the transition is known as the "angiogenic switch." Once the angiogenic switch is turned on, new vessels continue to form as long as the tumor grows. Furthermore, if the tumor shows rapid growth, the provision of blood can fail to keep up, and the oxygen and nutrient supply can be poor. This abnormality appears in areas of hypoxia within the tumor, which in turn stimulates further vessel formation. It also provides a route for the transport of tumor cells to distant sites where metastases can form [177]. Thus, angiogenesis is important for cancer proliferation and metastasis. Hypoxia plays a key role of regulating angiogenesis and hypoxia induces vascular endothelial growth factor (VEGF). Many pro-angiogenic regulators have been identified that either up-regulate or down-regulate angiogenesis. VEGF, fibroblast growth factor (FGF), TGF-α, and TGF-β up-regulate angiogenesis; while angiostatin, endostatin, thrombospondin-1, angiopoietin-2, interferon-α, and interleukin-12 down-regulate angiogenesis [174, 175, 178]. VEGF, in particular, is most important factor for tumor angiogenesis [174, 179-181].

VEGF Family Members

VEGF is a 34-46 kDa homodimeric glycoprotein and it is a ligand for VEGF receptor 1 (VEGFR 1) and VEGF receptor 2 (VEGFR 2) or Flk-1/KDR. VEGF family include VEGF (A, B, C, D, E), and placental growth factor (PIGF), especially, VEGF-C and VEGF-D are associated with lymphangiogenesis [182]. Expression of the VEGF is controlled by a number of factors mainly hypoxia. When the cancer cells are exposed to hypoxic condition, hypoxia-inducible factor-1α (HIF-1α) and HIF-2α binds with HIF-β in the nucleus. This complex interacts with the hypoxia response element (HRE), then cancer cells secrets the VEGF [183, 184]. VEGFR 2 is expressed on the endothelial cell membrane and VEGF binding to VEGFR 2 allows to form homodimer of VEGFR 2. VEGFR 2 dimers activate the tyrosine kinase or induce the autophosphorylation of the receptor VEGFR-2, thereby VEGFR 2 dimers mediates the biological activity through the phospholipase C (PLC)-protein kinase C (PKC)-MAPK signaling pathway [183, 185]. VEGF is one of the most important factor for proliferation and anti-apoptosis of vascular endothelial cells [186], vascular permeability [187], prevention of apoptosis on cancer cells [188], metastasis [189, 190], and the antitumor immune system [191] (Fig. **3**).

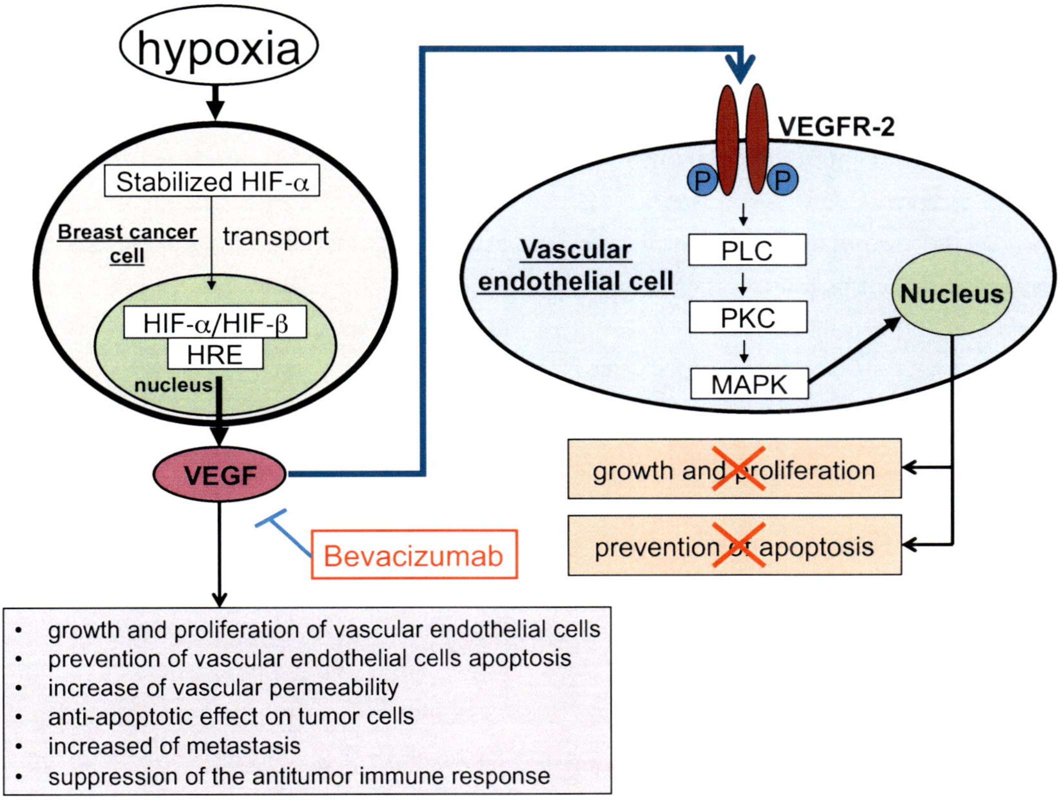

Fig. (3). Under hypoxic conditions, the transcription factors HIF-1α and HIF-2α are stabilized, and are transported to the nucleus where they interact with HIF-β. This complex then binds to the HRE, which stimulates VEGF gene transcription and VEGF protein is produced, then VEGF is secreted from the cancer cells [180, 181]. After the binding of VEGF to the VEGFR-2, which is expressed on the endothelial cell membrane, the homodimerization of the VEGF-2 receptor occurs. The effects of VEGF are then mediated by the activation of various intracellular signaling transduction pathways, such as the activation of receptor tyrosine kinase activity or the induction of autophosphorylation of the VEGFR-2, and this receptor mediated the biological action *via* the PLC-PKC-MAPK pathway [180, 182]. VEGF is one of the most important factor for proliferation and anti-apoptosis of vascular endothelial cells [186], vascular permeability [187], prevention of apoptosis on cancer cells [188], metastasis [189, 190], and the antitumor immune system [191].

Expression of VEGF in Breast Cancer

Numerous studies have reported the VEGF overexpression in tumors and the increased levels of VEGF in circulation in a number of human malignant tumors, such as breast cancer [192]. VEGF overexpression was reported to increase the malignant potential in tumor and to associate with the neovascularization [192-195], and a circulated VEGF concentration associated with disease progression or metastasis [196]. These data indicated that the VEGF overexpression is correlated with poor prognosis for malignant tumors including breast cancer [197-200]. Because VEGF plays a key role in cancer proliferation and metastasis, inhibiting VEGF activity should be a rational cancer treatment strategy. In basic studies, anti-VEGF monoclonal antibody inhibited tumor angiogenesis and suppressed the growth of tumors in animal xenograft models [201, 202]. From these data, it was suggested that inhibiting VEGF suppresses neovascularization and tumor proliferation. It was reported that VEGF avoids the apoptosis of vascular endothelial cells by increase the expression of the B-cell CLL/lymphoma 2 (Bcl-2), X-linked inhibitor of apoptosis protein (XIAP), and survivin in endothelial cells [203]. Hence VEGF induces the endothelial cells in the tumor vasculature to survive and tumor is supplied the blood continuously. Suppression of VEGF induces apoptosis to the endothelial cells and it is leading to disturb the tumor blood supply. Because angiogenesis and lymphangiogenesis are associated with tumor progression [204, 205], VEGF is essential factor for metastasis. In preclinical studies, anti-VEGF antibody can suppress metastasis in animal xenograft models, thus it seems that suppression of VEGF should inhibit metastases [189, 206]. Drugs targeting the VEGF system to promote the antitumor activity by such mechanisms are currently in development. One of the promising agents is bevacizumab which is anti-VEGF monoclonal antibody. Bevacizumab recognizes all isoforms of VEGF ligands and, it inhibits angiogenesis by suppression of VEGF signaling [207]. The efficacy of bevacizumab on breast cancer has been investigated in various clinical studies. In addition, small molecule oral TKIs, such as sunitinib and sorafenib, are also under investigation as new anti-angiogenic agents.

Bevacizumab

Combination Therapy of Bevacizumab and Conventional Chemotherapy for MBC

In a phase I/II study, pretreated MBC patients were administered with 3 to 20 mg/kg of bevacizumab [208]. The ORR was 9.3%. This trial recommended dose of 10 mg/kg, however, the efficacy of bevacizumab alone for breast cancer is not established by that trial. Thus, it is hypothesized that a combination of bevacizumab with chemotherapeutic agents should be more effectively [209, 210]. In a phase II study, pretreated MBC patients were treated with bevacizumab plus vinorelbine [211]. The RR was 34% and the TTP was 5.5 months. Furthermore, lower concentration of circulated VEGF was correlated with a longer TTP. In another phase II study, MBC patients were administered with bevacizumab plus docetaxel. The ORR was 52% and the PFS was 7.5 months [212]. In the phase III study, combination therapy of bevacizumab with capecitabine was conducted in pretreated with anthracycline or taxane in MBC patients [213]. The combination treatment statistically improved the RR (19.8% *vs* 9.1%, $P = 0.001$), but did not increase the PFS or the OS. That study clearly showed that bevacizumab had improved the clinical response, however, it did not improve the PFS or the OS. In the later stage of malignant tumor, another pro-angiogenic factor, including basic FGF, TGF-β, PIGF, platelet-derived endothelial cell growth factor (PD-ECGF) and pleiotrophin are secreted. Thus, the suppression of VEGF by bevacitzumab in the advanced stages of breast cancer should not be active because these pro-angiogenic factors induce tumor growth. From this mechanism, inhibiting of VEGF should be done in the early stages and bevacizumab should be used in first-line therapy for the MBC patients [199, 209].

First-Line Treatment with Bevacizumab in Combination with Conventional Chemotherapy for MBC

The phase III Eastern Cooperative Oncology Group 2100 (ECOG-E2100) study assessed combination first-line treatment of paclitaxel with bevacizumab in HER2-negative MBC patients [214]. Combination treatment statistically improved the ORR (36.9% *vs* 21.1%, $P < 0.001$) and the PFS (11.8 *vs* 5.9 months, $P < 0.001$); however, the combination therapy did not increase the OS (26.7 *vs* 25.2 months, P = 0.16). Although there was no improvement in the OS with ECOG-E2100 study, it showed improvement of activity for earlier stage MBC. The results of that trial led to accelerated approval of this regimen by the FDA and EMA, and subsequently in other countries. Two subsequent phase III first-line trials were undertaken in an attempt to validate the ECOG-E2100 study. The Avastin and Docetaxel (AVADO) trial assessed docetaxel with or without bevacizumab (7.5 or 15 mg/kg) in HER2-negative MBC as first-line treatment [215]. Combination treatment statistically improved the PFS (docetaxel plus placebo [D] = 8.1 months; docetaxel plus bevacizumab 7.5 mg/kg [DB7.5] = 9.0 months; and docetaxel plus bevacizumab 15 mg/kg [DB15] = 10.0 months) and the ORR (D = 46%; DB7.5 = 55%; and DB15 = 64%). OS was similar in all three treatment groups, with 31.9 months for D, 30.8 months for DB7.5, and 30.2 months for DB15. The AVADO trial showed that first-line combination treatment of docetaxel with bevacizumab statistically increased the PFS and the ORR compared with docetaxel monotherapy for MBC, but did not improve the OS. The Regimens in Bevacizumab for Breast Oncology (RIBBON)-1 trial was phase III study to compare the clinical activity and toxicity of bevacizumab in combination with several standard chemotherapeutic agents *vs* those agents plus placebo for first-line therapy in HER2-negative MBC patients [216]. In that trial, investigators selected capecitabine, taxane-based, or anthracycline-based chemotherapy before random assignment. Median PFS was improved for each bevacizumab combination, but did not improve the OS. The results of that trial showed a lack of direct clinical benefit and an increase in toxicity (such as bleeding, gastrointestinal perforation, and thromboembolic events), and failed to confirm the initial magnitude of PFS improvement noted in ECOG-E2100. As a result of those findings, on December 15, 2010, the FDA revoked the label of weekly paclitaxel plus bevacizumab for the first-line therapy of MBC [217]. However, the NCCN guidelines still include bevacizumab among combination regimens for stage IV metastatic or recurrent breast cancer, and it is suggested that the greatest efficacy appears in combination with paclitaxel [19]. On the other hand, European regulatory authorities came to a different conclusion than that of the FDA, and bevacizumab continues to be an accepted option for MBC [218]. The MO19391 Avastin Therapy for Advanced Breast Cancer (ATHENA) study is to further investigate the toxicity and efficacy of combination therapy of bevacizumab with taxane for MBC as a first-line treatment

[219]. The most frequent severe toxicity was neutropenia, and severe adverse events previously associated with bevacizumab included hypertension, arterial or venous thromboembolism, proteinuria, and bleeding. No new bevacizumab adverse events were observed. Median TTP was 9.5 months. The ORR was 52% in the intent-to-treat (ITT) population, and a further 33% achieved SD. It was concluded that the toxicity and anti-tumor effect of bevacizumab plus taxane treatment in this mega trial were consistent with results from other randomized first-line trials.

Triple-negative breast cancer (TNBC; estrogen receptor negative and progesterone receptor negative and HER2-negative) cells do not react to endocrine therapy or to anti-HER2 therapy, and the prognosis is poor [220]. Because chemotherapeutic agents are the only current therapeutic strategy, combination treatment of bevacizumab with chemotherapy is hypothesized to be active for TNBC. In a meta-analysis of three phase III studies of first-line bevacizumab treatment with TNBC, PFS was 8.1 months with bevacizumab *vs* 5.4 months with chemotherapy alone, and 1-year OS rates were 71% *vs* 65% [221]. Bevacizumab improved efficacy in subgroups of poor-prognosis patients with limited treatment options. Recently, the results of a phase II trial of first-line combination therapy of bevacizumab with nab-paclitaxel and carboplatin for triple-negative MBC were reported [222]. PFS was 9.2 months, CBR was 94%, and ORR was 85%, respectively. The regimen had an acceptable tolerabilty and the most common severe toxicities were neutropenia and thrombocytopenia. These data provide support for the combination treatment of bevacizumab with nab-paclitaxel and carboplatin in first-line TNBC treatment; however, as this was a trial with a small sample population, further studies of this combination are warranted.

The clinical trials of first-line combination therapy of bevacizumab with another molecularly targeted treatment have also been instigated. Preclinical studies have revealed a significant relationship between HER2 and VEGF [223, 224], and in animal models, superior anti-tumor activity was seen in combination of bevacizumab with trastuzumab [225]. From those data, a phase I trial of combination therapy of bevacizumab with trastuzumab was conducted [226]. The clinical activity (one CR and four PR) was seen in 56% patients, and the combination treatment had an acceptable tolerability. From this data, the recommended dosage was a 10 mg/kg of bevacizumab with a 4 mg/kg of trastuzumab and then 2 mg/kg. A phase II study assessed in first-line combination therapy of trastuzumab with bevacizumab in HER2-positive metastatic or locally relapsed breast cancer and surgically-unresectable breast cancer has also been conducted [227]. In that study, a clinical activity was demonstrated in 46% patients, all of them were a PR. These data suggested that the combination of bevacizumab with trastuzumab treatment is an active first-line treatment for HER2-positive MBC. The phase III Avastin (Bevacizumab) in Combination With Herceptin (Trastuzumab)/Docetaxel in Patients With HER2-Positive Metastatic Breast Cancer (AVEREL) study assessed docetaxel plus trastuzumab with or without bevacizumab in patients with HER2-positive, MBC or ABC [228]. Investigator-assessed PFS was 13.7 *vs* 16.5 months without bevacizumab and with bevacizumab groups, respectively (HR 0.82, P = 0.0775). The RR was 70% *vs* 74%, respectively (P = 0.3492). Febrile neutropenia and hypertension were more common with bevacizumab-containing group. High baseline plasma VEGF-A concentrations were related with greater bevacizumab response. Although combination of bevacizumab with docetaxel and trastuzumab did not significantly increase investigator-assessed PFS, the potential predictive value of plasma VEGF-A was found to be consistent with findings in HER2-negative MBC, warranting further evaluation. Efficacy outcomes from clinical trials of bevacizumab in MBC are summarized in Table **10**.

Effects of Bevacizumab in Neoadjuvant or Adjuvant Setting

In order to control micrometastasis by treating anti-angiogenic treatment at an early stage of breast cancer, clinical studies are currently investigating the efficacy of bevacizumab in a neoadjuvant or adjuvant treatment. Two randomized studies have assessed the combination of bevacizumab and conventional neoadjuvant chemotherapy. The phase III GeparQuinto trial randomized 1948 patients to treat neoadjuvant EC followed by docetaxel, with or without bevacizumab in HER2-negative breast cancer [229]. The pCR was 14.9% with chemotherapy alone, and 18.4% with chemothrapy plus bevacizumab (P = 0.04). In the triple negative group, pCR was 27.9% and 39.3% (P = 0.003), respectively. NSABPB-40 was a phase III study in patients with operable HER2-negative breast cancer in neoadjuvant setting. This study evaluated the pCR rate in combination of gemcitabine or capecitabine with docetaxel, followed by AC, and whether addition of bevacizumab to those chemotherapeutic agents would improve the pCR rate [230]. The combination of gemcitabine or capecitabine with docetaxel, as compared with docetaxel monotherapy, did not statistically improve the pCR (P = 0.69); however, the combination of bevacizumab statistically improved the pCR (28.2% without bevacizumab *vs* 34.5% with bevacizumab, P = 0.02). In those two phase III studies, the combination of bevacizumab with neoadjuvant chemotherapy significantly improved the pCR, which is considered to be a useful predictor of long-term outcome.

Table 10. Efficacy Outcomes from Clinical Trials of Bevacizumab in MBC Setting

Investigator (Trial)	Phase	Setting	Regimen	N	Results	Refs.
Cobleigh *et al.*	I/II	Pretreated	B	75	recommended dosage: 10mg/Kg ORR: 9.3%	[208]
Burstein *et al*	II	Pretreated	B+vinorelbine	56	RR: 34%, TTP: 5.5M	[211]
Ramaswamy *et al.*	II	First or second -line	B+DTX	27	ORR: 52%, PFS: 7.5M	[212]
Miller *et al.*	III	Pretreated	B+capecitabine *vs* capecitabine	232 230	RR: 19.8 *vs* 9.1% (*P* = 0.001) PFS: 4.86 *vs* 4.17M (HR 0.98) OS: 15.1 *vs* 14.5M	[213]
Miller *et al.* (ECOG-E2100)	III	First-line	B+PTX *vs* PTX	368 354	ORR: 36.9 *vs* 21.1% (*P*<0.001) PFS: 11.8 *vs* 5.9M (*P*<0.001) OS: 26.7 *vs* 25.2M (*P* = 0.16)	[214]
Miles *et al.* (AVADO)	III	First-line	B(15mg/Kg)+DTX *vs* B(7.5mg/Kg)+DTX *vs* placebo+DTX	247 248 241	ORR: 64 *vs* 55 *vs* 46% (B(15mg/Kg)+DTX *vs* placebo+DTX: *P*<0.001) PFS: 10.0 *vs* 9.0 *vs* 8.1M (B(15mg/Kg)+DTX *vs* placebo+DTX: *P*<0.001) OS: 30.2 *vs* 30.8 *vs* 31.9M	[215]
Robert *et al.* (RIBBON-1)	III	First-line	B+chemotherapy *vs* placebo+chemotherapy	cape cohort 615 Tax/Anthra cohort 622	PFS cape cohort increase from 5.7 to 8.6M (HR 0.69, *P*<0.001) Tax/Anthra cohort increase from 8.0 to 9.2M, (HR 0.64, *P*<0.001) OS: not significant	[216]
Smith *et al.* (ATHENA)	III	First-line	B+taxane-based chemotherapy	2251	ORR: 52%, TTP: 9.5M, OS: 14.6M	[219]
Gianni *et al.* (AVEREL)	III	First-line	B+T+DTX *vs* T+DTX	215 206	investigator-assessed PFS 16.5 *vs* 13.7M (HR 0.82, *P* = 0.0775) RR 74 *vs* 70% (*P* = 0.3492)	[228]

B: bevacizumab; DTX: docetaxel; PTX: paclitaxel; T: trastuzumab; ORR: overall response rate; RR: response rate; TTP: time-to-progression; PFS: progression-free survival; OS: overall survival; cape: capecitabne; HR: hazard ratio; Tax/Anthra: taxane/anthracycline.

In contrast, the BEATRICE study was the phase III study to assess the combination of bevacizumab with chemotherapeutic agents for TNBC in the adjuvant setting [231]. Invasive DFS events were shown 16% in the chemotherapy alone arm and 14% in the bevacizumab additional arm (HR 0.87, P = 0.18). The 3-year invasive DFS was 82.7% with chemotherapy alone and 83.7% with combination of bevacizumab with chemotherapy. No improvement in OS was seen between the arms (HR 0.84, P = 0.23). Combination treatment of bevacizumab with chemotherapy was increased rate of severe hypertension, severe cardiac events, and treatment discontinuation. On the basis of these data, bevacizumab cannot be recommended as adjuvant treatment for primary TNBC. Further follow-up is warranted to determine the potential activity of bevacizumab on OS. Efficacy outcomes of trasuzumab with chemotherapy in neoadjuvant or adjuvant setting are summarized in Table **11**.

Effects of Sunitinib in MBC Setting

Sunitinib (SU11248) is orally-administered, small-molecule multitargeted TKI which includes platelet-derived growth factor (PDGF-R), VEGF receptors, KIT (CD117) and RET which is important factor in tumor angiogenesis and proliferation [232-234]. In phase II study, pretreated with an anthracycline and a taxane patients treated with sunitinib 50 mg/day and the primary end point was ORR [235]. ORR was 11%, TTP was 10 weeks and OS was 38 weeks, and the

Table 11. Efficacy Outcomes from Clinical Trials of Bevacizumab in Early-Stage Breast Cancer

Investigator (Trial)	Phase	Setting	Regimen	N	Results	Refs.
von Minckwitz *et al.* (GeparQuinto trial)	III	Neoadjuvant	EC→DTX+B *vs* EC→DTX	956 969	pCR overall: 18.4 *vs* 14.9% (*P* = 0.04) TNBC: 39.3 *vs* 27.9% (*P* = 0.003)	[229]
Bear *et al.* (NSABP-B-40)	III	Neoadjuvant	B+chemotherapy *vs* chemothrapy	591 595	pCR: 34.5 *vs* 28.2% (*P* = 0.02)	[230]
Cameron *et al.* (BEATRICE)	III	Adjuvant	B+chemotherapy *vs* chemothrapy	1301 1230	Invasive DFS events 188 *vs.* 205 patients (HR 0.87, *P* = 0.18) 3-year Invasive DFS 83.7 *vs* 82.7% (HR 0.84, *P* = 0.23)	[231]

EC: epirubicin +cyclophosphamide; DTX: docetaxel; B: bevacizumab; pCR: pathological complete response; TNBC: triple negative breast cancer; DFS: disease-free survival; HR: hazard ratio.

toxicity was mild to moderate. Another phase II study was assessing the clinical activity of sunitinib (arm A) *vs* no treatment (arm B) with HER2-negative MBC patients [236]. PFS was 2.8 months in arm A and 3.1 months in arm B (P = 0.173), and arm A did not improve the OS (P = 0.749). Severe adverse events were observed in 69% in arm A, and only 11% in arm B. In the phase III trial, multicenter, randomized, open-label trial was compared the activity of sunitinib monotherapy and capecitabine for ABC [237]. The PFS was 2.8 months with sunitinib *vs* 4.2 months with capecitabine (HR 1.47, P = 0.002), OS was 15.3 months *vs* 24.6 months (HR 1.17, P = 0.35), and ORR was 11% *vs* 16% (P = 0.109), respectively. These data demonstrated that inferior efficacy was seen in sunitinib compared with capecitabine in ABC. Two phase III studies of combination therapy of sunitinib with chemotherapy were investigated. Bergh *et al.,* reported the results of sunitinib in combination with docetaxel *vs* docetaxel monotherapy in ABC as a first-line treatment [238]. The PFS was 8.6 months with sunitinib plus docetaxel *vs* 8.3 months with docetaxel monotherapy (HR 0.92, P = 0.265), median OS was 24.8 months *vs* 25.5 months (P = 0.904), and ORR was 55% *vs* 42% (P = 0.001), respectively. Crown *et al.,* conducted the phase III study of combination of sunitinib with capecitabine *vs* capecitabine alone in patients with previously treated MBC [239]. The PFS was 5.5 months with sunitinib plus capecitabine *vs* 5.9 months with capecitabine monotherapy (HR 1.22, P = 0.941). No statistical differences were observed in RR or OS between sunitinib plus capecitabine and capecitabine alone. From these data, it is evident that sunitinib monotherapy or the combination of sunitinib to chemotherapy does not improve the clinical activity for patients with ABC or MBC. Efficacy outcomes of sunitinib in MBC are summarized in Table **12**.

Effects of Sorafenib in MBC Setting

Preclinical studies have demonstrated that sorafenib, an oral small-molecule TKI, suppresses tumor proliferation and angiogenesis [240]. Moreno-Aspitia *et al.,* conducted phase II trial to evaluate efficacy and safety of sorafenib in pretreated MBC patients [241]. Although sorafenib monotherapy had an acceptable tolerability, this single agent did not demonstrate any clinical benefit. Recently, three phase II trial was reported to assess the clinical activity of the combination

Table 12. Efficacy Outcomes from Clinical Trials of Sunitinib in MBC Setting

Investigator (Trial)	Phase	Regimen	N	Results	Refs.
Burstein *et al.*	II	Sunitinib	64	ORR: 11%, TTP: 10 weeks, OS: 38 weeks	[235]
Wildiers *et al.*	II	Sunitinib *vs* No therapy	36 19	PFS 2.8 *vs* 3.1M (*P* = 0.173) OS: *P* = 0.749	[236]
Barrios *et al.*	III	Sunitinib *vs* Capecitabine	238 244	PFS 2.8 *vs* 4.2M (HR 1.47, *P* = 0.002) OS 15.3 *vs* 24.6M (HR 1.17, *P* = 0.350) ORR 11 *vs* 16% (*P* = 0.109)	[237]
Bergh *et al.*	III	Sunitinib+DTX *vs* DTX alone	296 297	PFS 8.6 *vs* 8.3M (HR 0.92, *P* = 0.265) OS 24.8 *vs* 25.5M (*P* = 0.904) ORR 55% *vs* 42% (*P* = 0.001)	[238]
Crown *et al.*	III	Sunitinib+capecitabine *vs* Capecitabine alone	217 215	PFS 5.5 *vs* 5.9M (HR 1.22, *P* = 0.941) OS 16.4 *vs* 16.5M (HR 0.99, *P* = 0.484) ORR 27 *vs* 22% (HR 1.27, *P* = 0.189)	[239]

DTX: docetaxel; ORR: overall response rate; TTP: time-to-progression; OS: overall survival; PFS: progression-free survival; HR: hazard ratio.

of sorafenib with chemotherapy. In one phase II study, patients were treated with capecitabine plus sorafenib or capecitabine plus placebo [242]. The median PFS was 6.4 months with capecitabine plus sorafenib *vs* 4.1 months with capecitabine plus placebo (HR 0.58, P = 0.001), however, there was no significant improvement for ORR and OS. The frequently toxicities in sorafenib arm were rash, diarrhea, mucosal inflammation, neutropenia, hypertention and HFS. Another phase II trial was conducted by Schwartzberg *et al.,* to evaluate adding the sorafenib to gemcitabine or capecitabine in ABC patients who was progressed during/after bevacizumab [243]. The median PFS was 3.4 months with sorafenib plus gemcitabine/capecitabine *vs* 2.7 months with placebo plus gemcitabine/ capecitabine (HR 0.65, P = 0.02), however, there was no significant improvement for ORR and OS. Combination therapy with sorafenib plus gemcitabine/ capecitabine had an acceptable tolerability with dose reductions. Gradishar *et al.,* also reported a phase IIb trial to assess the addition of the sorafenib to paclitaxel for HER2-negative locally recurrent or MBC as a first-line treatment [244]. Sorafenib and paclitaxel combination therapy improved ORR (P = 0.0468), but did not increase the PFS and OS in this study. Toxicity of the combination was manageable with dose reductions [244]. From these data, the addition of sorafenib to chemotherapy was active in patients with MBC. However, further study is needed to confirm the activity of sorafenib in breast cancer patients. The RESILIENCE trial is a multinational, randomized, phase III trial to assess the addition of sorafenib to first- or second-line capecitabine in advanced HER2-negative breast cancer [245], and this trial is underway. Efficacy outcomes of sorafenib in MBC are summarized in Table **13**.

Table 13. Efficacy Outcomes from Clinical Trials of Sorafenib in MBC Setting

Investigator (Trial)	Phase	Regimen	N	Results	Refs.
Moreno-Aspitia *et al.*	II	sorafenib	23	no patients experienced a PR or CR	[241]
Baselga *et al.*	II	capecitabine+sorafenib *vs* capecitabine+placebo	115 114	PFS 6.4 *vs* 4.1M (HR 0.58, *P* = 0.001) OS 22.2 *vs* 20.9M (HR 0.86, *P* = 0.42) ORR 38 *vs* 31% (*P* = 0.25)	[242]
Schwartzberg *et al.*	II	sorafenib+capecitabine or gemcitabine *vs* placebo+capecitabine or gemcitabine	81 79	PFS 3.4 *vs* 2.7M (HR 0.65, *P* = 0.02) OS 13.4 *vs* 11.4M (HR 1.01, *P* = 0.95) ORR 19.8 *vs* 12.7% (*P* = 0.235)	[243]
Gradishar *et al.*	II	PTX+sorafenib *vs* PTX+placebo	119 118	PFS 6.9 *vs* 5.6M (HR 0.788, *P* = 0.1715) OS 16.8 *vs*17.4M (HR 1.022, *P* = 0.904) ORR 67 *vs* 54% (*P* = 0.0468)	[244]

PTX: paclitaxel; PR: partial response; CR: complete response; PFS: progression-free survival; HR: hazard ratio; OS: overall survival; ORR: overall response rate.

CONCLUSION

HER2 blockade has reported in clinical benefit in MBC, adjuvant, and neoadjuvant, settings, and the development of dual HER2 blockade promises effective treatment options for HER2-overexpressing breast cancer patients; thus, clinical guidelines recommend HER2 blockade treatments for HER2-overexpressing breast cancer. In addition to dual HER2 blockade, numerous other agents, including mTOR/PI3K inhibitors, Akt inhibitors, Poly (ADP-ribose) polymerase (PARP) inhibitors, heat shock protein (HSP) 90 inhibitors, and IGF-1R inhibitors, are currently under investigation to increase the effect of treatment in patients with HER2 overexpressing breast cancer. In the near future, as when studies are completed, the role of anti-HER2 therapy in HER2-overexpressing breast cancer will become more clearly elucidated. On the other hand, the role of the anti-angiogenic agent bevacizumab in the treatment of MBC or early-stage breast cancer has not been clearly defined by the current studies, despite its promising results in the treatment of various other cancers such as NSCLC or colon cancer. Randomized trials of bevacizumab adding with chemotherapeutic agents for MBC have reported only modest improvements in PFS compare to chemotherapy alone with no OS advantage. Further studies are warranted to confirm whether long-term administration of bevacizumab will show significant improvement in MBC. In the early-stage breast cancer setting, the BETH (NSABP B-44) trial and the ECOG-E5103 trial are ongoing phase III studies in adjuvant setting for lymph node positive or lymph node negative with high risk breast cancer [246, 247]. The results of those trials are expected to determine the role of bevacizumab in an adjuvant setting for early-stage breast cancer. Moreover, small molecule oral TKIs including axitinib, pazopanib, motesanib *etc.* are under investigation as new anti-angiogenic agents [248]. Ongoing trials will be confirming a clear clinical activity for anti-angiogenic drugs in the therapeutic strategy of breast cancer. In the future, we may be able to develop biomarkers that may be useful to identify which patients well benefit from anti-HER2 or anti-angiogenic therapies, and we will thus be able to provide individualized therapy for breast cancer patients.

ACKNOWLEDGEMENTS

We would like to thank Izumi Kawaguchi and Eriko Matsuo for their invaluable help in completing this article.

CONFLICT OF INTEREST

The author confirms that this chapter contents have no conflict of interest.

REFERENCES

[1] Schlotter CM, Vogt U, Allgayer H, Brandt B. Molecular targeted therapies for breast cancer treatment. Breast Cancer Res 2008; 10(4): 211.

[2] Witton CJ, Reeves JR, Going JJ, Cooke TG, Bartlett JM. Expression of the HER1-4 family of receptor tyrosine kinases in breast cancer. J Pathol 2003; 200(3): 290-7.

[3] Koutras AK, Fountzilas G, Kalogeras KT, Starakis I, Iconomou G, Kalofonos HP. The upgraded role of HER3 and HER4 receptors in breast cancer. Crit Rev Oncol Hematol 2010; 74(2): 73-8.

[4] Olayioye MA, Neve RM, Lane HA, Hynes NE. The ErbB signaling network: receptor heterodimerization in development and cancer. EMBO J 2000; 19(13): 3159-67.

[5] Burgess AW, Cho HS, Eigenbrot C, Ferguson KM, Garrett TP, Leahy DJ, Lemmon MA, Sliwkowski MX, Ward CW, Yokoyama S. An open-and-shut case? Recent insights into the activation of EGF/ErbB receptors. Mol Cell 2003; 12(3): 541-52.

[6] Hynes NE, Lane HA. ERBB receptors and cancer: the complexity of targeted inhibitors. Nat Rev Cancer 2005; 5(5): 341-54.

[7] Cho HS, Leahy DJ. Structure of the extracellular region of HER3 reveals an interdomain tether. Science 2002; 297(5585): 1330-3.

[8] Ferguson KM, Berger MB, Mendrola JM, Cho HS, Leahy DJ, Lemmon MA. EGF activates its receptor by removing interactions that autoinhibit ectodomain dimerization. Mol Cell 2003; 11(2): 507-17.

[9] Ogiso H, Ishitani R, Nureki O, *et al.* Crystal structure of the complex of human epidermal growth factor and receptor extracellular domains. Cell 2002; 110(6): 775-87.

[10] Yarden Y, Sliwkowski MX. Untangling the ErbB signalling network. Nat Rev Mol Cell Biol 2001; 2(2): 127-37.

[11] Ghosh R, Narasanna A, Wang SE, *et al.* Trastuzumab has preferential activity against breast cancers driven by HER2 homodimers. Cancer Res 2011; 71(5): 1871-82.

[12] Sergina NV, Rausch M, Wang D, *et al.* Escape from HER-family tyrosine kinase inhibitor therapy by the kinase-inactive HER3. Nature 2007; 445(7126): 437-41.

[13] Atalay G, Cardoso F, Awada A, Piccart MJ. Novel therapeutic strategies targeting the epidermal growth factor receptor (EGFR) family and its downstream effectors in breast cancer. Ann Oncol 2003; 14(9): 1346-63.

[14] Lin NU, Winer EP. New targets for therapy in breast cancer: small molecule tyrosine kinase inhibitors. Breast Cancer Res 2004; 6(5): 204-10.

[15] Rosen LS, Ashurst HL, Chap L. Targeting signal transduction pathways in metastatic breast cancer: a comprehensive review. Oncologist 2010; 15(3): 216-35.

[16] Russo SM, Ove R. Molecular targets as therapeutic strategies in the management of breast cancer. Expert Opin Ther Targets 2003; 7(4): 543-57.

[17] Cho HS, Mason K, Ramyar KX, *et al.* Structure of the extracellular region of HER2 alone and in complex with the Herceptin Fab. Nature.2003; 421(6924): 756-60.

[18] Clynes RA, Towers TL, Presta LG, Ravetch JV. Inhibitory Fc receptors modulate *in vivo* cytotoxicity against tumor targets. Nat Med 2000; 6(4): 443-6.

[19] NCCN Clinical Practice Guidelines in Oncology (NCCN Guidelines)® Breast Cancer Version 1. 2014 Available from: http://www.nccn.org/professionals/physician_gls/pdf/breast.pdf [Cited: 30 Jan 2014].

[20] Baselga J, Tripathy D, Mendelsohn J, *et al.* Phase II study of weekly intravenous trastuzumab (Herceptin) in patients with HER2/neu-overexpressing metastatic breast cancer. Semin Oncol 1999; 26(4 Suppl 12): 78-83.

[21] Cobleigh MA, Vogel CL, Tripathy D, *et al.* Multinational study of the efficacy and safety of humanized anti-HER2 monoclonal antibody in women who have HER2-overexpressing metastatic breast cancer that has progressed after chemotherapy for metastatic disease. J Clin Oncol 1999; 17(9): 2639-48.

[22] Vogel CL, Cobleigh MA, Tripathy D, *et al.* Efficacy and safety of trastuzumab as a single agent in first-line treatment of HER2-overexpressing metastatic breast cancer. J Clin Oncol 2002; 20(3): 719-26.

[23] Baselga J, Carbonell X, Castañeda-Soto NJ, *et al.* Phase II study of efficacy, safety, and pharmacokinetics of trastuzumab monotherapy administered on a 3-weekly schedule. J Clin Oncol 2005; 23(10): 2162-71.

[24] Slamon DJ, Leyland-Jones B, Shak S, *et al.* Use of chemotherapy plus a monoclonal antibody against HER2 for metastatic breast cancer that overexpresses HER2. N Engl J Med 2001; 344(11): 783-92.

[25] Marty M, Cognetti F, Maraninchi D, *et al.* Randomized phase II trial of the efficacy and safety of trastuzumab combined with docetaxel in patients with human epidermal growth factor receptor 2-positive metastatic breast cancer administered as first-line treatment: the M77001 study group. J Clin Oncol 2005; 23(19): 4265-74.

[26] Pegram MD, Finn RS, Arzoo K, Beryt M, Pietras RJ, Slamon DJ. The effect of HER-2/neu overexpression on chemotherapeutic drug sensitivity in human breast and ovarian cancer cells. Oncogene 1997; 15(5): 537-47.

[27] Pegram M, Hsu S, Lewis G, *et al.* Inhibitory effects of combinations of HER-2/neu antibody and chemotherapeutic agents used for treatment of human breast cancers. Oncogene 1999; 18(13): 2241-51.

[28] Pegram MD, Konecny GE, O'Callaghan C, Beryt M, Pietras R, Slamon DJ. Rational combinations of trastuzumab with chemotherapeutic drugs used in the treatment of breast cancer. J Natl Cancer Inst 2004; 96(10): 739-49.

[29] Pietras RJ, Pegram MD, Finn RS, Maneval DA, Slamon DJ. Remission of human breast cancer xenografts on therapy with humanized monoclonal antibody to HER-2 receptor and DNA-reactive drugs. Oncogene 1998; 17(17): 2235-49.

[30] Pegram MD, Pienkowski T, Northfelt DW, *et al.* Results of two open-label, multicenter phase II studies of docetaxel, platinum salts, and trastuzumab in HER2-positive advanced breast cancer. J Natl Cancer Inst 2004; 96(10): 759-69.

[31] Robert N, Leyland-Jones B, Asmar L, *et al.* Randomized phase III study of trastuzumab, paclitaxel, and carboplatin compared with trastuzumab and paclitaxel in women with HER-2-overexpressing metastatic breast cancer. J Clin Oncol 2006; 24(18): 2786-92.

[32] Valero V, Forbes J, Pegram MD, *et al.* Multicenter phase III randomized trial comparing docetaxel and trastuzumab with docetaxel, carboplatin, and trastuzumab as first-line chemotherapy for patients with HER2-gene-amplified metastatic breast cancer (BCIRG 007 study): two highly active therapeutic regimens. J Clin Oncol 2011; 29(2): 149-56.

[33] Burstein HJ, Keshaviah A, Baron AD, *et al.* Trastuzumab plus vinorelbine or taxane chemotherapy for HER2-overexpressing metastatic breast cancer: the trastuzumab and vinorelbine or taxane study. Cancer 2007; 110(5): 965-72.

[34] Andersson M, Lidbrink E, Bjerre K, *et al.* Phase III randomized study comparing docetaxel plus trastuzumab with vinorelbine plus trastuzumab as first-line therapy of metastatic or locally advanced human epidermal growth factor receptor 2-positive breast cancer: the HERNATA study. J Clin Oncol 2011; 29(3): 264-71.

[35] Wagstaff AJ, Ibbotson T, Goa KL. Capecitabine: a review of its pharmacology and therapeutic efficacy in the management of advanced breast cancer. Drugs 2003; 63(2): 217-36.

[36] Fujimoto-Ouchi K, Sekiguchi F, Tanaka Y. Antitumor activity of combinations of anti-HER-2 antibody trastuzumab and oral fluoropyrimidines capecitabine/5'-dFUrd in human breast cancer models. Cancer Chemother Pharmacol 2002; 49(3): 211-6.

[37] Schaller G, Fuchs I, Gonsch T, *et al.* Phase II study of capecitabine plus trastuzumab in human epidermal growth factor receptor 2 overexpressing metastatic breast cancer pretreated with anthracyclines or taxanes. J Clin Oncol 2007; 25(22): 3246-50.

[38] Yamamoto D, Iwase S, Kitamura K, Odagiri H, Yamamoto C, Nagumo Y. A phase II study of trastuzumab and capecitabine for patients with HER2-overexpressing metastatic breast cancer: Japan Breast Cancer Research Network (JBCRN) 00 Trial. Cancer Chemother Pharmacol 2008; 61(3): 509-14.

[39] Yardley DA, Burris HA 3rd, Hanson S, *et al.* Weekly gemcitabine and trastuzumab in the treatment of patients with HER2-overexpressing metastatic breast cancer. Clin Breast Cancer 2009; 9(3): 178-83.

[40] Mini E, Nobili S, Caciagli B, Landini I, Mazzei T. Cellular pharmacology of gemcitabine. Ann Oncol 2006; 17 Suppl 5: v7-12.

[41] Wilks S, Puhalla S, O'Shaughnessy J, *et al.* Phase 2, multicenter, single-arm study of eribulin mesylate + trastuzumab as first-line therapy for locally recurrent or metastatic HER2-positive breast cancer. San Antonio Breast Cancer Symposium 2013 (abstr: P4-12-12)

[42] Romond EH, Perez EA, Bryant J, *et al.* Trastuzumab plus adjuvant chemotherapy for operable HER2-positive breast cancer. N Engl J Med 2005; 353(16): 1673-84.

[43] Gianni L, Dafni U, Gelber RD, *et al.* Herceptin Adjuvant (HERA) Trial Study Team. Treatment with trastuzumab for 1 year after adjuvant chemotherapy in patients with HER2-positive early breast cancer: a 4-year follow-up of a randomised controlled trial. Lancet Oncol 2011; 12(3): 236-44.

[44] Slamon D, Eiermann W, Robert N, *et al.* Breast Cancer International Research Group. Adjuvant trastuzumab in HER2-positive breast cancer. N Engl J Med 2011; 365(14): 1273-83.

[45] Joensuu H, Kellokumpu-Lehtinen PL, Bono P, *et al.* FinHer Study Investigators. Adjuvant docetaxel or vinorelbine with or without trastuzumab for breast cancer. N Engl J Med 2006; 354(8): 809-20.

[46] Goldhirsch A, Winer EP, Coates AS, *et al.* Panel members. Personalizing the treatment of women with early breast cancer: highlights of the St Gallen International Expert Consensus on the Primary Therapy of Early Breast Cancer 2013. Ann Oncol 2013; 24(9): 2206-23.

[47] Gonzalez-Angulo AM, Litton JK, Broglio KR, *et al.* High risk of recurrence for patients with breast cancer who have human epidermal growth factor receptor 2-positive, node-negative tumors 1 cm or smaller. J Clin Oncol 2009; 27(34): 5700-6.

[48] McArthur HL, Mahoney KM, Morris PG, *et al.* Adjuvant trastuzumab with chemotherapy is effective in women with small, node-negative, HER2-positive breast cancer. Cancer 2011; 117(24): 5461-8.

[49] Goldhirsch A, Gelber RD, Piccart-Gebhart MJ, *et al.* Herceptin Adjuvant (HERA) Trial Study Team. 2 years *versus* 1 year of adjuvant trastuzumab for HER2-positive breast cancer (HERA): an open-label, randomised controlled trial. Lancet 2013; 382(9897): 1021-8.

[50] Pivot X, Romieu G, Debled M, *et al.* PHARE trial investigators. 6 months *versus* 12 months of adjuvant trastuzumab for patients with HER2-positive early breast cancer (PHARE): a randomised phase 3 trial. Lancet Oncol 2013; 14(8): 741-8.

[51] Sawaki M, Tokudome N, Mizuno T, *et al.* Evaluation of trastuzumab without chemotherapy as a post-operative adjuvant therapy in HER2-positive elderly breast cancer patients: randomized controlled trial [RESPECT (N-SAS BC07)]. Jpn J Clin Oncol 2011; 41(5): 709-12.

[52] Mauri D, Pavlidis N, Ioannidis JP. Neoadjuvant *versus* adjuvant systemic treatment in breast cancer: a meta-analysis. J Natl Cancer Inst 2005; 97(3): 188-94.

[53] Untch M, Fasching PA, Konecny GE, *et al.* Pathologic complete response after neoadjuvant chemotherapy plus trastuzumab predicts favorable survival in human epidermal growth factor receptor 2-overexpressing breast cancer: results from the TECHNO trial of the AGO and GBG study groups. J Clin Oncol 2011; 29(25): 3351-7.

[54] Buzdar AU, Ibrahim NK, Francis D, *et al.* Significantly higher pathologic complete remission rate after neoadjuvant therapy with trastuzumab, paclitaxel, and epirubicin chemotherapy: results of a randomized trial in human epidermal growth factor receptor 2-positive operable breast cancer. J Clin Oncol 2005; 23(16): 3676-85.

[55] Buzdar AU, Valero V, Ibrahim NK, *et al.* Neoadjuvant therapy with paclitaxel followed by 5-fluorouracil, epirubicin, and cyclophosphamide chemotherapy and concurrent trastuzumab in human epidermal growth factor receptor 2-positive operable breast cancer: an update of the initial randomized study population and data of additional patients treated with the same regimen. Clin Cancer Res 2007; 13(1): 228-33.

[56] Steger G, Greil R, Jakesz R, *et al.* Finsl results of ABCSG-24, a randomized phase III study comparing epirubicin, docetaxel and capecitabine (EDC) to epirubicin and docetaxel (ED) as neoadjuvant treatment for early breast cancer and Comparing ED/EDC+ Trastuzumab (T) to ED/EDC as neoadjuvant treatment for early HER-2 positive breast cancer. Cancer Res 69, 2009 (suppl; abstr 1081).

[57] Gianni L, Eiermann W, Semiglazov V, *et al.* Neoadjuvant chemotherapy with trastuzumab followed by adjuvant trastuzumab *versus* neoadjuvant chemotherapy alone, in patients with HER2-positive locally advanced breast cancer (the NOAH trial): a randomised controlled superiority trial with a parallel HER2-negative cohort. Lancet 2010; 375(9712): 377-84.

[58] Untch M, Rezai M, Loibl S, Fasching PA, Huober J, Tesch H, Bauerfeind I, Hilfrich J, Eidtmann H, Gerber B, Hanusch C, Kühn T, du Bois A, Blohmer JU, Thomssen C, Dan Costa S, Jackisch C, Kaufmann M, Mehta K, von Minckwitz G. Neoadjuvant treatment with trastuzumab in HER2-positive breast cancer: results from the GeparQuattro study. J Clin Oncol 2010; 28(12): 2024-31.

[59] Pierga JY, Delaloge S, Espié M, Brain E, Sigal-Zafrani B, Mathieu MC, Bertheau P, Guinebretière JM, Spielmann M, Savignoni A, Marty M. A multicenter randomized phase II study of sequential epirubicin/cyclophosphamide followed by docetaxel with or without celecoxib or trastuzumab according to HER2 status, as primary chemotherapy for localized invasive breast cancer patients. Breast Cancer Res Treat 2010; 122(2): 429-37.

[60] Im SA, Lee KS, Ro J, Lee ES, Kwon Y, Ahn JH, Ahn JS, Kim JH, Kang HS, Shin KH, Noh DY, Park IA, Kim SB, Im YH, Ha SW. Phase II trial of preoperative paclitaxel, gemcitabine, and trastuzumab combination therapy in HER2 positive stage II/III breast cancer: the Korean Cancer Study Group BR 07-01. Breast Cancer Res Treat 2012; 132(2): 589-600.

[61] Buzdar A, Suman VJ, Meric-Bernstam F, Leitch AM, Ellis MJ, Boughey JC, Unzeitig GW, Royce M, Hunt K. ACOSOG Z1041 (Alliance): Definitive analysis of randomized neoadjuvant trial comparing FEC followed by paclitaxel plus trastuzumab (FEC → P+T) with paclitaxel plus trastuzumab followed by FEC plus trastuzumab (P+T → FEC+T) in HER2+ operable breast cancer. J Clin Oncol 31, 2013 (suppl; abstr 502).

[62] Valachis A, Mauri D, Polyzos NP, Chlouverakis G, Mavroudis D, Georgoulias V. Trastuzumab combined to neoadjuvant chemotherapy in patients with HER2-positive breast cancer: a systematic review and meta-analysis. Breast 2011; 20(6): 485-90.

[63] Schwartzberg LS, Tauer KW, Hermann RC, Nikolinakos PG, Houts AC. Phase I/II study of neoadjuvant carboplatin, eribulin mesylate, and trastuzumab (ECH) for operable HER2 positive (HER2+) breast cancer. J Clin Oncol 31, 2013 (suppl; abstr TPS659).

[64] ClinicalTrials.gov. Study of Neoadjuvant Carboplatin, Eribulin and Trastuzumab for Operable HER2 Positive Breast Cancer. Available from: http://clinicaltrials.gov/ct2/show/ NCT01388647?term = breast+cancer+trastuzumab+eribulin&rank = 2 [cited: 25th Nov 2013].

[65] Junttila TT, Li G, Parsons K, Phillips GL, Sliwkowski MX. Trastuzumab-DM1 (T-DM1) retains all the mechanisms of action of trastuzumab and efficiently inhibits growth of lapatinib insensitive breast cancer. Breast Cancer Res Treat 2011; 128(2): 347-56.

[66] Lewis Phillips GD, Li G, Dugger DL, Crocker LM, Parsons KL, Mai E, Blättler WA, Lambert JM, Chari RV, Lutz RJ, Wong WL, Jacobson FS, Koeppen H, Schwall RH, Kenkare-Mitra SR, Spencer SD, Sliwkowski MX. Targeting HER2-positive breast cancer with trastuzumab-DM1, an antibody-cytotoxic drug conjugate. Cancer Res 2008; 68(22): 9280-90.

[67] Kovtun YV, Audette CA, Ye Y, Xie H, Ruberti MF, Phinney SJ, Leece BA, Chittenden T, Blättler WA, Goldmacher *VS* Antibody-drug conjugates designed to eradicate tumors with homogeneous and heterogeneous expression of the target antigen. Cancer Res 2006; 66(6): 3214-21.

[68] Barok M, Tanner M, Köninki K, Isola J. Trastuzumab-DM1 causes tumour growth inhibition by mitotic catastrophe in trastuzumab-resistant breast cancer cells *in vivo*. Breast Cancer Res 2011; 13(2): R46.

[69] Krop IE, Beeram M, Modi S, Jones SF, Holden SN, Yu W, Girish S, Tibbitts J, Yi JH, Sliwkowski MX, Jacobson F, Lutzker SG, Burris HA. Phase I study of trastuzumab-DM1, an HER2 antibody-drug conjugate, given every 3 weeks to patients with HER2-positive metastatic breast cancer. J Clin Oncol 2010; 28(16): 2698-704.

[70] Burris HA 3rd, Rugo HS, Vukelja SJ, Vogel CL, Borson RA, Limentani S, Tan-Chiu E, Krop IE, Michaelson RA, Girish S, Amler L, Zheng M, Chu YW, Klencke B, O'Shaughnessy JA. Phase II study of the antibody drug conjugate trastuzumab-DM1 for the treatment of human epidermal growth factor receptor 2 (HER2)-positive breast cancer after prior HER2-directed therapy. J Clin Oncol 2011; 29(4): 398-405.

[71] Krop IE, LoRusso P, Miller KD, Modi S, Yardley D, Rodriguez G, Guardino E, Lu M, Zheng M, Girish S, Amler L, Winer EP, Rugo HS. A phase II study of trastuzumab emtansine in patients with human epidermal growth factor receptor 2-positive metastatic breast cancer who were previously treated with trastuzumab, lapatinib, an anthracycline, a taxane, and capecitabine. J Clin Oncol 2012; 30(26): 3234-41.

[72] Hurvitz SA, Dirix L, Kocsis J, Bianchi GV, Lu J, Vinholes J, Guardino E, Song C, Tong B, Ng V, Chu YW, Perez EA. Phase II randomized study of trastuzumab emtansine *versus* trastuzumab plus docetaxel in patients with human epidermal growth factor receptor 2-positive metastatic breast cancer. J Clin Oncol 2013; 31(9): 1157-63.

[73] Verma S, Miles D, Gianni L, Krop IE, Welslau M, Baselga J, Pegram M, Oh DY, Diéras V, Guardino E, Fang L, Lu MW, Olsen S, Blackwell K; EMILIA Study Group. Trastuzumab emtansine for HER2-positive advanced breast cancer. N Engl J Med 2012; 367(19): 1783-91.

[74] Geyer CE, Forster J, Lindquist D, Chan S, Romieu CG, Pienkowski T, Jagiello-Gruszfeld A, Crown J, Chan A, Kaufman B, Skarlos D, Campone M, Davidson N, Berger M, Oliva C, Rubin SD, Stein S, Cameron D. Lapatinib plus capecitabine for HER2-positive advanced breast cancer. N Engl J Med 2006; 355(26): 2733-43.

[75] ClinicalTrials.gov. A Study of Trastuzumab Emtansine (T-DM1) Sequentially With Anthracycline-Based Chemotherapy, As Adjuvant or Neoadjuvant Therapy for Patients With Early Stage HER2-Positive Breast Cancer. Available from: URL: http://clinicaltrials.gov/ct2/show/NCT01196052?term = NCT01196052&rank = 1 [Cited: 15th Dec 2013].

[76] ClinicalTrials.gov. A Study of Trastuzumab Emtansine *versus* Trastuzumab as Adjuvant Therapy in Patients With HER2-Positive Breast Cancer Who Have Residual Tumor in the Breast or Axillary Lymph Nodes Following Preoperative Therapy (KATHERINE). Available from: http://clinicaltrials.gov/ct2/show/NCT01772472?term = NCT01772472&rank = 1 [Cited: 15th Dec 2013].

[77] ClinicalTrials.gov. A Prospective, Randomized Multicenter, Open-label Comparison of Preoperative Trastuzumab Emtansine (T-DM1) With or Without Standard Endocrine Therapy *vs* Trastuzumab With Standard Endocrine Therapy Given for Twelve Weeks in Patients With Operable HER2+/HR+ Breast Cancer Within the ADAPT Protocol. (ADAPT; T-DM1). Available from: http://clinicaltrials.gov/ct2/show/NCT01745965?term = T-DM1+breast+cancer&rank = 5 [Cited: 15th Dec 2013].

[78] Ritter CA, Perez-Torres M, Rinehart C, Guix M, Dugger T, Engelman JA, Arteaga CL. Human breast cancer cells selected for resistance to trastuzumab *in vivo* overexpress epidermal growth factor receptor and ErbB ligands and remain dependent on the ErbB receptor network. Clin Cancer Res 2007; 13(16): 4909-19.

[79] Adams CW, Allison DE, Flagella K, Presta L, Clarke J, Dybdal N, McKeever K, Sliwkowski MX. Humanization of a recombinant monoclonal antibody to produce a therapeutic HER dimerization inhibitor, pertuzumab. Cancer Immunol Immunother 2006; 55(6): 717-27.

[80] Franklin MC, Carey KD, Vajdos FF, Leahy DJ, de Vos AM, Sliwkowski, MX. Insights into ErbB signaling from the structure of the ErbB2-pertuzumab complex. Cancer Cell 2004; 5(4): 317-28.

[81] Hughes JB, Berger C, Rødland MS, Hasmann M, Stang E, Madshus IH. Pertuzumab increases epidermal growth factor receptor down-regulation by counteracting epidermal growth factor receptor-ErbB2 heterodimerization. Mol Cancer Ther 2009; 8(7): 1885-92.

[82] Scheuer W, Friess T, Burtscher H, Bossenmaier B, Endl J, Hasmann M. Strongly enhanced antitumor activity of trastuzumab and pertuzumab combination treatment on HER2-positive human xenograft tumor models. Cancer Res 2009; 69(24): 9330-6.

[83] Agus DB, Gordon MS, Taylor C, Natale RB, Karlan B, Mendelson DS, Press MF, Allison DE, Sliwkowski MX, Lieberman G, Kelsey SM, Fyfe G. Phase I clinical study of pertuzumab, a novel HER dimerization inhibitor, in patients with advanced cancer. J Clin Oncol 2005; 23(11): 2534-43.

[84] Cortes J, Baselga J, Petrella T, Gelmon K, Fumoleau P, Verma S, Pivot X, Ross G, Szado T, Gianni L. Pertuzumab monotherapy following trastuzumab-based treatment: activity and tolerability in patients with advanced HER2 positive breast cancer. J Clin Oncol 46, 2009. (suppl; abstr 1022).

[85] Gianni L, Lladó, A, Bianchi G, Cortes J, Kellokumpu-Lehtinen PL, Cameron DA, Miles D, Salvagni S, Wardley A, Goeminne JC, Hersberger V, Baselga J. Open-label, phase II, multicenter, randomized study of the efficacy and safety of two dose levels of Pertuzumab, a human epidermal growth factor receptor 2 dimerization inhibitor, in patients with human epidermal growth factor receptor 2-negative metastatic breast cancer. J Clin Oncol 2010; 28(7): 1131-7.

[86] Hubbard, SR. EGF receptor inhibition: attacks on multiple fronts. Cancer Cell 2005; 7(4): 287-8.

[87] Portera CC, Walshe JM, Rosing DR, Denduluri N, Berman AW, Vatas U, Velarde M, Chow CK, Steinberg SM, Nguyen D, Yang SX, Swain SM. Cardiac toxicity and efficacy of trastuzumab combined with pertuzumab in patients with [corrected] human epidermal growth factor receptor 2-positive metastatic breast cancer. Clin Cancer Res 2008; 14(9): 2710-6.

[88] Baselga J, Gelmon KA, Verma S, Wardley A, Conte P, Miles D, Bianchi G, Cortes J, McNally VA, Ross GA, Fumoleau P, Gianni L. Phase II trial of pertuzumab and trastuzumab in patients with human epidermal growth factor receptor 2-positive metastatic breast cancer that progressed during prior trastuzumab therapy. J Clin Oncol 2010; 28(7): 1138-44.

[89] Cortés J, Fumoleau P, Bianchi GV, Petrella TM, Gelmon K, Pivot X, Verma S, Albanell J, Conte P, Lluch A, Salvagni S, Servent V, Gianni L, Scaltriti M, Ross GA, Dixon J, Szado T, Baselga J. Pertuzumab monotherapy after trastuzumab-based treatment and subsequent reintroduction of trastuzumab: activity and tolerability in patients with advanced human epidermal growth factor receptor 2-positive breast cancer. J Clin Oncol 2012; 30(14): 1594-600.

[90] Baselga J, Cortés J, Kim SB, Im SA, Hegg R, Im YH, Roman L, Pedrini JL, Pienkowski T, Knott A, Clark E, Benyunes MC, Ross G, Swain SM; CLEOPATRA Study Group. Pertuzumab plus trastuzumab plus docetaxel for metastatic breast cancer. N Engl J Med 2012; 366(2): 109-19.

[91] Swain SM, Kim SB, Cortés J, Ro J, Semiglazov V, Campone M, Ciruelos E, Ferrero JM, Schneeweiss A, Knott A, Clark E, Ross G, Benyunes MC, Baselga J. Pertuzumab, trastuzumab, and docetaxel for HER2-positive metastatic breast cancer (CLEOPATRA study): overall survival results from a randomised, double-blind, placebo-controlled, phase 3 study. Lancet Oncol 2013; 14(6): 461-71.

[92] ClinicalTrials.gov. A study of a combination of trastuzumab and capecitabine with or without pertuzumab in patients with HER2-positive metastatic breast cancer (PHEREXA). Available from: http://clinicaltrials.gov/ct2/show/NCT01026142?term = pertuzumab+breast+cancer&rank = 7 [Cited: 22th Dec 2013].

[93] ClinicalTrials.gov. A Study of Pertuzumab in Combination With Herceptin (Trastuzumab) And Vinorelbine in First Line in Patients With Metastatic or Locally Advanced HER2-Positive Breast Cancer. Available from: http://clinicaltrials.gov/ct2/show/NCT01565083?term = NCT01565083&rank = 1 [Cited: 22th Dec 2013].

[94] Datko FM, D'Andrea G, Dickler MN, Goldfarb SB, Theodoulou M, Lake D, Fornier MN, Shanu Modi S, Fasano J, Comen EA, Gajria D, Moynahan ME, Traina TA, Chen M, Hamilton N, Patil S, Chandarlapaty S, Hudis C, Dang CT. Phase II study of pertuzumab, trastuzumab, and weekly paclitaxel in patients with HER2-overexpressing metastatic breast cancer (MBC). J Clin Oncol 31, 2013 (suppl; abstr 606).

[95] Miller K, Gianni L, Andre F, Dieras V, Mahtani RL, Harbeck N, Huang JE, Shih T, Choi Y, Burris HA III. A phase Ib/II trial of trastuzumab-DM1 (T-DM1) with pertuzumab (P) for women with HER2-positive, locally advanced or metastatic breast cancer (BC) who were previously treated with trastuzumab (T). J Clin Oncol 28, 2010 (suppl; abstr 1012).

[96] Diéras V, Harbeck N, Albain K, Burris H, Awada A, Crivellari D, Andre F, Choi YJ, Huang J, Miller KD. A phase Ib/II trial of trastuzumab-DM1 with pertuzumab for patients with HER2-Positive, locally advanced or metastatic breast cancer: interim efficacy and safety results. Cancer Res 70, 2010 (suppl; abstr P3-14-01).

[97] ClinicalTrials.gov. A study of trastuzumab emtansine (T-DM1) plus pertuzumab/pertuzumab placebo *versus* trastuzumab [herceptin] plus a taxane in patients with metastatic breast cancer (MARIANNE). Available from: http://clinicaltrials.gov/ct2/show/NCT01120184?term = MARIANNE&rank = 3 [Cited: 22th Dec 2013].
[98] Nahta R, Esteva FJ. Herceptin: mechanisms of action and resistance. Cancer Lett 2006; 232(2): 123-38.
[99] Gianni L, Pienkowski T, Im YH, Roman L, Tseng LM, Liu MC, Lluch A, Staroslawska E, de la Haba-Rodriguez J, Im SA, Pedrini JL, Poirier B, Morandi P, Semiglazov V, Srimuninnimit V, Bianchi G, Szado T, Ratnayake J, Ross G, Valagussa P. Efficacy and safety of neoadjuvant pertuzumab and trastuzumab in women with locally advanced, inflammatory, or early HER2-positive breast cancer (NeoSphere): a randomised multicentre, open-label, phase 2 trial. Lancet Oncol 2012; 13(1): 25-32.
[100] ClinicalTrials.gov. A Study of pertuzumab in addition to chemotherapy and herceptin (trastuzumab) as adjuvant therapy in patients with HER2-positive primary breast cancer. Available from: http://clinicaltrials.gov/ct2/show/NCT01358877?term = NCT01358877&rank = 1 [Cited: 22th Jan 2014].
[101] De Mattos-Arruda L, Cortes J. Use of pertuzumab for the treatment of HER2-positive metastatic breast cancer. Adv Ther 2013; 30(7): 645-58.
[102] Lackey KE. Lessons from the drug discovery of lapatinib, a dual ErbB1/2 tyrosine kinase inhibitor. Curr Top Med Chem 2006; 6(5): 435-60.
[103] Xia W, Mullin RJ, Keith BR, Liu LH, Ma H, Rusnak DW, Owens G, Alligood KJ, Spector NL. Anti-tumor activity of GW572016: a dual tyrosine kinase inhibitor blocks EGF activation of EGFR/erbB2 and downstream Erk1/2 and AKT pathways. Oncogene 2002; 21(41): 6255-63.
[104] Nagata Y, Lan KH, Zhou X, Tan M, Esteva FJ, Sahin AA, Klos KS, Li P, Monia BP, Nguyen NT, Hortobagyi GN, Hung MC, Yu D. PTEN activation contributes to tumor inhibition by trastuzumab, and loss of PTEN predicts trastuzumab resistance in patients. Cancer Cell 2004; 6(2): 117-27.
[105] Nahta R, Yuan LX, Zhang B, Kobayashi R, Esteva FJ. Insulin-like growth factor-I receptor/human epidermal growth factor receptor 2 heterodimerization contributes to trastuzumab resistance of breast cancer cells. Cancer Res 2005; 65(23): 11118-28.
[106] Xia W, Husain I, Liu L, Bacus S, Saini S, Spohn J, Pry K, Westlund R, Stein SH, Spector NL. Lapatinib antitumor activity is not dependent upon phosphatase and tensin homologue deleted on chromosome 10 in ErbB2-overexpressing breast cancers. Cancer Res 2007; 67(3): 1170-5.
[107] Nahta R, Yuan LX, Du Y, Esteva FJ. Lapatinib induces apoptosis in trastuzumab-resistant breast cancer cells: effects on insulin-like growth factor I signaling. Mol Cancer Ther 2007; 6(2): 667-74.
[108] Scaltriti M, Rojo F, Ocaña A, Anido J, Guzman M, Cortes J, Di Cosimo S, Matias-Guiu X, Ramon y Cajal S, Arribas J, Baselga J. Expression of p95HER2, a truncated form of the HER2 receptor, and response to anti-HER2 therapies in breast cancer. J Natl Cancer Inst 2007; 99(8): 628-38.

[109] Vogel C, Chan A, Gril B, Kim SB, Kurebayashi J, Liu L, Lu YS, Moon H. Management of ErbB2-positive breast cancer: insights from preclinical and clinical studies with lapatinib. Jpn J Clin Oncol 2010; 40(11): 999-1013.

[110] Blackwell KL, Pegram MD, Tan-Chiu E, Schwartzberg LS, Arbushites MC, Maltzman JD, Forster JK, Rubin SD, Stein SH, Burstein HJ. Single-agent lapatinib for HER2-overexpressing advanced or metastatic breast cancer that progressed on first- or second-line trastuzumab-containing regimens. Ann Oncol 2009; 20(6): 1026-31.

[111] Gomez HL, Doval DC, Chavez MA, Ang PC, Aziz Z, Nag S, Ng C, Franco SX, Chow LW, Arbushites MC, Casey MA, Berger MS, Stein SH, Sledge GW. Efficacy and safety of lapatinib as first-line therapy for ErbB2-amplified locally advanced or metastatic breast cancer. J Clin Oncol 2008; 26(18): 2999-3005.

[112] Di Leo A, Gomez HL, Aziz Z, Zvirbule Z, Bines J, Arbushites MC, Guerrera SF, Koehler M, Oliv C, Stein SH, Williams LS, Dering J, Finn RS, Press MF. Phase III, double-blind, randomized study comparing lapatinib plus paclitaxel with placebo plus paclitaxel as first-line treatment for metastatic breast cancer. J Clin Oncol 2008; 26(34): 5544-52.

[113] Konecny GE, Pegram MD, Venkatesan N, Finn R, Yang G, Rahmeh M, Untch M, Rusnak DW, Spehar G, Mullin RJ, Keith BR, Gilmer TM, Berger M, Podratz KC, Slamon DJ. Activity of the dual kinase inhibitor lapatinib (GW572016) against HER-2-overexpressing and trastuzumab-treated breast cancer cells. Cancer Res 2006; 66(3): 1630-9.

[114] Xia W, Gerard CM, Liu L, Baudson NM, Ory TL, Spector NL. Combining lapatinib (GW572016), a small molecule inhibitor of ErbB1 and ErbB2 tyrosine kinases, with therapeutic anti-ErbB2 antibodies enhances apoptosis of ErbB2-overexpressing breast cancer cells. Oncogene 2005; 24(41): 6213-21.

[115] Blackwell KL, Burstein HJ, Storniolo AM, Rugo HS, Sledge G, Aktan G, Ellis C, Florance A, Vukelja S, Bischoff J, Baselga J, O'Shaughnessy J. Overall survival benefit with lapatinib in combination with trastuzumab for patients with human epidermal growth factor receptor 2-positive metastatic breast cancer: final results from the EGF104900 Study. J Clin Oncol 2012; 30(21): 2585-92.

[116] Guarneri V, Frassoldati A, Bottini A, Cagossi K, Bisagni G, Sarti S, Ravaioli A, Cavanna L, Giardina G, Musolino A, Untch M, Orlando L, Artioli F, Boni C, Generali DG, Serra P, Bagnalasta M, Marini L, Piacentini F, D'Amico R, Conte P. Preoperative chemotherapy plus trastuzumab, lapatinib, or both in human epidermal growth factor receptor 2-positive operable breast cancer: results of the randomized phase II CHER-LOB study. J Clin Oncol 2012; 30(16): 1989-95.

[117] Rimawi MF, Mayer IA, Forero A, Nanda R, Goetz MP, Rodriguez AA, Pavlick AC, Wang T, Hilsenbeck SG, Gutierrez C, Schiff R, Osborne CK, Chang JC. Multicenter phase II study of neoadjuvant lapatinib and trastuzumab with hormonal therapy and without chemotherapy in patients with human epidermal growth factor receptor 2-overexpressing breast cancer: TBCRC 006. J Clin Oncol 2013; 31(14): 1726-31.

[118] Baselga J, Bradbury I, Eidtmann H, Di Cosimo S, de Azambuja E, Aura C, Gómez H, Dinh P, Fauria K, Van Dooren V, Aktan G, Goldhirsch A, Chang TW, Horváth Z, Coccia-Portugal M, Domont J, Tseng LM, Kunz G, Sohn JH, Semiglazov V, Lerzo G, Palacova M,

Probachai V, Pusztai L, Untch M, Gelber RD, Piccart-Gebhart M; NeoALTTO Study Team. Lapatinib with trastuzumab for HER2-positive early breast cancer (NeoALTTO): a randomised, open-label, multicentre, phase 3 trial. Lancet 2012; 379(9816): 633-40.

[119] Carey LA, Berry DA, Ollila D, Harris L, Krop IE, Weckstein D, Henry NL, Anders CK, Cirrincione C, Winer EP, Perou CM, Hudis C. Clinical and translational results of CALGB 40601: A neoadjuvant phase III trial of weekly paclitaxel and trastuzumab with or without lapatinib for HER2-positive breast cancer. J Clin Oncol 31, 2013 (suppl; abstr 500).

[120] Holmes FA, Espina V, Liotta LA, Nagarwala YM, Danso M, McIntyre KJ, Osborne CR, Anderson T, Krekow L, Blum JL, Pippen J, Florance A, Mahoney J, O'Shaughnessy JA. Pathologic complete response after preoperative anti-HER2 therapy correlates with alterations in PTEN, FOXO, phosphorylated Stat5, and autophagy protein signaling. BMC Res Notes 2013; 6: 507.

[121] Untch M, Loibl S, Bischoff J, Eidtmann H, Kaufmann M, Blohmer JU, Hilfrich J, Strumberg D, Fasching PA, Kreienberg R, Tesch H, Hanusch C, Gerber B, Rezai M, Jackisch C, Huober J, Kühn T, Nekljudova V, von Minckwitz G; German Breast Group (GBG); Arbeitsgemeinschaft Gynäkologische Onkologie-Breast (AGO-B) Study Group. Lapatinib *versus* trastuzumab in combination with neoadjuvant anthracycline-taxane-based chemotherapy (GeparQuinto, GBG 44): a randomised phase 3 trial. Lancet Oncol 2012; 13(2): 135-44.

[122] Robidoux A, Tang G, Rastogi P, Geyer CE Jr, Azar CA, Atkins JN, Fehrenbacher L, Bear HD, Baez-Diaz L, Sarwar S, Margolese RG, Farrar WB, Brufsky AM, Shibata HR, Bandos H, Paik S, Costantino JP, Swain SM, Mamounas EP, Wolmark N. Lapatinib as a component of neoadjuvant therapy for HER2-positive operable breast cancer (NSABP protocol B-41): an open-label, randomised phase 3 trial. Lancet Oncol 2013; 14(12): 1183-92.

[123] ClinicalTrials.gov. ALTTO (Adjuvant Lapatinib And/Or Trastuzumab Treatment Optimisation) Study; BIG 2-06/N063D. Available from: http://clinicaltrials.gov/ct2/show/NCT00490139?term = ALTTO&rank = 1 [Cited: 29th Dec 2013].

[124] Gril B, Palmieri D, Bronder JL, Herring JM, Vega-Valle E, Feigenbaum L, Liewehr DJ, Steinberg SM, Merino MJ, Rubin SD, Steeg PS. Effect of lapatinib on the outgrowth of metastatic breast cancer cells to the brain. J Natl Cancer Inst 2008; 100(15): 1092-103.

[125] Lin NU, Diéras V, Paul D, Lossignol D, Christodoulou C, Stemmler HJ, Roché H, Liu MC, Greil R, Ciruelos E, Loibl S, Gori S, Wardley A, Yardley D, Brufsky A, Blum JL, Rubin SD, Dharan B, Steplewski, K, Zembryki D, Oliva C, Roychowdhury D, Paoletti P, Winer EP. Multicenter phase II study of lapatinib in patients with brain metastases from HER2-positive breast cancer. Clin Cancer Res 2009; 15(4): 1452-9.

[126] Metro G, Foglietta J, Russillo M, Stocchi L, Vidiri A, Giannarelli D, Crinò L, Papaldo P, Mottolese M, Cognetti F, Fabi A, Gori S. Clinical outcome of patients with brain metastases from HER2-positive breast cancer treated with lapatinib and capecitabine. Ann Oncol 2011; 22(3): 625-30.

[127] Ro J, Park S, Kim S, Kim TY, Im YH, Rha SY, Chung JS, Moon H, Santillana S. Clinical outcomes of HER2-positive metastatic breast cancer patients with brain metastasis treated with lapatinib and capecitabine: an open-label expanded access study in Korea. BMC Cancer 2012; 12: 322.

[128] Bachelot T, Romieu G, Campone M, Diéras V, Cropet C, Dalenc F, Jimenez M, Le Rhun E, Pierga JY, Gonçalves A, Leheurteur M, Domont J, Gutierrez M, Curé H, Ferrero JM, Labbe-Devilliers C. Lapatinib plus capecitabine in patients with previously untreated brain metastases from HER2-positive metastatic breast cancer (LANDSCAPE): a single-group phase 2 study. Lancet Oncol 2013; 14(1): 64-71.

[129] Rabindran SK, Discafani CM, Rosfjord EC, Baxter M, Floyd MB, Golas J, Hallett WA, Johnson BD, Nilakantan R, Overbeek E, Reich MF, Shen R, Shi X, Tsou HR, Wang YF, Wissner A. Antitumor activity of HKI-272, an orally active, irreversible inhibitor of the HER-2 tyrosine kinase. Cancer Res 2004; 64(11): 3958-65.

[130] Wong KK, Fracasso PM, Bukowski RM, Lynch TJ, Munster PN, Shapiro GI, Jänne PA, Eder JP, Naughton MJ, Ellis MJ, Jones SF, Mekhail T, Zacharchuk C, Vermette J, Abbas R, Quinn S, Powell C, Burris HA. A phase I study with neratinib (HKI-272), an irreversible pan ErbB receptor tyrosine kinase inhibitor, in patients with solid tumors. Clin Cancer Res 2009; 15(7): 2552-8.

[131] Burstein HJ, Sun Y, Dirix LY, Jiang Z, Paridaens R, Tan AR, Awada A, Ranade A, Jiao S, Schwartz G, Abbas R, Powell C, Turnbull K, Vermette J, Zacharchuk C, Badwe R. Neratinib, an irreversible ErbB receptor tyrosine kinase inhibitor, in patients with advanced ErbB2-positive breast cancer. J Clin Oncol 2010; 28(8): 1301-7.

[132] Martin M, Bonneterre J, Geyer CE Jr, Ito Y, Ro J, Lang I, Kim SB, Germa C, Vermette J, Wang K, Wang K, Awada A. A phase two randomised trial of neratinib monotherapy *versus* lapatinib plus capecitabine combination therapy in patients with HER2+ advanced breast cancer. Eur J Cancer 2013; 49(18): 3763-72.

[133] Awada A, Dirix L, Manso Sanchez L, Xu B, Luu T, Diéras V, Hershman DL, Agrapart V, Ananthakrishnan R, Staroslawska E. Safety and efficacy of neratinib (HKI-272) plus vinorelbine in the treatment of patients with ErbB2-positive metastatic breast cancer pretreated with anti-HER2 therapy. Ann Oncol 2013; 24(1): 109-16.

[134] Chow LW, Xu B, Gupta S, Freyman A, Zhao Y, Abbas R, Vo Van ML, Bondarenko I. Combination neratinib (HKI-272) and paclitaxel therapy in patients with HER2-positive metastatic breast cancer. Br J Cancer 2013; 108(10): 1985-93.

[135] ClinicalTrials.gov. Study evaluating neratinib plus paclitaxel *vs* trastuzumab plus paclitaxel in ErbB-2 positive advanced breast cancer (NEFERTT). Available from: http://clinicaltrials.gov/ct2/show/NCT00915018?term = NCT00915018&rank = 1 [Cited: 30th Dec 2013].

[136] ClinicalTrials.gov. Study evaluating the effects of neratinib after adjuvant trastuzumab in women with early stage breast cancer (ExteNET). Available from: http://clinicaltrials.gov/ct2/show/NCT00878709?term = NCT00878709&rank = 1 [Cited: 30th Dec 2013].

[137] Li D, Ambrogio L, Shimamura T, Kubo S, Takahashi M, Chirieac LR, Padera RF, Shapiro GI, Baum A, Himmelsbach F, Rettig WJ, Meyerson M, Solca F, Greulich H, Wong KK. BIBW2992, an irreversible EGFR/HER2 inhibitor highly effective in preclinical lung cancer models. Oncogene 2008; 27(34): 4702-11.

[138] Minkovsky N, Berezov A. BIBW-2992, a dual receptor tyrosine kinase inhibitor for the treatment of solid tumors. Curr Opin Investig Drugs 2008; 9(12): 1336-46.

[139] Canonici A, Pedersen K, Browne B, McDermott M, Walsh N, Crown J, O'Donovan N. Effect of afatinib alone and in combination with trastuzumab in HER2-positive breast cancer cell lines. J Clin Oncol 31, 2013 (suppl; abstr 632).

[140] Yap TA, Vidal L, Adam J, Stephens P, Spicer J, Shaw H, Ang J, Temple G, Bell S, Shahidi M, Uttenreuther-Fischer M, Stopfer P, Futreal A, Calvert H, de Bono JS, Plummer R. Phase I trial of the irreversible EGFR and HER2 kinase inhibitor BIBW 2992 in patients with advanced solid tumors. J Clin Oncol 2010; 28(25): 3965-72.

[141] Lin NU, Winer EP, Wheatley D, Carey LA, Houston S, Mendelson D, Munster P, Frakes L, Kelly S, Garcia AA, Cleator S, Uttenreuther-Fischer M, Jones H, Wind S, Vinisko R, Hickish T. A phase II study of afatinib (BIBW 2992), an irreversible ErbB family blocker, in patients with HER2-positive metastatic breast cancer progressing after trastuzumab. Breast Cancer Res Treat 2012; 133(3): 1057-65.

[142] Harbeck N, Im SA, Huang CS, Im YH, Xu B, Hurvitz SA, Lee KS, Ahn JH, Mehta AO, Arora SR, Sun Q, Qin S, Jacob LA, Jassem J, Staroslawka E, Sufliarsky J, Wojtukiewicz JM, Lahogue A, Uttenreuther-Fischer MM, Piccart-Gebhart MJ, the LUX-Breast 1 Study Group. LUX-breast 1: Randomized, phase III trial of afatinib and vinorelbine *versus* trastuzumab and vinorelbine in patients with HER2-overexpressing metastatic breast cancer (MBC) failing one prior trastuzumab treatment. J Clin Oncol 30, 2012 (suppl; abstr TPS649).

[143] Hickish T, Tseng LM, Mehta AO, Tsang J, Kovalenko N, Udovitsa D, Pelling K, Uttenreuther-Fischer MM, Huang CS, LUX-Breast 2 Study Group. LUX-breast 2: Phase II, open-label study of oral afatinib in HER2-overexpressing metastatic breast cancer (MBC) patients (pts) who progressed on prior trastuzumab (T) and/or lapatanib (L). J Clin Oncol 30, 2012 (suppl; abstr TPS651).

[144] Joensuu H, Kaci MO. LUX-breast 3: Randomized phase II study of afatinib alone or with vinorelbine *versus* investigator's choice of treatment in patients (pts) with HER2-positive breast cancer (BC) with progressive brain metastases (BM) after trastuzumab or lapatinib-based therapy. J Clin Oncol 30, 2012 (suppl; abstr TPS647).

[145] Geuna E, Montemurro F, Aglietta M, Valabrega G. Potential of afatinib in the treatment of patients with HER2-positive breast cancer. Breast Cancer (Dove Med Press) 2012; 4: 131-7.

[146] Borders EB, Bivona C, Medina PJ. Mammalian target of rapamycin: biological function and target for novel anticancer agents. Am J Health Syst Pharm 2010; 67(24): 2095-106.

[147] Wullschleger S, Loewith R, Hall MN. TOR signaling in growth and metabolism. Cell 2006; 124(3): 471-84.

[148] Sabatini DM. mTOR and cancer: insights into a complex relationship. Nat Rev Cancer 2006; 6(9): 729-34.

[149] Alessi DR, Deak M, Casamayor A, Caudwell FB, Morrice N, Norman DG, Gaffney P, Reese CB, MacDougall CN, Harbison D, Ashworth A, Bownes M. 3-Phosphoinositide-dependent protein kinase-1 (PDK1): structural and functional homology with the Drosophila DSTPK61 kinase. Curr Biol 1997; 7(10): 776-89.
[150] Stephens L, Anderson K, Stokoe D, Erdjument-Bromage H, Painter GF, Holmes AB, Gaffney PR, Reese CB, McCormick F, Tempst P, Coadwell J, Hawkins PT. Protein kinase B kinases that mediate phosphatidylinositol 3,4,5-trisphosphate-dependent activation of protein kinase B. Science 1998; 279(5351): 710-4.
[151] Vivanco I, Sawyers CL. The phosphatidylinositol 3-Kinase AKT pathway in human cancer. Nat Rev Cancer 2002; 2(7): 489-501.
[152] Inoki K, Li Y, Zhu T, Wu J, Guan KL. TSC2 is phosphorylated and inhibited by Akt and suppresses mTOR signaling. Nat Cell Biol 2002; 4(9): 648-57.
[153] Manning BD, Tee AR, Logsdon MN, Blenis J, Cantley LC. Identification of the tuberous sclerosis complex-2 tumor suppressor gene product tuberin as a target of the phosphoinositide 3-kinase/akt pathway. Mol Cell 2002; 10(1): 151-62.
[154] Vander Haar E, Lee SI, Bandhakavi S, Griffin TJ, Kim DH. Insulin signalling to mTOR mediated by the Akt/PKB substrate PRAS40. Nat Cell Biol 2007; 9(3): 316-23.
[155] Hay N, Sonenberg N. Upstream and downstream of mTOR. Genes Dev. 2004; 18(16): 1926-45.
[156] Jacinto E, Loewith R, Schmidt A, Lin S, Rüegg MA, Hall A, Hall MN. Mammalian TOR complex 2 controls the actin cytoskeleton and is rapamycin insensitive. Nat Cell Biol 2004; 6(11): 1122-8.
[157] LoRusso PM. Mammalian target of rapamycin as a rational therapeutic target for breast cancer treatment. Oncology 2013; 84(1): 43-56.
[158] Cantley LC, Neel BG. New insights into tumor suppression: PTEN suppresses tumor formation by restraining the phosphoinositide 3-kinase/AKT pathway. Proc Natl Acad Sci USA 1999; 96(8): 4240-5.
[159] Cully M, You H, Levine AJ, Mak TW. Beyond PTEN mutations: the PI3K pathway as an integrator of multiple inputs during tumorigenesis. Nat Rev Cancer 2006; 6(3): 184-92.
[160] Liu P, Cheng H, Roberts TM, Zhao JJ. Targeting the phosphoinositide 3-kinase pathway in cancer. Nat Rev Drug Discov 2009; 8(8): 627-44.
[161] Sarbassov DD, Ali SM, Kim DH, Guertin DA, Latek RR, Erdjument-Bromage H, Tempst P, Sabatini DM. Rictor, a novel binding partner of mTOR, defines a rapamycin-insensitive and raptor-independent pathway that regulates the cytoskeleton. Curr Biol 2004; 14(14): 1296-302.
[162] Raymond E, Alexandre J, Faivre S, Vera K, Materman E, Boni J, Leister C, Korth-Bradley J, Hanauske A, Armand JP. Safety and pharmacokinetics of escalated doses of weekly intravenous infusion of CCI-779, a novel mTOR inhibitor, in patients with cancer. J Clin Oncol 2004; 22(12): 2336-47.
[163] Chan S, Scheulen ME, Johnston S, Mross K, Cardoso F, Dittrich C, Eiermann W, Hess D, Morant R, Semiglazov V, Borner M, Salzberg M, Ostapenko V, Illiger HJ, Behringer D, Bardy-Bouxin N, Boni J, Kong S, Cincotta M, Moore L. Phase II study of temsirolimus (CCI-779), a novel inhibitor of mTOR, in heavily pretreated patients with locally advanced or metastatic breast cancer. J Clin Oncol 2005; 23(23): 5314-22.

[164] Wolff AC, Lazar AA, Bondarenko I, Garin AM, Brincat S, Chow L, Sun Y, Neskovic-Konstantinovic Z, Guimaraes RC, Fumoleau P, Chan A, Hachemi S, Strahs A, Cincotta M, Berkenblit A, Krygowski M, Kang LL, Moore L, Hayes DF. Randomized phase III placebo-controlled trial of letrozole plus oral temsirolimus as first-line endocrine therapy in postmenopausal women with locally advanced or metastatic breast cancer. J Clin Oncol 2013; 31(2):195-202.

[165] Ellard SL, Clemons M, Gelmon KA, Norris B, Kennecke H, Chia S, Pritchard K, Eisen A, Vandenberg T, Taylor M, Sauerbrei E, Mishaeli M, Huntsman D, Walsh W, Olivo M, McIntosh L, Seymour L. Randomized phase II study comparing two schedules of everolimus in patients with recurrent/metastatic breast cancer: NCIC Clinical Trials Group IND.163. J Clin Oncol 2009; 27(27): 4536-41.

[166] Berns K, Horlings HM, Hennessy BT, Madiredjo M, Hijmans EM, Beelen K, Linn SC, Gonzalez-Angulo AM, Stemke-Hale K, Hauptmann M, Beijersbergen RL, Mills GB, van de Vijver MJ, Bernards R. A functional genetic approach identifies the PI3K pathway as a major determinant of trastuzumab resistance in breast cancer. Cancer Cell 2007; 12(4): 395-402.

[167] Lu CH, Wyszomierski SL, Tseng LM, Sun MH, Lan KH, Neal CL, Mills GB, Hortobagyi GN, Esteva FJ, Yu D. Preclinical testing of clinically applicable strategies for overcoming trastuzumab resistance caused by PTEN deficiency. Clin Cancer Res 2007; 13(19): 5883-8.

[168] Morrow PK, Wulf GM, Ensor J, Booser DJ, Moore JA, Flores PR, Xiong Y, Zhang S, Krop IE, Winer EP, Kindelberger DW, Coviello J, Sahin AA, Nuñez R, Hortobagyi GN, Yu D, Esteva FJ. Phase I/II study of trastuzumab in combination with everolimus (RAD001) in patients with HER2-overexpressing metastatic breast cancer who progressed on trastuzumab-based therapy. J Clin Oncol 2011; 29(23): 3126-32.

[169] Andre F, Campone M, O'Regan R, Manlius C, Massacesi C, Sahmoud T, Mukhopadhyay P, Soria JC, Naughton M, Hurvitz SA. Phase I study of everolimus plus weekly paclitaxel and trastuzumab in patients with metastatic breast cancer pretreated with trastuzumab. J Clin Oncol 2010; 28(34): 5110-5.

[170] Jerusalem G, Fasolo A, Dieras V, Cardoso F, Bergh J, Vittori L, Zhang Y, Massacesi C, Sahmoud T, Gianni L. Phase I trial of oral mTOR inhibitor everolimus in combination with trastuzumab and vinorelbine in pre-treated patients with HER2-overexpressing metastatic breast cancer. Breast Cancer Res Treat 2011; 125(2): 447-55.

[171] O'Regan R, Ozguroglu M, Andre F, Toi M, Jerusalem GHM, Wilks S, Isaacs C, Xu B, Masuda N, Arena FP, Yardley DA, Yap YS, Mukhopadhyay P, Douma S, El-Hashimy M, Taran T, Sahmoud T, Lebwohl DE, Gianni L. Phase III, randomized, double-blind, placebo-controlled multicenter trial of daily everolimus plus weekly trastuzumab and vinorelbine in trastuzumab-resistant, advanced breast cancer (BOLERO-3). J Clin Oncol 31, 2013 (suppl; abstr 505).

[172] Hurvitz SA, Andre F, Burris HA, Toi M, Buyse ME, Sahmoud T, Mukhopadhyay P, Massacesi C, Taran T, Ko J, Rupin M. BOLERO-1: A randomized, phase III, double-blind, placebo-controlled multicenter trial of everolimus in combination with trastuzumab and paclitaxel as first-line therapy in women with HER2-positive (HER2+), locally advanced or metastatic breast cancer (BC). J Clin Oncol 30, 2012 (suppl; abstr TPS648).

[173] Bergers G, Benjamin LE. Tumorigenesis and the angiogenic switch. Nat Rev Cancer 2003; 3(6): 401-10.
[174] Jain, RK. Molecular regulation of vessel maturation. Nat Med 2003; 9(6): 685-93.
[175] Carmeliet P. Mechanisms of angiogenesis and arteriogenesis. Nat Med 2000; 6(4): 389-95.
[176] Brown LF, Guidi AJ, Schnitt SJ, Van De Water L, Iruela-Arispe ML, Yeo TK, Tognazzi K, Dvorak HF. Vascular stroma formation in carcinoma *in situ*, invasive carcinoma, and metastatic carcinoma of the breast. Clin Cancer Res 1999; 5(5): 1041-56.
[177] Neufeld G, Kessler O, Vadasz Z, Gluzman-Poltorak Z. The contribution of proangiogenic factors to the progression of malignant disease: role of vascular endothelial growth factor and its receptors. Surg Oncol Clin N Am 2001; 10(2): 339-56.
[178] Sledge GW Jr, Miller KD. Angiogenesis and antiangiogenic therapy. Curr Probl Cancer 2002; 26(1): 1-60.
[179] Ferrara N, Gerber HP, LeCouter J. The biology of VEGF and its receptors. Nat Med 2003; 9(6): 669-76.
[180] Lewis NL, Meropol NJ. Development of new agents for the treatment of advanced colorectal cancer. Clin Colorectal Cancer 2003; 3(3): 154-64.
[181] Yancopoulos GD, Davis S, Gale NW, Rudge JS, Wiegand SJ, Holash J. Vascular-specific growth factors and blood vessel formation. Nature 2000; 407(6801): 242-8.
[182] Gu Y, Qi X, Guo S. Lymphangiogenesis induced by VEGF-C and VEGF-D promotes metastasis and a poor outcome in breast carcinoma: a retrospective study of 61 cases. Clin Exp Metastasis 2008; 25(7): 717-25.
[183] Shibuya M. Structure and function of VEGF/VEGF-receptor system involved in angiogenesis. Cell Struct Funct 2001; 26(1): 25-35.
[184] Fox SB, Generali DG, Harris AL. Breast tumour angiogenesis. Breast Cancer Res 2007; 9(6): 216.
[185] Takahashi T, Ueno H, Shibuya M. VEGF activates protein kinase C-dependent, but Ras-independent Raf-MEK-MAP kinase pathway for DNA synthesis in primary endothelial cells. Oncogene 1999; 18(13): 2221-30.
[186] Nör JE, Christensen J, Mooney DJ, Polverini PJ. Vascular endothelial growth factor (VEGF)-mediated angiogenesis is associated with enhanced endothelial cell survival and induction of Bcl-2 expression. Am J Pathol 1999; 154(2): 375-84.
[187] Houck KA, Ferrara N, Winer J, Cachianes G, Li B, Leung DW. The vascular endothelial growth factor family: identification of a fourth molecular species and characterization of alternative splicing of RNA. Mol Endocrinol 1991; 5(12): 1806-14.
[188] Pidgeon GP, Barr MP, Harmey JH, Foley DA, Bouchier-Hayes DJ. Vascular endothelial growth factor (VEGF) upregulates BCL-2 and inhibits apoptosis in human and murine mammary adenocarcinoma cells. Br J Cancer 2001; 85(2): 273-8.
[189] Kanai T, Konno H, Tanaka T, Baba M, Matsumoto K, Nakamura S, Yukita A, Asano M, Suzuki H, Baba S. Anti-tumor and anti-metastatic effects of human-vascular-endothelial-growth-factor-neutralizing antibody on human colon and gastric carcinoma xenotransplanted orthotopically into nude mice. Int J Cancer 1998; 77(6): 933-6.
[190] Okamoto K, Oshika Y, Fukushima Y, Yoshimura M, Ohnishi Y, Tokunaga T, Hashimoto T, Hatanaka H, Tomii Y, Yoshida Y, Miura S, Tsuchida T, Kijima H, Yamazaki H, Nakamura M, Ueyama Y. Inhibition of liver metastasis of colon cancer by *in vivo* administration of anti-vascular endothelial growth factor antibody. Oncol Rep 1999; 6(3): 553-6.

[191] Gabrilovich D, Ishida T, Oyama T, Ran S, Kravtsov V, Nadaf S, Carbone DP. Vascular endothelial growth factor inhibits the development of dendritic cells and dramatically affects the differentiation of multiple hematopoietic lineages *in vivo*. Blood 1998; 92(11): 4150-66.

[192] Brown LF, Berse B, Jackman RW, Tognazzi K, Guidi AJ, Dvorak HF, Senger DR, Connolly JL, Schnitt SJ. Expression of vascular permeability factor (vascular endothelial growth factor) and its receptors in breast cancer. Hum Pathol 1995; 26(1): 86-91.

[193] Nakasaki T, Wada H, Shigemori C, Miki C, Gabazza EC, Nobori T, Nakamura S, Shiku H. Expression of tissue factor and vascular endothelial growth factor is associated with angiogenesis in colorectal cancer. Am J Hematol 2002; 69(4): 247-54.

[194] Takahashi Y, Kitadai Y, Bucana CD, Cleary KR, Ellis LM. Expression of vascular endothelial growth factor and its receptor, KDR, correlates with vascularity, metastasis, and proliferation of human colon cancer. Cancer Res 1995; 55(18): 3964-8.

[195] Fujii T, Sudo T, Sueyoshi S, Tanaka T, Fujita H, Shirouzu K, Ban S, Toyonaga A, Kato S, Yamana H. Clinicopathologic study of neovascularization and VEGF expression in superficial esophageal carcinoma. Int J Oncol 2002; 21(6): 1181-7.

[196] Karayiannakis AJ, Bolanaki H, Syrigos KN, Asimakopoulos B, Polychronidis A, Anagnostoulis S, Simopoulos C. Serum vascular endothelial growth factor levels in pancreatic cancer patients correlate with advanced and metastatic disease and poor prognosis. Cancer Lett 2003; 194(1): 119-24.

[197] Gasparini G, Toi M, Gion M, Verderio P, Dittadi R, Hanatani M, Matsubara I, Vinante O, Bonoldi E, Boracchi P, Gatti C, Suzuki H, Tominaga T. Prognostic significance of vascular endothelial growth factor protein in node-negative breast carcinoma. J Natl Cancer Inst 1997; 89(2): 139-47.

[198] Linderholm B, Lindh B, Tavelin B, Grankvist K, Henriksson R. p53 and vascular-endothelial-growth-factor (VEGF) expression predicts outcome in 833 patients with primary breast carcinoma. Int J Cancer 2000; 89(1): 51-62.

[199] Relf M, LeJeune S, Scott PA, Fox S, Smith K, Leek R, Moghaddam A, Whitehouse R, Bicknell R, Harris AL. Expression of the angiogenic factors vascular endothelial cell growth factor, acidic and basic fibroblast growth factor, tumor growth factor β-1, platelet-derived endothelial cell growth factor, placenta growth factor, and pleiotrophin in human primary breast cancer and its relation to angiogenesis. Cancer Res 1997; 57(5): 963-9.

[200] Toi M, Inada K, Suzuki H, Tominaga T. Tumor angiogenesis in breast cancer: its importance as a prognostic indicator and the association with vascular endothelial growth factor expression. Breast Cancer Res Treat 1995; 36(2): 193-204.

[201] Borgström P, Gold DP, Hillan KJ, Ferrara N. Importance of VEGF for breast cancer angiogenesis *in vivo*: implications from intravital microscopy of combination treatments with an anti-VEGF neutralizing monoclonal antibody and doxorubicin. Anticancer Res 1999; 19(5B): 4203-14.

[202] Kim KJ, Li B, Winer J, Armanini M, Gillett N, Phillips HS, Ferrara N. Inhibition of vascular endothelial growth factor-induced angiogenesis suppresses tumour growth *in vivo*. Nature 1993; 362(6423): 841-4.

[203] Ferrara N. VEGF: an update on biological and therapeutic aspects. Curr Opin Biotechnol 2000; 11(6): 617-24.

[204] Greenlee RT, Hill-Harmon MB, Murray T, Thun M. Cancer statistics. CA Cancer J Clin 2001; 51(1): 15-36.

[205] Weidner N, Semple JP, Welch WR, Folkman J. Tumor angiogenesis and metastasis-correlation in invasive breast carcinoma. N Engl J Med 1991; 324(1): 1-8.

[206] Melnyk O, Zimmerman M, Kim KJ, Shuman M. Neutralizing anti-vascular endothelial growth factor antibody inhibits further growth of established prostate cancer and metastases in a pre-clinical model. J Urol 1999; 161(3): 960-3.

[207] Presta LG, Chen H, O'Connor SJ, Chisholm V, Meng YG, Krummen L, Winkler M, Ferrara N. Humanization of an anti-vascular endothelial growth factor monoclonal antibody for the therapy of solid tumors and other disorders. Cancer Res 1997; 57(20): 4593-9.

[208] Cobleigh MA, Langmuir VK, Sledge GW, Miller KD, Haney L, Novotny WF, Reimann JD, Vassel A. A phase I/II dose-escalation trial of bevacizumab in previously treated metastatic breast cancer. Semin Oncol 2003; 30(5 Suppl 16): 117-24.

[209] Fujii T, Takahashi H, Namoto Matsubayashi R, Inoue Y, Takenaka M, Toh U, Kage M, Yamana H, Shirouzu K. First-line treatment of metastatic breast cancer: focus on bevacizumab. Clin Med 2009; 1: 583-93.

[210] Sweeney CJ, Miller KD, Sissons SE, Nozaki S, Heilman DK, Shen J, Sledge GW Jr. The antiangiogenic property of docetaxel is synergistic with a recombinant humanized monoclonal antibody against vascular endothelial growth factor or 2-methoxyestradiol but antagonized by endothelial growth factors. Cancer Res 2001; 61(8): 3369-72.

[211] Burstein HJ, Chen YH, Parker LM, Savoie J, Younger J, Kuter I, Ryan PD, Garber JE, Chen H, Campos SM, Shulman LN, Harris LN, Gelman R, Winer EP. VEGF as a marker for outcome among advanced breast cancer patients receiving anti-VEGF therapy with bevacizumab and vinorelbine chemotherapy. Clin Cancer Res 2008; 14(23):7871-7.

[212] Ramaswamy B, Elias AD, Kelbick NT, Dodley A, Morrow M, Hauger M, Allen J, Rhoades C, Kendra K, Chen HX, Eckhardt SG, Shapiro CL. Phase II trial of bevacizumab in combination with weekly docetaxel in metastatic breast cancer patients. Clin Cancer Res 2006; 12(10): 3124-9.

[213] Miller KD, Chap LI, Holmes FA, Cobleigh MA, Marcom PK, Fehrenbacher L, Dickler M, Overmoyer BA, Reimann JD, Sing AP, Langmuir V, Rugo HS. Randomized phase III trial of capecitabine compared with bevacizumab plus capecitabine in patients with previously treated metastatic breast cancer. J Clin Oncol 2005; 23(4): 792-9.

[214] Miller K, Wang M, Gralow J, Dickler M, Cobleigh M, Perez EA, Shenkier T, Cella D, Davidson NE. Paclitaxel plus bevacizumab *versus* paclitaxel alone for metastatic breast cancer. N Engl J Med 2007; 357(26): 2666-76.

[215] Miles DW, Chan A, Dirix LY, Cortés J, Pivot X, Tomczak P, Delozier T, Sohn JH, Provencher L, Puglisi F, Harbeck N, Steger GG, Schneeweiss A, Wardley AM, Chlistalla A, Romieu G. Phase III study of bevacizumab plus docetaxel compared with placebo plus docetaxel for the first-line treatment of human epidermal growth factor receptor 2-negative metastatic breast cancer. J Clin Oncol 2010; 28(20): 3239-47.

[216] Robert NJ, Diéras V, Glaspy J, Brufsky AM, Bondarenko I, Lipatov ON, Perez EA, Yardley DA, Chan SY, Zhou X, Phan SC, O'Shaughnessy J. RIBBON-1: randomized, double-blind, placebo-controlled, phase III trial of chemotherapy with or without bevacizumab for first-line treatment of human epidermal growth factor receptor 2-negative, locally recurrent or metastatic breast cancer. J Clin Oncol 2011; 29(10): 1252-60.

[217] FDA CENTER FOR DRUG EVALUATION AND RESEARCH, Memorandum to the File BLA 125085 Avastin (bevacizumab)2010. Available from: http://www.fda.gov/downloads/drugs/drugsafety/postmarketdrugsafetyinformationforpatientsandproviders/ucm237171.pdf [Cited: 4th Feb 2014].

[218] Montero AJ, Escobar M, Lopes G, Glück S, Vogel C. Bevacizumab in the treatment of metastatic breast cancer: friend or foe? Curr Oncol Rep 2012; 14(1): 1-11.

[219] Smith IE, Pierga JY, Biganzoli L, Cortés-Funes H, Thomssen C, Pivot X, Fabi A, Xu B, Stroyakovskiy D, Franke FA, Kaufman B, Mainwaring P, Pienkowski T, De Valk B, Kwong A, González-Trujillo JL, Koza I, Petrakova K, Pereira D, Pritchard KI; ATHENA Study Group. First-line bevacizumab plus taxane-based chemotherapy for locally recurrent or metastatic breast cancer: safety and efficacy in an open-label study in 2,251 patients. Ann Oncol 2011; 22(3): 595-602.

[220] Sørlie T, Perou CM, Tibshirani R, Aas T, Geisler S, Johnsen H, Hastie T, Eisen MB, van de Rijn M, Jeffrey SS, Thorsen T, Quist H, Matese JC, Brown PO, Botstein D, Eystein Lønning P, Børresen-Dale AL. Gene expression patterns of breast carcinomas distinguish tumor subclasses with clinical implications. Proc Natl Acad Sci USA 2001; 98(19): 10869-74.

[221] Miles DW, Diéras V, Cortés J, Duenne AA, Yi J, O'Shaughnessy J. First-line bevacizumab in combination with chemotherapy for HER2-negative metastatic breast cancer: pooled and subgroup analyses of data from 2447 patients. Ann Oncol 2013; 24(11): 2773-80.

[222] Hamilton E, Kimmick G, Hopkins J, Marcom PK, Rocha G, Welch R, Broadwater G, Blackwell K. Nab-paclitaxel/bevacizumab/carboplatin chemotherapy in first-line triple negative metastatic breast cancer. Clin Breast Cancer 2013; 13(6): 416-20.

[223] Klos KS, Wyszomierski SL, Sun M, Tan M, Zhou X, Li P, Yang W, Yin G, Hittelman WN, Yu D. ErbB2 increases vascular endothelial growth factor protein synthesis *via* activation of mammalian target of rapamycin/p70S6K leading to increased angiogenesis and spontaneous metastasis of human breast cancer cells. Cancer Res 2006; 66(4): 2028-37.

[224] Konecny GE, Meng YG, Untch M, Wang HJ, Bauerfeind I, Epstein, M, Stieber P, Vernes JM, Gutierrez J, Hong K, Beryt M, Hepp H, Slamon DJ, Pegram MD. Association between HER-2/neu and vascular endothelial growth factor expression predicts clinical outcome in primary breast cancer patients. Clin Cancer Res 2004; 10(5): 1706-16.

[225] Scheuer W, Friess T, Hasmann M. Enhanced antitumour effect by combination of HER2-targeting antibodies with bevacizumab in a human breast cancer xenograft model. Eur J Cancer 4, 2006 (suppl; abstr 213).

[226] Pegram MD, Yeon C, Ku NC, Gaudreault J, Slamon D. Phase I combined biological therapy of breast cancer using two humanized monoclonal antibodies directed against HER2 proto-oncogene and vascular endothelial growth factor (VEGF). Breast Cancer Res Treat 88, 2004. (Suppl; abstr 3039).

[227] Pegram M, Chan D, Dichmann RA, Tan-Chiu E, Yeon C, Durna L, Lin LS, Slamon D. Phase II combined biological therapy targeting the HER2 proto-oncogene and the vascular endothelial growth factor using trastuzumab (T) and bevacizumab (B) as first line treatment of HER2-amplified breast cancer. Breast Cancer Res Treat 100, 2006 (suppl; abstr 301).

[228] Gianni L, Romieu GH, Lichinitser M, Serrano SV, Mansutti M, Pivot X, Mariani P, Andre F, Chan A, Lipatov O, Chan S, Wardley A, Greil R, Moore N, Prot S, Pallaud C, Semiglazov V. AVEREL: a randomized phase III Trial evaluating bevacizumab in combination with docetaxel and trastuzumab as first-line therapy for HER2-positive locally recurrent/metastatic breast cancer. J Clin Oncol 2013; 31(14): 1719-25.

[229] von Minckwitz G, Eidtmann H, Rezai M, Fasching PA, Tesch H, Eggemann H, Schrader I, Kittel K, Hanusch C, Kreienberg R, Solbach C, Gerber B, Jackisch C, Kunz G, Blohmer JU, Huober J, Hauschild M, Fehm T, Müller BM, Denkert C, Loibl S, Nekljudova V, Untch M; German Breast Group; Arbeitsgemeinschaft Gynäkologische Onkologie-Breast Study Groups. Neoadjuvant chemotherapy and bevacizumab for HER2-negative breast cancer. N Engl J Med 2012; 366(4): 299-309.

[230] Bear HD, Tang G, Rastogi P, Geyer CE Jr, Robidoux A, Atkins JN, Baez-Diaz L, Brufsky AM, Mehta RS, Fehrenbacher L, Young JA, Senecal FM, Gaur R, Margolese RG, Adams PT, Gross HM, Costantino JP, Swain SM, Mamounas EP, Wolmark N. Bevacizumab added to neoadjuvant chemotherapy for breast cancer. N Engl J Med 2012; 366(4): 310-20.

[231] Cameron D, Brown J, Dent R, Jackisch C, Mackey J, Pivot X, Steger GG, Suter TM, Toi M, Parmar M, Laeufle R, Im YH, Romieu G, Harvey V, Lipatov O, Pienkowski T, Cottu P, Chan A, Im SA, Hall PS, Bubuteishvili-Pacaud L, Henschel V, Deurloo RJ, Pallaud C, Bell R. Adjuvant bevacizumab-containing therapy in triple-negative breast cancer (BEATRICE): primary results of a randomised, phase 3 trial. Lancet Oncol 2013; 14(10): 933-42.

[232] Abrams TJ, Lee LB, Murray LJ, Pryer NK, Cherrington JM. SU11248 inhibits KIT and platelet-derived growth factor receptor beta in preclinical models of human small cell lung cancer. Mol Cancer Ther 2003; 2(5):471-8.

[233] Mendel DB, Laird AD, Xin X, Louie SG, Christensen JG, Li G, Schreck RE, Abrams TJ, Ngai TJ, Lee LB, Murray LJ, Carver J, Chan E, Moss KG, Haznedar JO, Sukbuntherng J, Blake RA, Sun L, Tang C, Miller T, Shirazian S, McMahon G, Cherrington JM. *In vivo* antitumor activity of SU11248, a novel tyrosine kinase inhibitor targeting vascular endothelial growth factor and platelet-derived growth factor receptors: determination of a pharmacokinetic/pharmacodynamic relationship. Clin Cancer Res 2003; 9(1): 327-37.

[234] Kim DW, Jo YS, Jung HS, Chung HK, Song JH, Park KC, Park SH, Hwang JH, Rha SY, Kweon GR, Lee SJ, Jo KW, Shong M. An orally administered multitarget tyrosine kinase inhibitor, SU11248, is a novel potent inhibitor of thyroid oncogenic RET/papillary thyroid cancer kinases. J Clin Endocrinol Metab 2006; 91(10):4070-6.

[235] Burstein HJ, Elias AD, Rugo HS, Cobleigh MA, Wolff AC, Eisenberg PD, Lehman M, Adams BJ, Bello CL, DePrimo SE, Baum CM, Miller KD. Phase II study of sunitinib malate, an oral multitargeted tyrosine kinase inhibitor, in patients with metastatic breast cancer previously treated with an anthracycline and a taxane. J Clin Oncol 2008; 26(11):1810-6.

[236] Wildiers H, Fontaine C, Vuylsteke P, Martens M, Canon JL, Wynendaele W, Focan C, De Greve J, Squifflet P, Paridaens R. Multicenter phase II randomized trial evaluating antiangiogenic therapy with sunitinib as consolidation after objective response to taxane chemotherapy in women with HER2-negative metastatic breast cancer. Breast Cancer Res Treat 2010; 123(2): 463-9.

[237] Barrios CH, Liu MC, Lee SC, Vanlemmens L, Ferrero JM, Tabei T, Pivot X, Iwata H, Aogi K, Lugo-Quintana R, Harbeck N, Brickman MJ, Zhang K, Kern KA, Martin M. Phase III randomized trial of sunitinib *versus* capecitabine in patients with previously treated HER2-negative advanced breast cancer. Breast Cancer Res Treat 2010; 121(1): 121-31.

[238] Bergh J, Bondarenko IM, Lichinitser MR, Liljegren A, Greil R, Voytko NL, Makhson AN, Cortes J, Lortholary A, Bischoff J, Chan A, Delaloge S, Huang X, Kern KA, Giorgetti C. First-line treatment of advanced breast cancer with sunitinib in combination with docetaxel *versus* docetaxel alone: results of a prospective, randomized phase III study. J Clin Oncol 2012; 30(9): 921-9.

[239] Crown JP, Diéras V, Staroslawska E, Yardley DA, Bachelot T, Davidson N, Wildiers H, Fasching PA, Capitain O, Ramos M, Greil R, Cognetti F, Fountzilas G, Blasinska-Morawiec M, Liedtke C, Kreienberg R, Miller WH Jr, Tassell V, Huang X, Paolini J, Kern KA, Romieu G. Phase III trial of sunitinib in combination with capecitabine *versus* capecitabine monotherapy for the treatment of patients with pretreated metastatic breast cancer. J Clin Oncol 2013; 31(23): 2870-8.

[240] Wilhelm SM, Adnane L, Newell P, Villanueva A, Llovet JM, Lynch M. Preclinical overview of sorafenib, a multikinase inhibitor that targets both Raf and VEGF and PDGF receptor tyrosine kinase signaling. Mol Cancer Ther 2008; 7(10): 3129-40.

[241] Moreno-Aspitia A, Morton RF, Hillman DW, Lingle WL, Rowland KM Jr, Wiesenfeld M, Flynn PJ, Fitch TR, Perez EA. Phase II trial of sorafenib in patients with metastatic breast cancer previously exposed to anthracyclines or taxanes: North Central Cancer Treatment Group and Mayo Clinic Trial N0336. J Clin Oncol 2009; 27(1): 11-5.

[242] Baselga J, Segalla JG, Roché H, Del Giglio A, Pinczowski H, Ciruelos EM, Filho SC, Gómez P, Van Eyll B, Bermejo B, Llombart A, Garicochea B, Durán MÁ, Hoff PM, Espié M, de Moraes AA, Ribeiro RA, Mathias C, Gil Gil M, Ojeda B, Morales J, Kwon Ro S, Li S, Costa F. Sorafenib in combination with capecitabine: an oral regimen for patients with HER2-negative locally advanced or metastatic breast cancer. J Clin Oncol 2012; 30(13): 1484-91.

[243] Schwartzberg LS, Tauer KW, Hermann RC, Makari-Judson G, Isaacs C, Beck JT, Kaklamani V, Stepanski EJ, Rugo HS, Wang W, Bell-McGuinn K, Kirshner JJ, Eisenberg P, Emanuelson R, Keaton M, Levine E, Medgyesy DC, Qamar R, Starr A, Ro SK, Lokker NA, Hudis CA. Sorafenib or placebo with either gemcitabine or capecitabine in patients with HER-2-negative advanced breast cancer that progressed during or after bevacizumab. Clin Cancer Res 2013; 19(10): 2745-54.

[244] Gradishar WJ, Kaklamani V, Sahoo TP, Lokanatha D, Raina V, Bondarde S, Jain M, Ro SK, Lokker NA, Schwartzberg L. A double-blind, randomised, placebo-controlled, phase 2b study evaluating sorafenib in combination with paclitaxel as a first-line therapy in patients with HER2-negative advanced breast cancer. Eur J Cancer 2013; 49(2): 312-22.

[245] Baselga J, Costa F, Gomez H, Hudis CA, Rapoport B, Roche H, Schwartzberg LS, Petrenciuc O, Shan M, Gradishar WJ. A phase 3 tRial comparing capecitabinE in combination with SorafenIb or pLacebo for treatment of locally advanced or metastatIc HER2-Negative breast CancEr (the RESILIENCE study): study protocol for a randomized controlled trial. Trials 2013; 14: 228.

[246] Clinicaltrials.gov. BETH Study: Treatment of HER2 positive breast cancer with chemotherapy plus trastuzumab *vs* chemotherapy plus trastuzumab plus bevacizumab Available from: http://clinicaltrials.gov/ct2/show/NCT00625898?term = bevacizumab+AND+breast+cancer+AND+adjuvant&rank = 6 [Cited: 9th March 2009].

[247] Clinicaltrials.gov. Doxorubicin, cyclophosphamide, and paclitaxel with or without bevacizumab in treating patients with lymph node-positive or high-risk, lymph node-negative breast cancer Available from: http://clinicaltrials.gov/ct2/show/NCT00433511? term = bevacizumab+AND+breast+cancer+AND+adjuvant&rank = 6 [Cited: 9th March 2009].

[248] Mackey JR, Kerbel RS, Gelmon KA, McLeod DM, ChiaSK, Rayson D, Verma S, Collins LL, Paterson AH, Robidoux A, Pritchard KI. Controlling angiogenesis in breast cancer: a systematic review of anti-angiogenic trials. Cancer Treat Rev 2012; 38(6): 673-88.

CHAPTER 5

Purinergic Modulation and CD39/ENTPD1 in Cancer

Lili Feng[1,2], Elliot B. Tapper[1], Xiaofeng Sun[1], Marina Gehring[1], Simon C. Robson[1] and Yan Wu[*,1]

[1]Division of Gastroenterology, Department of Medicine, Beth Israel Deaconess Medical Center, Harvard Medical School, Boston, MA, USA; and [2]Department of Hematology, Provincial Hospital Affiliated to Shandong University, Jinan, P.R. China

Abstract: Multiple, pleiotropic functional traits are acquired by transformed cells during progression to the neoplastic state. These include genomic instability with several defined mutations that are associated with uncontrolled proliferation, resistance to cell death with induction of immortality, altered cellular metabolism, loss/inactivation of tumor suppressor responses, evasion of immune surveillance, induction of angiogenesis with vascular perturbation, and activation of cell invasiveness resulting in metastasis. A better understanding of any overlapping pathogenetic mechanisms underpinning several of these properties would facilitate development of novel and more effective modalities to treat cancer. Dissecting out the molecular basis for these unique properties of malignancy has already resulted in the discovery and development of novel anticancer drugs.

Extracellular nucleotides and nucleosides have been recently identified as crucial signal mediators in the tumor microenvironment and are known to specifically interact with purinergic receptors. These cellular activation processes provoke different intracellular signaling transduction pathways, termed as "purinergic signaling". Ectonucleotidases, especially those of CD39/ENTPD family, regulate pericellular levels of pro-inflammatory adenosine 5'-triphosphate (ATP) to ultimately generate antagonistic anti-inflammatory nucleosides such as adenosine thereby tightly modulating purinergic signaling. Such regulated cascades of purinergic signaling have been shown to participate in many of the above fundamental pathophysiological processes in the context of inflammation and immune responses within the tumor microenvironment.

In this chapter, we review several purinergic mechanisms involved in cancer. We specifically highlight the discovery and development and the potential uses of drugs targeting ectonucleotidases that would be applicable to cancer therapy. We further discuss recent advances using purinergic modulation in cancer therapy and consider several of the therapeutic obstacles that would need to be overcome.

***Corresponding Author Yan Wu:** Beth Israel Deaconess Medical Center, Harvard Medical School, 3 Blackfan Circle, Rm601, Boston, MA 02215, USA. Tel. 617-735-2924; Fax. 617-735-2930;
E-mail: ywu@bidmc.harvard.edu

Atta-ur-Rahman / M. Iqbal Choudhary (Eds.)

Keywords: Adenosine, adjunctive therapy, ATP, cancer therapy, CD39, CD73, ectonucleotidases, purine-based drugs.

AT A GLANCE

- Purinergic mechanisms appear to play distinct and opposing roles in the biology of transplanted and autochthonous tumors.
- ATP-mediated type 2 purinergic (P2) receptor signaling is crucial in augmenting antitumor immune responses; whereas adenosine-P1 receptor signaling attenuates or suppresses immunity.
- CD39/ENTPD1 is the dominant and rate-limiting ectoenzyme for extracellular ATP phosphohydrolysis to adenosine and one of the master switches in the purinergic system.
- In the tumor microenvironment, the balance of extracellular nucleotide- *vs* nucleoside-initiated purinergic signaling dictates biology and integrates those specific metabolic changes associated with cell growth, inflammation and immunity.
- Chronic inflammation with scarring predisposes to malignancy and this process is associated with the perturbation of purinergic mechanisms.
- CD39 activity and downstream purinergic signaling pathways are novel therapeutic targets that hold great promise as adjunctive anticancer therapies.

INTRODUCTION

ATP and Other Purinergic Mediators

Indispensable throughout evolution, nucleotides such as adenosine triphosphate (ATP) are highly conserved in all organisms. As the well-recognized universal energy currency of the cell, intracellular ATP is an absolute requirement for the maintenance of cell metabolism and intracellular signals. At steady state, ATP concentration in the cytosol is at the millimolar (mM) range (3 to 10 mM), whereas it is thought to be around 10 nanomolar (nM) in the extracellular microenvironment [1]. As such, there is a 10^6-fold gradient in this process of ATP efflux. Cells actively release ATP in response to tissue damage and cellular stress. Even small leaks of ATP from the intracellular space elicit relatively dramatic elevations of extracellular ATP concentrations and therefore modulate purinergic signaling [1].

Extracellular purines are tremendously important metabolic signals. Since the first description of ATP as a specific signaling molecule, it has been well documented that extracellular nucleotides and the derivatives function as "signal transmitters" that induce intracellular signaling transduction through interaction with specific membrane purinergic receptors (purinoceptors) [2, 3]. This process termed "purinergic signaling" has been shown to participate in many physiological and pathological processes, regulating cell growth, metabolism, angiogenesis, inflammation and immunity.

Purinergic Systems

Purinergic systems have three essential components: extracellular nucleotides and their sources, specific receptors for these molecular transmitters (or derived products such as adenosine diphosphate (ADP) and adenosine), and ectonucleotidases that hydrolyze nucleotides (to nucleosides) [4]. Each of these has important effects on purinergic signal transduction, leading to critical changes in cellular responses.

We discuss these elements separately.

Release of Extracellular Nucleotides and Cellular Sources

ATP release can occur virtually from all cell types. Multiple mechanisms underlying ATP release by stressed, injured, or stimulated cells have been reported and these are either well-regulated or uncontrolled [5]. For example, synaptic vesicles release both ATP and neurotransmitters upon fusion with the cell membrane [6]. Lysosomes mediate ATP release by way of exocytosis [7-9]. Apoptotic or inflammatory cells release ATP through various types of membrane channels/efflux pathways, including connexin and pannexin hemichannels [10,

11], maxi-anion channels [12], volume-regulated anion channels [13], and the type 2 purinergic (P2) receptors P2X4 and P2X7 [14]. Finally, direct, uncontrolled ATP leakage can occur, whether at the center of rapidly proliferating solid tumors which become necrotic as proliferating cells outstrip the vascular supply or from the disrupted membranes of dying tumor cells treated with radiation or chemotherapy [15-17].

Purinergic Receptors

Purinergic receptors are broadly distributed on the cell surface of virtually all cell types. The precise actions of extracellular nucleotides or nucleosides are determined by the receptor(s) with which these mediators interact. These differ mainly by alterations in ligand binding affinity and cell/tissue distribution. Nearly all biological processes can be modulated by purinergic receptors, *e.g.* cell growth and metabolism, angiogenesis, platelet activation, and inflammatory and immune responses [18].

In 1978, Burnstock proposed a taxonomy for purinergic receptors that described two distinct subclasses: type 1 purinergic (P1) receptors are selective for adenosine, whereas type 2 purinergic (P2) receptors specifically bind ATP (as well as other nucleoside tri and diphosphates) [19]. To date, four P1 receptors (A1, A2A, A2B, and A3), seven ionotropic P2X receptors (P2X1-7), and eight metabotropic P2Y receptors (P2Y1, 2, 4, 6, 11-14) have been cloned and characterized [20, 21]. Different subtypes in the P2 and P1 receptor families often mediate opposing physiological functions by initiating different downstream signaling cascades. Any given cell type expresses a broad-spectrum of purinergic receptors. As different purinergic receptors express differential agonist affinity and specificity, the relative pericellular purine concentrations regulate distinct cellular functions in both health and disease [22-24].

P2X receptors are ATP-gated ion channels for Na^+, K^+ and Ca^{2+}. The diversity of P2X receptor function is tremendous. The infertility of P2X1 null male mice, for example, is a consequence of defective P2X1 signaling in the ductus deferens [25]. P2X2, 4, and 6 are the most abundant subunits found in neurons [26]. P2X3 expression is limited to a subgroup of afferent neurons. By forming a heteromeric channel with P2X2, P2X3 fully executes the transmission of nociception by ATP [27-29]. P2X4, distributed in various tissues, is mainly involved in modulation of epithelial and endothelial function, controlling ciliary function and calcium flux [23]. Moreover, several P2X receptors (inclusive of P2X1-4 and 7) have been shown to associate with lipid rafts [30-33]. Among the P2X receptors, P2X7 is the most extensively characterized subtype, and has critical roles in many fundamental pathophysiological processes (including inflammation, immunity, and carcinogenesis) [34].

P2Y receptors are seven-transmembrane-domain G protein-coupled receptors (GPCRs) [3]. These can be further divided into five Gq/11-coupled subtypes (P2Y1, 2, 4, 6 and 11) and three Gi/o-coupled subtypes (P2Y12-14). In general, elicitation of Gq/11-coupled P2Y receptors often induces Ca^{2+} release from the intracellular stores, through activation of phospholipase C (PLC) and inositol triphosphate (IP3) pathways; whereas Gi/o-coupled P2Y subtypes modulate ion channel function *via* the inhibition of adenylyl cyclase activity [35].

In addition, adenylate cyclase can be stimulated by P2Y1 by Gs protein [3, 36, 37]. Alterations in cytoplasmic cyclic AMP (cAMP) levels, in turn, impact protein kinase A (PKA) activity. Finally, P2Y receptors are ubiquitously expressed on hematopoietic cells. Indeed, P2Y2 is the major P2 receptor subtype responsible for recruitment and activation of neutrophils, dendritic cells (DCs), and macrophages at the inflammatory sites [38]. Beneficial effects of P2 receptor antagonists have been noted in various pathological conditions, including stroke and vascular inflammatory diseases [39, 40].

P1 receptors are also GPCRs, each of which has downstream signaling pathways of tremendous importance to both health and disease. A2A and A2B subtypes possess high adenosine binding affinity, whereas A1 and A3 receptors have low affinity. A2B activates PLC through the Gq protein [41]. A1 activation also stimulates PLC, by suppressing adenylate cyclase, thereby decreasing intracellular cAMP levels [42]. A3 signaling differentially impacts normal *vs* tumor cells [42, 43].

In normal cells, A3 activation is linked to NF-κB signaling to further drive production of growth factors. By contrast, in tumor cells, A3 agonists result in NF-κB and Wnt signaling-mediated apoptosis and tumor growth inhibition. Finally, all P1 receptor signals have been coupled to the mitogen-activated protein kinase (MAPK) pathway (inclusive of extracellular signal-regulated kinase 1 and 2 (ERK1/2), JUN N-terminal kinase (JNK), and p38) [44]. Important functional implications of P1 receptors have been implicated in numerous essential pathophysiological processes, *e.g.* vascular integrity and immunomodulation [45].

Ectonucleotidases

Ectonucleotidases are an essential regulatory component of purinergic signaling. By scavenging extracellular nucleotides, ectonucleotidase activity maintains the physiological 10^6-fold ATP gradient between the intracellular and extracellular compartment and thereby tightly controls purinergic responses.

To date, eight different ectonucleoside triphosphate diphosphohydrolase (ENTPDase) subtypes of the CD39 family have been identified (ENTPD1-8, each with distinct cellular location and catalytic properties). ENTPD1, 2, 3, and 8 are prototypical plasma membrane-associated enzymes with an extracellular catalytic site. Properties that are shared by CD39/ENTPD1 and other ectonucleotidases include localization in membrane lipid rafts [46] and the regulation of cellular signaling pathways [47].

Wu *et al.,* found that CD39 could directly interact with Ran-binding protein M (RanBPM), a membrane scaffolding protein with GTPase activity [48]. Distinct phosphohydrolytic activities among ENTPDase subtypes are, in large part, as a result of substantial differences in their sequences as well as in secondary, tertiary and quaternary structures [49, 50]. Beyond that, these have distinct preferences for substrates and divalent cations, hydrolyze nucleoside triphosphates at varying rates, and generate different products [51]. Micromolar levels of Ca^{2+} or Mg^{2+} ions are absolutely requisite for these four cell surface-located ectoenzymes to exert maximal activity. CD39/ENTPD1, with a preference of Mg^{2+} over Ca^{2+}, equally degrades ATP and ADP. ENTPD2, originally identified as an ecto-ATPase, favors hydrolysis of nucleoside triphosphates and also prefers Mg^{2+} over Ca^{2+} [51]. In contrast, ENTPD3 and 8 preferentially metabolize ATP over ADP and are in favor of Ca^{2+} over Mg^{2+} [52-54]. ENTPD5 and 6 are intracellularly located and, after being heterologously expressed, can be secreted. Finally, ENTPD4 and 7 are found entirely within cells [55].

CD39 is the rate-limiting enzyme in the nucleotide to adenosine hydrolytic cascade, but other ectoenzymes participate in a major way in purine metabolism [56]. These include amongst others CD73 (ecto-5'-nucleotidase; or Nt5e) which degrades AMP to adenosine and the adenosine deaminases (ADAs) which further hydrolyze adenosine to inosine. The conversion of ATP into AMP can be reversed by the action of extracellular soluble kinases such as adenylate kinase (AK). However, AMP conversion to adenosine seems to be largely reversible only within cells, as catalyzed by adenosine kinase after adenosine transporter-mediated adenosine uptake [57].

These ectoenzymes are inextricably linked by the dynamic substrate concentrations and resultant feedback loops. The first evidence in this regard was reported by Camici *et al.,* in 1985 [58, 59]. The authors noted that ATP and ADP could potently inhibit CD73 enzymatic activity in a competitive manner. Furthermore, this group found that the inhibition by ADP was more effective than ATP, albeit both functioned at low micromolar ranges. In 1986, Gordon and colleagues also observed that the higher the initial ATP concentration, the slower the appearance of adenosine. This suggested a "feed-forward inhibition" of CD73 by ADP [60]. This was further corroborated by the recent observation that loss of CD39 bioactivity causes the accumulation of ATP and ADP and results in local "feed-forward inhibition" of CD73 function, in turn inhibiting adenosine generation [61]. At the same time, increased ecto-ATPDase activity shifts the adenine nucleotide composition towards increased AMP, which is a substrate for CD73 to generate adenosine [62]. The result is a compensatory upregulation of CD73, which implied significant demand for conversion of ATP/ADP into adenosine [63].

The two major cell types expressing CD39 and/or CD73 are the vascular endothelium and immune system [64-69]. CD39 is expressed by many types of activated hematopoietic cells including B cells, natural killer (NK) and NKT cells, activated T cell subsets, monocytes/macrophages, and leukocytes. CD73, on the other hand, is expressed by activated B cells but neither naive T cells nor follicular DCs [57]. Indeed, CD73 has been suggested as a phenotypic marker of effector memory T helper type 17 (Th17) cells to monitor inflammatory response [70]. Similarly, dual expression of CD39 and CD73 distinguishes $CD4^+Foxp3^+$ regulatory T (Treg) cells from other T cells [71, 72]. More importantly, this dual expression, *via* production of adenosine, provides a novel immunosuppressive mechanism that is independent of conventional inhibitory cytokines [34, 73, 74]. $Foxp3^-CD39^+$ cells are able to mitigate TGF-β-induced conversion of $Foxp3^-CD39^-$ cells into Tregs (iTregs) [75]. Additionally, expression of CD39 is also observed on pre-existing $CD4^+CD44^+CD62L^-Foxp3^-$ memory T cells (inclusive of T helper type 1 (Th1), type 2 (Th2), and Th17 subsets), accompanied by elevated alloreactivity. NKT cells coexpress CD39 and CD73, whereas NK cells only contain CD39 [76]. Finally, expression of CD39 and/or CD73, which is regulated by hypoxia, has also been observed on many types of tumor cells [18-21, 35, 38, 45, 77-85].

Other than the enzymatic activity-dependent actions of CD39 and CD73, these ectonucleotidases may function independently of their ectoenzymatic activities. As an example, CD39 directly associates with RanBPM whereas CD73 has the capacity to both transmit strong activation signals in T cells upon antibody ligation and may serve as a cell adhesion molecule [48, 86]. More recently, it has been shown that blocking monoclonal antibodies (mAbs) against CD73 inhibit primary tumor growth and metastasis in mice, in both CD73 enzymatic activity-dependent and -independent manners. The underlying mechanism of this effect involves clustering and internalization of the CD73 protein, which does not require cross-linking of CD73 mAbs [87].

CANCER AND PURINERGIC MECHANISMS

The specific tumor microenvironment is critical for tumorigenesis. Chronic inflammation predisposes malignancy. Putative links between inflammation and cancer have been corroborated by countless epidemiological studies [88], since the first observation in the 19th century by Rudolf Virchow of the accumulation of cancers in chronically inflamed tissues. Mechanistic roles of chronic inflammation in tumorigenesis have been better characterized during the past decade [89, 90].

As critical components of tumor progression, tumor-infiltrating inflammatory cells participate in malignant transformation of premalignant cells as well as proliferation, survival, and migration of cancer cells [91]. Tumor cells also release inflammatory mediators that activate and recruit leukocytes to tumor vascular endothelium, driving production of angiogenic, chemotactic, and growth factors as well as proteolytic enzymes. These processes will, in turn, promote recruitment of additional inflammatory cells thereby supporting tumor growth and metastasis [90]. In summary, tumors often develop mechanisms to evade the host antitumor immune system and instead use it to their own advantage to survive, proliferate, and spread [92].

Numerous important signal mediators, including extracellular ATP and adenosine, provide essential local milieu for cancer development, which is further governed by reciprocal and dynamic tumor-host interactions. In recent years, there has been an increasing focus on the role of purinergic signaling and the potential as a therapeutic target in a large variety of diseases inclusive of cancer. Because of the broad-spectrum of P2 and P1 receptor expression on both tumor bulk and host tissues, purinergic signaling that integrates distinct cellular changes/responses has been explicitly ascribed to virtually all aspects of cancer biology. In general, ATP is thought to be pro-inflammatory whereas adenosine is anti-inflammatory.

In this section, we will summarize key findings delineating the purinergic mechanisms underpinning select aspects of carcinogenesis. A few concepts should be clarified at the outset. First, since ATP is an upstream signal released by inflammatory or damaged tumor cells and as CD73 function and adenosine generation is dependent on CD39, we will focus on discussing fundamental molecular mechanisms underlying modulation of tumor biology by ATP-P2 receptor/CD39 signaling. Second, as the majority of research investigations to date have utilized transplanted tumor models (either xenograft or syngenic), we will focus on how purinergic modulation impacts transplanted tumor biology (post malignant transformation), and also review the limited, albeit very important studies on autochthonous tumor development (premalignant and malignant transformation). Third, though these cancer aspects will be discussed in separate subsections for clearer presentation, the following concepts should always be kept in mind: i) each property of the tumor is certainly not independent as crosstalk among these different elements are indispensable for functions; ii) pericellular ATP/adenosine would impact any cell capable of sensing purine alterations, regardless of the cellular sources of purines. Therefore, ATP/adenosine effects may be autocrine or paracrine, as determined by the differential expression pattern of CD39/CD73 on a given cell type; iii) purinergic signaling can act alone or synergistically with other oncogenic signaling pathways (*e.g.* hypoxia, growth factors, chemokines, and toxins) to modulate cellular responses.

Intrinsic Tumor Responses

Virtually all types of cancer cells possess more than one functional purinergic receptor that efficiently sense changes in purine concentrations within the local milieu. As a consequence, such purinergic signals can activate multiple intracellular pathways that control intrinsic properties of the tumor cells, including metabolism and growth.

Tumor Metabolism

Cell metabolism is fundamental to cell growth. In normal differentiated tissues, cell metabolism is largely dependent upon the availability of nutrients. In the presence of oxygen, normal cells metabolize glucose to CO_2 *via* oxidative phosphorylation to maximize production of the energy currency ATP. When oxygen is scarce, cells switch to anaerobic glycolysis to generate lactate and produce ATP. Proliferating or cancer cells, on the other hand, regardless of the availability of oxygen, primarily rely on glycolytic metabolism that converts most glucose to lactate leading to rapid production of ATP [93]. Termed the "Warburg effect", this metabolic phenomenon serves to provide essential building blocks supporting rapid cell division. Activation of oncogenic signaling, such as Ras and PI3K-AKT-mTOR, has been shown to drive changes in metabolism and has been implicated in the regulation of aspects of the "Warburg effect" [94, 95].

Many recent innovative anticancer therapeutic avenues have been focusing on targeting the key regulators in tumor metabolism. Several groups have successfully developed clinically promising inhibitors for glutaminase 1 (GLS1), a glutaminase isoform that is highly upregulated in cancer cells. Similarly, modulating the activity of pyruvate kinase M2 (PKM2), a glycolytic enzyme that is frequently elevated in tumors, by targeted inhibition might also result in antitumor therapeutic effects. Furthermore, several groups have developed fatty acid synthase (FASN) inhibitors to target tumorigenesis. Many inhibitors for hypoxia-inducible factor (HIF) and HIF targets, are also potential anticancer drugs. Early phase clinical trial data show that blocking lactate production using dichloroacetate (DCA) also inhibits HIF-1α signaling and activates p53, ultimately suppressing tumor angiogenesis in glioblastoma patients.

Glycolysis inhibitors are also of interest in anticancer therapy. For instance, FX11, a selective suppressor of lactate dehydrogenase A (LDH-A) activity, is among the most advanced inhibitors of tumor metabolism in clinical trials (Phase II). It is known that metformin, commonplace in the medical therapy of insulin resistance, inhibits mitochondrial complex I, thereby decreasing ATP production. Lack of ATP subsequently stimulates LKB1-AMPK pathways and blocks gluconeogenesis, leading to lower blood glucose concentrations, improved sensitivity to insulin and diminished insulin production. Metformin has been well documented to improve cancer patient survival and also perturb cancer stem cells (CSCs). However, it is unclear whether metformin improves cancer clinical outcomes by lowering blood glucose levels and insulin/insulin-like growth factor production or by directly targeting cancer cells. Nevertheless, the scope of promising interventions for disrupting tumor metabolism that leverage purinergic mechanisms is broad and ranges from the investigational to those possibilities that are now readily available [96].

Our studies have linked purinergic signaling with metabolic pathways in premalignant and tumor cells. Sun *et al.* for example, recently demonstrated how metabolic pathways are altered to meet the continuous demands of constitutively proliferating premalignant hepatocytes, as a result of aberrant activation of ATP-P2Y2 receptor signaling [97]. Specifically, in the CD39 null mouse, elevated extracellular ATP (ranging from 10 to 100 μM) facilitates anabolic pathways by way of altering expression/activity of several critical glycolytic switch enzymes (*e.g.* PKM2 and LDH-A) as well as by abrogating autophagy, a fundamentally catabolic process in the liver. These changes are associated with disruptions in multiple genes involved in mitochondrial biogenesis and regulation (*e.g.* mitochondrial uncoupling protein (UCP) 2). The end result of these processes push cells substantively towards glycolysis.

UCP2 is an important player in this process. UCP2 controls both reactive oxidative species (ROS) production and mitochondrial ATP biosynthesis [98]. Disruptions in these processes dictate the fate of cells through reprogramming proliferative and glycolytic pathways. Elevated UCP2 levels have been noted in some cancers [99, 100], with putative roles in both impaired tumor suppression and chemoresistance, mediated largely *via* diverting metabolic signals [100, 101]. Other recent findings have elucidated several molecular underpinnings of the critical contributions of UCP2 to metabolic transformation of cancer cells [98]. Owing to UCP2's indispensable role in the maintenance of mitochondrial homeostasis, the lethality of altered mitochondrial uncoupling has limited identification of the downstream components.

Recently, p53 is recognized as a downstream target of UCP2's uncoupling activity in cancer cells [101]. p53 signaling can be altered by intracellular ROS levels, which are determined by UCP2 function. Whether p53 provokes anti-oxidant or pro-oxidant responses is mainly dependent upon the oxidative stress levels. UCP2-driven aberrant p53 signals are an encouraging opportunity for novel anticancer strategies [98].

Additionally, an important study by Fang *et al.,* has further unraveled an essential role for ENTPD5 in mediating the "Warburg effect" in cancer cells. Heightened levels of ENTPD5, an UDPase located on endoplasmic reticulum (ER), have been noted in several human malignancy models, including both cell lines and tumor specimens [102]. ENTPD5 not only facilitates protein folding *via* driving N-glycosylation, but also in concert with cytidine monophosphate kinase-1 and adenylate kinase-1, orchestrates an ATP metabolism cycle hydrolyzing ATP to AMP [102]. The latter process tightly modulates the PTEN (phosphatase and tensin homolog) and PI3K-AKT pathways providing a novel compensatory mechanism driving aerobic glycolysis [102]. Moreover, combined suppression of ENTPD5 and PTEN markedly inhibits tumor growth (both *in vitro* and *in vivo*), associated with increased ER stress and diminished growth factor receptor expression. These novel findings support the targeting of ENTPD5 as a potential therapy in cancer [102].

Tumor Growth

The established roles of extracellular ATP *vs* adenosine in tumor growth are in large part reciprocal, either tumor-promoting or tumoricidal. These responses are largely determined by the specific expression/activation of P2 and P1 receptor subtypes, which impact the cellular machinery of proliferation, apoptotic/necrotic/autophagic death, and differentiation.

Proliferative Activities

P2Y1 receptor activation is shown to be pro-proliferative in human thyroid cancer [103]. More generalized tumor-promoting activity has also been suggested for the P2Y2 receptor in melanoma, squamous cell carcinoma, breast, lung, thyroid, and liver cancer cells [104-109]. Recently, extracellular ATP has been reported to inactivate Forkhead Box O (FoxO) transcription factors and drive cell cycle progression through the P2Y2-mediated PI3K-AKT pathway in MCF-7 breast cancer cells [110]. In studies exposing human lung cancer A549 cells to radiation, P2Y6 and P2Y12 receptor signaling activates cellular DNA repair machinery and facilitates cell survival through an ERK1/2 pathway mechanism [109, 111, 112]. In 132N1 astrocytoma cells, P2Y6-provoked PKC activation abrogates tumor necrosis factor (TNF)-induced apoptosis [113], while P2Y12 signaling activates Ca^{2+} signals to regulate cell proliferation and differentiation [114].

In addition, accumulation of ATP/ADP in the local tumor microenvironment may result in activation of platelets. P2Y1 and P2Y12 activation by ADP promotes thrombosis [36]. Thrombosis, in turn, leads to further tumor ischemia/necrosis and thus a positive feedback loop of ATP release which, together with platelet-derived growth factor release, stimulates tumor growth.

A2A and A2B receptors are generally thought to promote tumor cell proliferation. Their activation has been reported to stimulate proliferation of lung, pancreatic, intestinal, and prostate cancer cells [115-117]. Adenosine also enhances chemoresistance of chronic lymphocytic leukamia cells through this mechanism [118]. Moreover, A1 receptor function has also been shown to be required for proliferation of MDA-MB-468 breast cancer cells [119] and poorly differentiated HT-29 human colon cancer cells [120].

Tumoricidal Actions

The anti-neoplastic activity of ATP was first described by Rapaport *et al.,* in 1983 [121]. The authors demonstrated that *in vitro* supplementation of exogenous ATP could block growth of pancreatic and colon cancer cells, by promoting cell-cycle arrest at S phase. Since then, cytotoxic actions of ATP on tumors have been extensively exploited in the laboratory setting using both *in vitro* experimentation systems and *in vivo* animal models. Chiefly, all types of tumor cells express one or several purinergic receptor subtypes that differentially sense alterations in extracellular ATP/adenosine levels, and thereby initiate distinct downstream intracellular signaling regulatory networks to dictate the cell fate - growth, quiescence, or death [104, 122-125].

Amongst these P2 receptors, P2X7 has been labeled as the “death receptor”. This P2X7 has been associated with ATP-evoked tumor cell death in many types of cancer, namely colon cancer, melanoma [65, 126, 127], squamous cell carcinomas [128], glioma [129], cervical cancer [130], and endometrial cancer [131]. P2X7 activation leads to membrane pore formation and cytoskeletal re-organization, often leading to tumor cell apoptosis.

Indeed, low level or defective P2X7 expression have been linked to cancer development by allowing escape from the P2X7 controlled pro-apoptotic mechanism [132]. P2X7 receptor expression as a diagnostic biomarker and/or therapeutic target has been explicitly explored not only in solid tumors [131], but also in haematologic malignancies [133].

Feng *et al.,* showed that high levels of exogenous purines, inclusive of ATP, ADP, and adenosine, all effectively and dose-dependently inhibit cell proliferation and induce apoptotic/necrotic cell death in murine B16/F10 melanoma and MCA38 colon cancer cells [65]. Thereafter, Bian *et al.,* linked the concentration-dependent ATP-P2X7 triggered autophagic cell death to two downstream signaling axes - the PI3K-AKT pathway and the AMPK-PRAS40-mTOR signaling. These two signaling pathways, synergistic but independent, are not modulated by Ca^{2+} signaling [127]. The clinical import of P2X7 signaling is becoming increasingly clear. Induction of ATP-P2X7-mediated apoptosis has also been indicated as a novel chemoprevention strategy for epithelial cancers [134]. In human breast cancer cells, upregulation of microRNA (miR)-150 is found to inhibit P2X7 expression and function, thereby driving cell growth and aggressive phenotype [132]. In glioma, P2X7 blockade also exerts a growth-promoting effect, concurrent with upregulated expression levels of epithelial growth factor receptor (EGFR), HIF-1α, and vascular endothelial growth factor (VEGF) [135]. P2X7 activation elicited by high extracellular ATP alone, or in combination with cholesterol-lowing drugs statins, decreases phosphorylated AKT levels in the nuclei, thereby inhibiting cancer cell growth. This is largely mediated through interactions of P2X7 with several protein/lipid phosphatases including PTEN [136-138]. These findings speak to potential anticancer therapeutic strategies using purinergic modulation alone or in combination with other oncogenic pathway inhibitors.

Activation of multiple purinergic receptor subtypes slow tumor cell growth, through a combined action of induction of apoptosis and differentiation. Tumoricidal functions of P2X5/P2X7 and/or P2Y11 receptors have been documented in both hormone refractory prostate cancer (PC-3) and high-grade bladder cancer (HT-1376) cells [105, 139, 140]. P2Y receptor subtypes are also implicated in cancer biology. Namely, P2Y1 and P2Y2 signaling can both alter intracellular cAMP levels (*via* adenylyl cyclase) and elevate intracellular Ca^{2+} concentrations (*via* PLC pathway). Accordingly, these proteins can significantly impact cell proliferation [114]. Indeed, anti-proliferative activity has been observed for both P2Y1 and P2Y2 in melanoma A375, colon cancer and oesophageal cancer cells [106, 141-144]. Collectively, cytotoxic effects of extracellular ATP on most neuroblastoma cell lines appear to be largely mediated *via* P2X7, P2Y2, and P2Y6 receptors.

Adenosine has also been shown to limit cell growth in some cancer types *via* activation of distinct P1 receptors. In human colon cancer (Caco-2) and hepatoma (HepG2) cells, A2A signaling decreases expression of anti-apoptotic protein BCL-XL while increasing pro-apoptotic factor BH3 interacting-domain (BID) which could ultimately lead to cancer cell death [118, 145]. When combined with a phosphodiesterase inhibitor (to maximize intracellular cAMP levels), A2A receptor agonists provoke death of multiple myeloma and diffuse large cell lymphoma [146]. As to A1 and A3 receptors, considerable evidence directly links their activation to tumor cell killing [147]. Activation of A1 receptor induces apoptosis in CW2 human colon cancer cells (mediated *via* caspase-3, -8 and -9) [148] and mouse glioblastoma [149]. A3 signaling has been demonstrated to inhibit growth of a wide range of cancer cell types, including human lymphoma, melanoma, prostate, lung, colon, and neural cancer cells, and murine hepatocellular carcinoma (HCC) cells [150-160]. The underlying mechanisms suggested are varied: induction of G0 or G1 cell cycle arrest, upregulation of pro-apoptotic genes with concurrent reduction of anti-apoptotic genes, or inhibition of the Wnt pathway [150-160].

These ambiguities amongst purinoreceptor functionalities in tumor growth (summarized in Tables **1** and **2**) have yet to be fully explained. Further study is required and ought to consider the role of concurrent activation of distinct, yet opposite, intracellular signals, and/or relative differences in the levels of extracellular ATP/adenosine.

As control nodes for extracellular ATP metabolism, ectonucleotidases CD39 and/or CD73 (to a lesser extent) play pivotal and direct roles in tumor growth. Both have been shown to be overexpressed on several types of cancer cells. For instance, CD39 is the dominant ectonucleotidase on human melanocytes, and melanoma cells and differentiated human melanomas overexpress CD39 [161]. Heightened CD39 expression is also found in some newly developed human hematological malignant cell lines, such as BALM-25 (derived from acute lymphoblastic leukemia) [162], MedB-1 (derived from large B-cell lymphoma) [163], and chronic lymphocytic leukemia cell lines [164, 165]. Cancer cells

Table 1. P2 Receptors and Impact on Cancer Cell Growth

Receptor	Cancer Type	Cell Line	Impact on Cell Growth	References
P2X5	Prostate cancer	PC-3	↓	[139]
	Bladder cancer	HT-1376	↓	[105]
P2X7	Colon cancer	MCA38, HCT8	↓	[65, 106,127,141,142]
	Melanoma	B16/F10, A375	↓	[65, 106,127,141,142]
	Squamous cell carcinoma	A431	↓	[128]
	Glioma	U-138MG, U-251MG	↓	[129,135]
	Cervical cancer	hECE, CaSki	↓	[130]
	Endometrial cancer	Tissue only	↓	[131]
	Prostate cancer	PC-3	↓	[139]
	Bladder cancer	HT-1376	↓	[105]
	Breast cancer	MDA-MB-231, MCF-7	↓	[132]
P2Y1	Melanoma	A375	↓	[106,141,142]
	Colon cancer	HCT8	↓	[106,141,142]
	Thyroid cancer	ARO	↑	[103]
P2Y2	Melanoma	A375	↓	[106]
	Colon cancer	HCT8, HT29	↓	[106,141,142,143]
	Oesophageal cancer	Kyse-140	↓	[144]
	Prostate cancer	HT-1376	↑	[105]
	Melanoma	A375	↑	[106]
	Squamous cell carcinoma	A431	↑	[107]
	Breast cancer	MCF-7	↑	[108]
	Lung cancer	A549	↑	[109]
	Breast cancer	MCF-7	↑	[110]
P2Y6	Lung cancer	A549	↑	[109,112]
	Astrocytoma	132N1	↑	[113]
P2Y11	Prostate cancer	PC-3	↓	[139]
	Bladder cancer	HT-1376	↓	[105]
P2Y12	Lung cancer	A549	↓	[111]

Note: ↓: Tumor-killing function. ↑: Tumor-promoting function.

Table 2. P1 Adenosine Receptors and Impact on Cancer Cell Growth

Receptor	Cancer Type	Cell Line	Impact on Cell Growth	References
A1	Colon cancer	CW2	↓	[148]
	Glioblastoma	Gl261	↓	[149]
	Breast cancer	MDA-MB-468	↑	[119]
	Colon cancer	HT-29	↑	[120]
A2A	Lung adenocarcinoma	PC9	↑	[115]
	Pancreatic cancer	BON-1	↑	[116]
	Intestinal cancer	KRJ-I	↑	[116]
	Prostate cancer	PC-3, DU145, and LNCaP	↑	[117]
	Colon cancer	Caco-2	↓	[118,145]
	Hepatoma	HepG2	↓	[145]
	Multiple myeloma	MM.1S	↓	[146]
	Lymphoma	SU-DHL6	↓	[146]
A2B	Lung adenocarcinoma	PC9	↑	[115]
	Pancreatic cancer	BON-1	↑	[116]
	Intestinal cancer	KRJ-I	↑	[116]
	Prostate cancer	PC-3	↑	[117]
A3	Lymphoma	Nb2-11C	↓	[150]
	Melanoma	A375	↓	[151]
	Prostate cancer	DU-145, PC3, LNcap-FGC10	↓	[152]
	Colon cancer	HCT-116	↓	[153]
	Melanoma	B16-F10	↓	[153]
	Hepatoma	N1S1	↓	[154]

Note: ↓: Tumor-killing function. ↑: Tumor-promoting function.

overexpressing CD73 include bladder cancer [166], leukemia [167], glioma [168], glioblastoma [169], melanoma [170], ovarian [165], thyroid [171], esophageal [172], gastric [173], colon [174], prostate, breast [175], and endometrial cancer [85].

Recently, Clayton *et al.,* discovered that exosomes from diverse cancer cell types (HT1376 bladder, Caco2 colon, and DU145 and PC3 prostate cancer cells) coexpress CD39 and CD73 and display high ectonucleotidase activity [176]. Coexpression of CD39 and CD73 on cancer cells or derived exosomes suggest that cancer cells could produce adenosine from extracellular substrates in an autocrine fashion.

Taken together, CD39 and/or CD73, expressed on both tumor and host immune or other cells, have been demonstrated to have potent influences, either directly or indirectly, on tumor growth. These actions are modulated by multiple purinergic mechanisms that initiate different, sometimes opposing, cellular responses. The final outcome is dictated by the balance of these divergent cellular functions. These aspects will be discussed in further detail throughout this section.

Host Adaptations and Responses

Purinergic elements expressed by almost all types of host cells critically control the host adaptations and responses, *e.g.* angiogenic and immune responses in the local tumor microenvironment.

Angiogenesis

Tumor angiogenesis, *de novo* formation of tumor-associated blood vessels, is vitally important to the development, malignant transformation, rapid growth, and progression of solid tumors. It has also become a major target for cancer therapeutics [177-180]. The capacity for tumor growth above the size of 2-3 mm^3 is determined by the availability of oxygen and nutrients [181, 182]. Enhanced angiogenesis can be noted during early carcinogenesis. Hypoxic conditions during proliferation drive cancer cells to produce pro-angiogenic proteins, including VEGF, basic fibroblast growth factor (bFGF), TGF-β, and interleukin-8 (IL-8) [183-185]. Besides indispensable vascular ECs, several other cell types in supporting roles also greatly contribute to angiogenesis. Monocytes/macrophages can secrete angiogenic factors and metalloproteases to facilitate EC migration and new vessel growth [186]. Vascular smooth muscle cells facilitate vascular endothelial maturation and pericytes protect the nascent, *de novo* formed EC-lined tubes [187]. Accessory and stromal cells are also linked to tumor angiogenesis, yet the sources of these cells are still not clear.

When cancer cells undergo ischemia, the associated release of angiogenic mediators (*e.g.* ATP and other chemoattractants) promotes angiogenesis. Further intratumoral accumulation of adenosine is another key driver of tumor angiogenesis. Purinergic signaling modulates growth, function, and migration of all cell types associated with tumor angiogenesis, and is a fundamental player in this crucial process dictating cancer development.

With the growing importance of angiogenesis in cancer biology, it is worthwhile to exploit mechanisms of extracellular nucleotide/nucleoside metabolism and action, in order to limit angiogenesis thereby blocking tumor growth and potentially preventing metastasis and associated cancer mortality [188].

Vascular Endothelial Cells (ECs)

Vascular ECs, the key player in angiogenesis, express broad-spectrum P2 receptors including P2Y1, P2Y2, P2Y11, P2X4, and P2X7 [189] as well as A2A and A2B adenosine receptors [190-192].

P2Y receptors, well-established integral modulators of blood flow [193], have been recognized as important regulators of EC function [194, 195]. Several elegant mechanistic studies demonstrate the abilities of endothelial P2Y receptors to drive angiogenesis *vis-a-vis* EC motility, mitogenic responses, and vascular permeability [196-198]. Extracellular ATP is considered as a vasoactive mediator. It can activate P2Y1/2 expressed on vascular ECs to promote release of additional vasoactive mediators including ATP, nitric oxide (NO), and prostacyclin [199-201]. Consequently, through an autocrine, positive feedback mechanism these effects boost vasoactive and angiogenic responses [202].

P2Y2 receptor contains an extracellular integrin-binding domain RGD (arginine-glycine-aspartic acid). RGD has been shown, in human K562 erythroleukemia cells, to interact with integrins $\alpha v\beta 3$ and $\alpha v\beta 5$, both key players in modulating vascular EC functionality and angiogenesis [203]. Activation of P2Y2 transactivates VEGFR-2, suggesting crosstalk among signals for extracellular nucleotides (specifically ATP and UTP *via* a GPCR) and growth factors (*via* receptor tyrosine kinase; RTK) [204].

Buvinic *et al.,* noted that synergy between P2Y1 (an ADP receptor) and EGFR signaling enhances cell proliferation [205]. Rumjahn *et al.,* reported that extracellular nucleotide-initiated angiogenic responses are mediated through convergent elicitation of P2Y1 receptor and subsequent VEGFR-2 signaling in ECs [206]. Beldi *et al.,* explicitly delineate how, in the hepatic microenvironment, alterations in extracellular nucleotide fluxes (ATP, UTP, and ADP) tightly control the crosstalk between P2Y2 and VEGFR-2 signaling in both hepatocytes and liver sinusoidal endothelial cells (LSECs) to control the release of mitogenic factors. As critical mediators of LSEC and hepatocyte proliferation, these mitogenic factors (including VEGF, HGF, and IL-6) further govern the success of the well-regulated, multistep liver regeneration process. Moreover, colocalization of VEGFR-2 and P2Y receptors is also noted in endothelial caveolae [195, 207-210], allowing for sufficient pro-angiogenic signaling activation, even with stimulation by small amounts of agonists.

P2X4 is a highly expressed P2X subtype in ECs [189]. It is thought that P2X4 plays a key role in regulation of EC responses to changes in blood flow and sheer stress and thereby controls blood flow-dependent processes including angiogenesis and vascular remodeling [211]. In human umbilical vein endothelial cells (HUVECs), ATP-P2X4 signaling mediates biotinylated thymosin β-4 (Tβ4)-stimulated cell migration [212]. P2X7 also plays important, yet paradoxical, roles in angiogenesis. Persistent P2X7 activation drives primary human monocytes to vigorously release VEGF, dependent on calcium signals and linked to ROS production [213]. However, transient P2X7 activation by high ATP levels exerts direct cytotoxicity on ECs limiting tumor angiogenesis [65].

Of note, adenosine-mediated A2A and A2B receptor signaling has been extensively demonstrated to directly enhance EC proliferation and pro-angiogenic factor secretion, driving tumor angiogenesis [190-192].

Finally, owing to the complexity of signal transduction networks, suppression of an element often activates other compensatory pathways, chiefly by perturbing crucial negative feedback loops. Genetic knock down/out systems might develop strong compensatory effects, since knockdown of a specific receptor subtype could lead to a compensatory activation of other subtype functions [214]. As an example, P2X7 deficiency is shown to induce compensatory elevations of P2X4 [127, 215] and P2X1 [216].

Monocytes/Macrophages

Blood mononuclear cell populations, and derived cells including tissue macrophages, are also involved in modulation of angiogenesis [217]. Monocytes/macrophages possess several P2/P1 receptors. Upregulation of P2X7 receptor mRNA in monocytes has been observed upon the differentiation to macrophages [218]. In macrophages, activation of P2X7 receptor signaling by high levels of ATP has been linked to several downstream MAPKs (such as ERK1/2 and p38). These signals play important roles in numerous pathophysiological responses *e.g.* inflammation and tissue remodeling [218], possibly mediated through the production of inflammatory mediators (inclusive of tissue factor that has been implicated in thrombotic disorders, angiogenesis, and metastasis) [219]. Clark *et al.,* recently documented that A1 signaling transduction in peripherally-derived monocytes stimulates VEGF release to further impact EC function [220].

Vascular Smooth Muscle Cells, Accessory and Stromal Cells

Vascular smooth muscle cells express P2X receptors that mediate extracellular ATP-initiated vasoconstrictor responses [221]. These cells also possess a variety of P2Y and P1 receptors to control the vascular tonus [221, 222]. In human coronary smooth muscle cells, ATP-induced growth suppression is mediated *via* the P2X1-transcription factor NR4A1 signaling axis [223]. Activation of A2A, A2B, and A3 receptors in these cells is able to drive release of pro-angiogenic mediators including growth factors and cytokines [224, 225]. Paradoxically, adenosine is also shown to suppress proliferation of rat and human aortic smooth muscle cells *via* A2B receptor signaling transduction [226]. Additionally, accessory and stromal cells are also capable to metabolize pericellular ATP thereby participating in tumor angiogenesis.

In principle, CD39 and/or CD73 modulate and control these ATP- or adenosine-mediated angiogenic responses, through tightly regulating the local pericellular ATP/adenosine levels within the tumor microenvironment. Being critical for EC growth and function, CD39 is absolutely requisite for angiogenesis [227, 228]. Deletion of CD39 has been shown to abrogate growth of transplanted tumors in various types in mice, largely due to defective angiogenesis [72, 229]. Vascular cells expressing CD39 also boost angiogenesis by scavenging cytotoxic extracellular ATP [65], leading to the production of adenosine that is able to promote tumor angiogenesis through activation of A2A receptor on ECs [21]. In addition, CD39 also protects macrophages from ATP-P2X7 elicited cell death [230].

Loss of CD39 leads to perturbed chemotactic and mitogenic responses of ECs, monocytes/macrophages, and pericytes, and impaired integrin expression, as well as defective release of angiogenic factors and mitogens. This dysfunction is the result, at least in part, of disordered P2Y receptor signaling [227, 231, 232]. Finally, CD39 expression on vascular smooth muscle cell also plays a critical role in cell migration [233].

More recently, host cell expression of CD73 has been shown to drive angiogenic responses *in vivo* such as tube formation and EC migration [234]. Furthermore, ENTPD2 activity appears to also play a critical role in tumor progression through ADP production, which recruits platelets to the tumor site and thereby regulates angiogenesis and tumor growth [235].

Innate and Adaptive Immune Responses

An effective immune system, inclusive of both innate and adaptive systems, is required for clearance of the invading tumor cells. Simultaneously, the inflammatory tumor microenvironment, endowed by both innate and adaptive immune cells, possesses a bifunctional feature: this is either stimulatory or inhibitory for cancer cells. The purinergic system, expressed on multiple inflammatory and immune cells, plays an indispensable role in inflammation [236] and antitumor immune responses [4, 237].

Extracellular ATP in Innate Immunity

In general, high extracellular ATP levels have immune stimulatory effects and boost innate responses. Accumulated pericellular ATP levels within the tumor function as chemoattractants to recruit virtually all innate immune cells towards the tumor. Purinergic responses also subsequently induce pro-inflammatory cytokine release by these cells.

Damaged cells/tissues release endogenous "danger signals" (termed damage-associated molecular pattern molecules (DAMPs)). Innate immune cells appear to sense these soluble molecules and then become fully activated [238]. One unique feature shared by all DAMPs is their complete absence under physiological conditions and rapid accumulation in the extracellular milieu upon cell damage. The high levels of ATP released by necrotic cells [79] are actually potent DAMPs [38]. Chemotherapy-induced ATP release by tumor cells is also able to trigger immunogenic cell death [17, 239-241].

Beyond the role as a danger signal, high extracellular ATP levels perform other antitumor actions mediated through multiple molecular mechanisms [1]. ATP can also act as a "find-me" signal to initiate and drive efficient clearance of apoptotic cells by phagocytes [242].

Based on persuasive *in vitro* and *in vivo* evidence, P2Y2 and P2X7 are the major P2 receptor subtypes mediating ATP-induced pro-inflammatory responses. Indeed, P2Y2 is essential for recruitment and function of inflammatory cells at the inflammation sites, namely the release of pro-inflammatory mediators (*e.g.* elastase, interleukin-33 (IL-33), and mononcyte chemoattractant protein-1 (MCP-1/CCL2)) [38]. In addition, upon binding P2X7 receptor expressed on monocytes/macrophages, ATP activates the NLRP3 inflammasome, and as a consequence, promotes production of pro-inflammatory cytokine interleukin-1β (IL-1β) [243]. In brief, ATP's effects are complex and occasionally contradictory; ATP is also reported to block the synthesis of pro-inflammatory cytokines interleukin-12 (IL-12) and TNF-α in macrophages [82].

Extracellular ATP in Adaptive Immunity

As DCs that trigger T-cell costimulation and specific immune-cell activation are key players linking the host innate and adaptive responses against cancer, we will discuss these elements in more detail. The danger signals released by activated, injured, or dying tumor cells - including ATP - are perceived by DCs and then elicit an effective antitumor response (*e.g.* adjunctive vaccine effect). Indeed, ATP modulates DC maturation [244], migration, and function [123], and plays a critical role in signal amplification during T-cell activation [245-247]. Tumor-derived ATP acts on the P2X7 receptor present on DCs to evoke the NLRP3/ASC/caspase-1 inflammasome, thereby driving IL-1β production. IL-1β subsequently fosters the maturation of IFNγ-producing $CD8^+$ cytotoxic T lymphocytes (CTLs), conferring maximal cytotoxicity towards tumor cells. These novel findings support the potential for ATP-P2X7 signaling as a potent adjuvant in cancer chemotherapy treatment [240].

As recently shown using the murine experimental autoimmune encephalomyelitis (EAE), binding of IL-27 to its receptor on DCs limits Th1 and Th17 cell generation and EAE development [248]. This is mediated in large part through induction of intrinsic CD39 expression/activity that impedes ATP-dependent NLRP3 inflammasome activation *via* clearance of pericellular ATP [249]. Additionally, IL-27 released by DCs upon exposure to supernatants of apoptotic cancer cells has the capacity to activate $CD39^+CD69^+$ Tregs thereby decreasing myelotoxicity [250]. On the contrary, ATP is also able to perturb DC maturation and capability of recruiting and evoking Th1 cell responses [80, 81].

Furthermore, ATP can also directly drive Th-cell differentiation towards highly pro-inflammatory populations Th1 and Th17 [1], thereby augmenting antitumor immunity. A subset of human Th17 cells, so called “supTh17”, can also display immune suppressive function *in vitro*. We recently found that, in contrast to "pathogenic" Th17 cells, these supTh17 cells express high levels of CD39 and exhibit enzymatic activity, capable of metabolizing exogenous ATP to adenosine thereby exerting immunosuppressive activity [251]. Additionally, ATP-P2X7 signaling further boosts antitumor immune responses by inducing Treg apoptosis [252, 253].

Adenosinergic Modulation of Antitumor Immunity

As a potent immunosuppressant, through multiple P1 receptor signaling pathways, adenosine converts the inflammatory and immune cell functions to confer a hostile tumor microenvironment [21, 147, 254]. Adenosine generation is heightened under hypoxic conditions, as in the necrotic center of high-grade tumors. As a key molecule maintaining oxygen homeostasis, HIF-1 is responsible for hypoxia-driven responses [255]. Hypoxia seems to regulate CD73 expression, given that the CD73 gene promoter contains a binding site for the HIF-1 transcription factor [256]. Recently, HIF-1 has been implicated in modulation of adenosine production and subsequent downstream signals [255, 257].

Adenosine in general, has suppressive effects on the host innate and adaptive immunity [258, 259]. As Gs-coupled receptors, A2A and A2B play essential roles in adenosine-induced immunosuppression in a cAMP-dependent manner. Adenosine-A2A signaling blocks function of activated NK cells, the first line in the tumor immune surveillance program against malignant cells [260]. Beyond that, binding of adenosine to A2A and A2B could control adaptive immune responses in many ways: induction of tolerogenic DC differentiation and secretion of inhibitory cytokines such as interleukin-10 (IL-10) and TGF-β [261]; and potent suppression of effector T-cell proliferation, cytokine production, and cytotoxic activity [262-266].

In addition, A2A signaling also promotes intratumor immune-suppressive Treg accumulation [21, 254]. A2B activation stimulates the expansion of another important immune suppressor myeloid-derived suppressor cells (MDSCs) and intrinsic release of angiogenic factors [21, 254], ultimately facilitating tumor growth. Moreover, adenosine also skews T-cell differentiation towards Th type 2 (Th2) cells and Tregs that are thought to suppress antitumor immunity [267].

Cellular sources of adenosine are many and include tumor cells, immunosuppressor cells, and the tumor-vasculature, each coexpressing CD39 and CD73. In order to promote the antitumor responses, it is of great importance to inhibit adenosine production by way of blocking CD39 and/or CD73 [268]. $CD39^{+}CD73^{+}$ Tregs, that mediate potent immunosuppression operational *via* adenosine-mediated pathways [73], are upregulated in most human malignancies. NK cell-mediated antitumor functions, both *in vitro* and *in vivo*, are also susceptible to direct Treg suppression [269]. Many well-conducted studies have illustrated the role of tumor-infiltrating $CD39^{+}$ Tregs in promoting immunosuppression by suppressing NK tumor-killing activity and scavenging tumoricidal ATP while supplying adenosine [56, 72].

Genetic deletion of CD39 is shown to result in defective angiogenesis and slower tumor growth in several syngenic murine cancer models, concurrent with substantively decreased migratory potential of inflammatory cells [72, 229, 232, 270]. Hence, blockade of CD39 may have favorable outcomes in cancer by restoring antitumor immune responses.

Invasion and Metastasis

Besides local growth, tumor cells often spread by "metastasis", which is the dissemination of a cancer from its primary tissue/organ to other distant location(s) through circulation or direct seeding. It is a complex, multistep process and tumor-host interactions are vital during these processes.

In order to attain invasive and metastatic characteristics, tumor cells must first acquire the ability to secrete cytokines, chemokines, and matrix degrading enzymes. These drivers of metastasis are either intrinsic such as genetic mutations or extrinsic *e.g.* hypoxia. It has been reported that breast cancer cells can be driven to extrude nucleoside diphosphate kinase (sNDPK-B), locally converting ADP to ATP.

ATP and derivatives then further activate endothelial P2Y receptor signaling thereby modulating blood flow and vascular permeability and ultimately initiating the metastatic process [206, 271-273]. In cancer cells, ATP-P2Y2-mediated MAPK ERK1/2 and p38 signaling activates epithelial-mesenchymal transition (EMT)/invasion-related genes to facilitate migratory, invasive, and metastatic capacities of these cells [274-276].

Additionally, in ECs, synergy between P2Y2 and integrin signaling confers maximal adhesive activity for circulating tumor cells to adhere [277]. Moreover, tumor cells can stimulate platelets to release adenine nucleotides, which also act on P2Y2 receptor expressed by ECs to promote cancer cell survival and breach the endothelial barrier to allow cancer cell transendothelial migration [278]. P2Y1 activation mediates glioma cell mobility and migration through the alteration of intracellular Ca^{2+} levels suggesting yet another mechanistic link between activated purinergic receptor and functional responses [279]. These findings imply that pharmacological modulation of P2Y2- or P2Y1-dependent signaling pathways may serve as novel therapeutic options to lower aggressiveness and slow metastasis of tumors.

P2X7, too, has been linked to tumor metastasis in many cancer types. Pro-invasive roles of P2X7 signaling have been suggested in breast cancer where activation of this receptor increases cell motility and extracellular matrix infiltration as well as levels of cathepsins [280, 281]. In patients with papillary thyroid carcinoma, upregulated P2X7 expression was suggested as a biomarker for lymph node metastasis [282]. P2X7-mediated signaling also modulates migration of PC-9 human lung cancer cells [283].

Elevated expression and activity of CD39 and/or CD73 has also been linked to more aggressive clinical behaviors, higher tumor grade, and higher metastatic potentials of several cancer types [118, 171, 175, 270, 284-287]. Tumor cells coexpressing CD39/CD73 can generate adenosine that promotes metastatic behavior through A2A and A2B receptors. A2A blocks incoming antitumor T lymphocytes to protect cancer cells and facilitate tumor metastasis [265]. Select tumors are endowed with high adenosine generation capability and abundant expression of A2B. In these cells, adenosine-provoked A2B signaling would cause PKA pathway-mediated reductions in prenylation and cell membrane localization of Rap1B, thereby increasing cell scattering and invasive potential [288]. To the contrary, actions by A3 receptor, which is intrinsically expressed on tumor cells, are anti-metastatic. Interestingly, muscle cells have the capacity to secrete natural/endogenous A3 receptor agonists, which are stable, non-hydrolyzable, and exert systemic anticancer and chemoprotective activity, underlying the scarcity of muscle metastases [153].

The specific role of CD39 in tumor invasion and metastasis has been evaluated. Tumor cell adhesion has been linked to ecto-ATPDases, either directly *via* intrinsic enzymatic activity, or indirectly *via* both integrin-dependent and-independent adhesion pathways. Pharmacological inhibition of CD39 is shown to enhance the adhesive interactions between neutrophils and ECs [161]. Interactions of CD39 with adhesion molecules influence P2 receptor activation thereby regulating cell adhesion. In human ECs, ATP-evoked P2 receptor signaling enhances intracellular calcium levels. This pathway would lead to subsequent cytoskeletal and cell contact rearrangements, as well as phosphorylation of several integrin signaling components, including focal adhesionkinase (FAK), paxillin, and proline-rich tyrosine kinase 2 (Pyk2) [55]. Wild type ECs exhibit robust phosphorylation of FAK, whereas the integrin-mediated FAK activation is defective in CD39 null cells. As such, deletion of CD39 results in differential P2 receptor desensitization, which impedes the activity and function of integrins [229].

Another study has shown that RanBPM forms a molecular complex with CD39 on cell membrane. This interaction has the potential to regulate ENTPDase catalytic activity [48]. RanBPM is also associated with integrin and modulates integrin function [289]. Furthermore, within the "immunological synapse", CD39 on DCs is essential for the maintenance of proper synergies among signaling transduction for integrins, ATP, and chemokines [71].

CD73 generally promotes tumor metastasis, possibly by stimulating chemotaxis. Indeed, resistance to melanoma metastasis is noted with CD73 null mice [268, 290]. This phenomenon is thought to be as a result of CD73 loss in both hematopoietic and nonhematopoietic cells. CD73 deficiency might limit lymphocyte trafficking to the distant sites by decreasing cell adhesive and migratory abilities to/through the endothelium that are dependent of CD73-generated adenosine [290]. However, severe combined immunodeficiency (SCID) mice still preserve CD73-mediated pro-metastatic functions [291]. Moreover, intrinsic CD73 expression by tumor cells is also found to facilitate metastasis, yet the underlying molecular mechanism remains unclear [292].

In vivo mechanistic studies on tumor metastasis overall are very limited, owing to difficulties in examining the complex multievent metastatic process using a single animal model. For example, in humans, dissemination through the lymphatic system is an important feature of breast cancer biology. Tumor cells within lymph nodes provide a cell reservoir for future lethal metastases, and therefore, lymph node status in breast cancer patients is a critical factor for clinical decision-making.

By contrast, although mouse models for breast cancer metastasis can be easily induced by tumor cell injection and xenograft transplantation [293, 294], unfortunately, metastatic target sites in these models are always lungs. This discrepancy may be due to much less efficient lymphatic system in mice. Meanwhile, for human lung cancer, metastatic target organs include lung (contralateral side), adrenal glands, bones, and brain. However, in animal models of lung cancer metastasis, irrespective of injection method, metastasis often occurs to mediastinal lymph nodes and systemic metastases are extremely uncommon [295].

The molecular underpinnings of why and how tumors undergo metastases are not fully understood. Recent studies have highlighted the importance of tumor microenvironment, in which communication between tumor cells and the host occurs [296, 297]. Specifically, inflammation and host immune responses that chiefly contribute to the metastatic process are critical aspects that athymic nude mouse models lack [296, 297]. To date, cancer drugs specifically targeting metastasis are still lacking. This is, in large part, due to lack of clinically relevant preclinical animal models for drug development (*e.g.* testing the efficacy, effectiveness, and safety), which is always imperative before clinical trials.

Over the past decade, our laboratory has been devoted to the development of innovative small animal models for studying tumor metastases in distinct organs. As for melanoma and colon cancers, the most common initial site of tumor spread is to the liver, causing substantive morbidity and mortality in such patients. Our strategy is to dissect the multistep metastatic process using these separate models by way of different injection/implantation routes.

For example, we directly implant/inject mouse colon tumor tissues and dispersed cells into mouse colonic wall and into the liver *via* portal vein infusion (or splenic injection), respectively. We can then investigate cancer metastasis at different steps, *i.e.* how the primary cancer cells grow locally and invade into circulation, as well as how the circulating cancer cells colonize and expand at the target organ *e.g.* liver. By engineering tumor cell lines to express bioluminescence markers, we can better trace metastatic cancer cells using state-of-the-art non-invasive imaging techniques for small animals. These models closely resemble human colon cancer metastases [72, 270] (and unpublished data in Robson lab).

Utilizing such unique, clinically relevant metastasis animal models, we have delineated the pro-metastatic roles of CD39 expressed on the vasculature and immune cells. Jackson *et al.,* showed that loss of CD39 markedly blocks melanoma growth and metastasis to the lungs [229]. More recently, Sun and Wu *et al.,* demonstrated that metastases of melanoma and colon cancer cells in the liver are abrogated in CD39 null mice [72].

Multiple CD39-dependent mechanisms have been established, including defective EC functions, increased EC death, and enhanced tumor clearance activity of NK cells secondary to decreased Treg suppressive function [65, 72, 229, 270]. In addition, the decreased metastatic behavior of tumor cells in CD39 null liver has also been attributed to impaired EC-tumor crosstalk and decreased adhesive and invasive activities, accompanied by lowered expression of adhesion molecules such as integrins and cadherins [229, 232] (and unpublished data in Robson lab). These in-depth *in vivo* data manifest the striking anti-metastatic growth effects of CD39 blockade, suggesting promising molecular target in cancer therapy.

Perspectives and Future Therapies

Carcinogenesis is a very complicated dynamic multi-event process comprising opposing and multilevel host-cancer interactions depending on the clinical stage. These include: i) Tumor-host interactions may involve reciprocal crosstalk, *viz.*, tumor cells release several signaling molecules including ATP. These interactions are simultaneously capable of enhancing VEGF levels to facilitate angiogenesis, promote cell proliferation and inflammation, allow for immune system escape, assist in cell matrix infiltration, invasion, and metastasis to distant sites and neovascularization [298, 299]. Inversely, ECs can also produce growth factors and inflammatory cytokines driving tumor cell growth and inflammation. ii) Low levels of chronic inflammation are known to drive early tumor angiogenesis in premalignant tissues thereby promoting malignant transformation and enabling invasive behavior; heightened pro-inflammatory responses, on the other hand are required for efficient clearance of malignant cells. These issues may underscore the paradoxical finding recently noted of increased susceptibility to autochthonous liver cancer formation in aged CD39 null mice [97].

Given the broad-spectrum expression of purinoreceptors, multiple receptors expressed on different cell types might be simultaneously elicited by a given extracellular nucleotide or nucleoside or other signal. It is difficult to determine the end result of these complex cellular responses using any *in vitro* systems or animal models that are genetically modified for purinergic receptors. The unique CD39 mutant murine model has provided a powerful and useful tool for the study of purinergic modulation in cancer biology.

THERAPEUTIC APPROACH AND POSSIBLE TARGETS

Experimental data indicate that activity/function of ectonucleotidases and/or purinergic receptors can be modulated by bioactive pharmacological compounds, blocking monoclonal antibodies (mAbs), or genetic modifications, thereby altering a given purinergic response. Purine-based drugs, either alone or in combination with currently available anticancer modalities, have been tested using preclinical animal models.

In this section, we will highlight the discovery, development, and potential clinical applications of purine-based drugs in cancer therapy. We will also discuss recent advances targeting purinergic modulation as innovative cancer therapeutics and the hurdles that need to be overcome.

Targeting Pericellular Nucleotide/Nucleoside Levels in Cancer Therapy

Several clinical trials have evaluated the benefits of direct supplementation of exogenous ATP in treating patients with non-small cell lung carcinoma (NSCLC). The detailed safety and pharmacokinetics and pharmacodynamics profiles as well as precise mechanisms of action still remain largely elusive. These studies have shown that intravenous injection of ATP fails to cause tumor regression, but successfully mitigates against a range of systemic symptoms associated with advanced malignancies including weight loss [126, 300-302].

There are limits to using systematic infusion of ATP. Extracellular ATP metabolism is such a dynamic process generating multiple intermediates that may exert distinct/opposing functions on many types of cells/tissues. Several approaches, including both *in vitro* luciferase assays and *in vivo* imaging of luciferase indicator mice, have been established to measure the levels and depositions of ATP and derived nucleotides/nucleosides [124, 303]. Currently, there are no non-invasive tools for monitoring these parameters after ATP infusion in the clinical setting.

Secondly, as ATP concentrations in local extracellular microenvironment or in circulation are constantly and precisely controlled and sustained, achieving consistent tumoricidal levels is very difficult. Even when the desired final ATP concentrations are very low, dilution effect *via* delivery route to the designated tissues/organs must be considered. It is also unclear what original concentration is needed to achieve and maintain the desired levels in the final destination for a certain time period that is sufficient to exert their optimal activity/function.

Accordingly, to harness purinergic signaling for adjunctive cancer therapy, we must focus on the intrinsic mechanisms that include ectonucleotidase expression/function as well as ATP release. Control of the local extracellular ATP-adenosine repertoire through regulating expression/activity of ectonucleotidases, especially the master switch molecule CD39, to ultimately govern the purinergic signals within the designated path, might provide the key to development of successful anticancer purinergic modalities that would greatly benefit cancer patients.

Targeting Purinergic Receptors in Cancer Therapy

The anticancer therapeutic effects of drugs targeting purinergic receptors have been widely explored. As a key pro-apoptosis modulator, P2X7-mediated effects provide a novel pharmacological modality for cancer therapy. Induction of intrinsic tumor P2X7 expression leads to tumor cell death, suggestive of the therapeutic utility of P2X7 agonists in cancer treatments [104]. Conversely, P2X7 inhibition by the putative antagonist brilliant blue G (BBG) promotes glioma cell growth [135]. More recently, high ATP levels are reported to induce tumor cell death *via* P2X7 integrated AMPK-PRAS40-mTOR and PI3K-AKT signaling pathways [65, 127].

These well-delineated molecular mechanisms provide a further rationale for the potential utility of purine-based drugs in management of cancer. However, P2X7 receptor antagonism, *e.g.* by emodin (1,3,8-trihydroxy-6-methylanthraquinone; previously shown to contain anticancer properties) or the cholesterol-lowing drug atorvastatin, is able to attenuate ATP-driven invasive and metastatic potentials of human cancer cells [304-306].

In addition, several selective agonists to P2Y1 (*e.g.* methylthioadenosine-5-diphosphate (2-methylthio-ADP) and the ADP analogue MRS2365) and P2Y2, and an antagonist to P2Y12 have been shown to inhibit tumor growth [106, 144, 307, 308]. However, exploration of pharmacological modulation of P2 receptors as innovative approaches or neoadjuvants for anticancer therapy has been limited to *in vitro* studies, largely lacking *in vivo* evidence.

In parallel, the potential therapeutic values of anti-adenosinergic modalities targeting P1 receptors have also been tested in treating cancer. These mediators are operational, in large part, *via* inhibiting immune evasion mechanisms in preclinical animal models. Suppression of A2A receptor in antitumor T cells by antagonists such as caffeine, or by gene silencing using small interfering RNAs (siRNAs), markedly improves effectiveness in blocking tumor growth, limiting metastases, and preventing neovascularization of these cells [265]. Inhibition of A2A and/or A2B receptors on $CD73^+$ tumor cells drastically decreases the metastatic potential, *via* both immunological and non-immunological mechanisms [309, 310]. And also, blockade of A2B on DCs enhances DC activation and chemokine receptor CXCR3-dependent antitumor responses, thereby hindering growth of bladder and breast cancers [311]. Moreover, hypoxia is able to increase A2B expression on colon cancer cells, seemingly promoting cell growth. In turn, A2B is responsible for the release of an array of pro-angiogenic cytokines under hypoxic conditions [312]. Inactivation of the immunosuppressive A2A and A2B receptors (*via* genetic deletion or pharmacological blockade) can prevent hypoxia-mediated inhibition of tumor-infiltrating antitumor T cells, and resultantly lead to complete tumor necrosis [265, 313, 314].

Selective agonists for A3 receptor, specifically CF101 and CF102, were found to enhance anti-inflammatory and anticancer responses in both xenograft and syngenic mouse models. Orally administered CF101 (also known as IB-MECA) efficaciously suppresses tumor growth at the primary sites as well as liver metastases of CT-26 colon cancer cells [315]. Oral administration of Cl-IB-MECA, a synthetic selective A3 agonist with high affinity, to melanoma-bearing mice substantially slows the development of tumor metastases in the lungs [316]. CF102 blocks HCC Hep3B cell growth [317], *via* deregulation of Wnt and NF-κB signaling pathways [154]. Truncated thio-Cl-IB-MECA, a novel A3 antagonist, has been shown to effectively inhibit both T24 bladder and lung cancer cell growth *via* induction of growth arrest and apoptosis [318, 319].

Targeting Ectonucleotidases in Cancer Therapy

Blockade of CD39 and/or CD73 could improve targeted cancer therapies not only by specifically labeling overexpressed tumor antigens but also by blocking adenosine-dependent immune evasion in malignancies, providing novel anticancer treatment options [320]. Several pharmacological inhibitors and blocking mAbs of ectonucleotidases have been developed and tested using both *in vitro* and *in vivo* experimentation systems. To name a few: the inhibitory compounds include ARL67156 (for CD39), polyoxometalate (POM)-1 (potent for CD39 and ENTPD3; much weaker for ENTPD2), POM-6 (for ENTPD2 and 3), PSB06126 (for ENTPD3), PSB069 (for ENTPD1-3), and adenosine 5'-(α, β-methylene) diphosphate (APCP; for CD73).

Inhibition of CD39 bioactivity using ARL67156 is capable of partially overcoming T cell hyporesponsiveness, thereby restoring antitumor immunity [262]. Amongst all these inhibitors, POM-1 shows the highest selectivity for CD39 (with an IC50 at 2.6 μM) [321] and displays potent antitumor activity towards melanoma and colon cancers in a recent preclinical investigation [72]. The antitumor effect of POM-1 in CD39-expressing wild type mice was comparable to that seen with CD39 deficiency. Moreover, administration of POM-1 in tumor-bearing CD39 null mice did not impact metastatic tumor growth, suggesting that the tumor-killing actions of POM-1 in wild type mice were indeed mediated *via* specific inhibition of host CD39 functionality [72]. Minimal *in vivo* toxicity was noted with the optimal short-term treatment strategy for POM-1 (daily intraperitoneal injection at 5 mg/kg for 10 days). In contrast, growth of hepatic metastases of MC-26 colon cancer cells was markedly increased in transgenic mice over-expressing CD39, as compared to wild type or CD39 null mice [270].

Immunotherapeutics targeting CD39 to boost antitumor immune responses have also been actively pursued. Two mAbs against human CD39 (clones BY40 and BA54G) have been recently developed by Bastid and colleagues. Both antibodies specifically bind human CD39 thereby efficiently blocking CD39 enzymatic activity [56]. The BY40 clone is able to restore $CD39^+$ Treg-suppressed CD4 and CD8 T cell proliferation *in vitro* [56], implicating their potential in re-establishing antitumor immunity. However, *in vivo* efficacy and safety of BY40 remains to be extensively tested in preclinical animal models. Although it fails to block ectonucleotidase activity *in vitro,* the 5F2 anti murine CD39 mAb produced in Robson laboratory exhibits potent anti-thrombotic effects *in vivo*, putatively *via* clearance of CD39 from cell surface by internalization (unpublished data in Robson lab). *In vivo* testing of this mAb clone in tumor models is of great interest and is ongoing.

Because of the availability of several blocking mAbs to both mouse and human CD73, many studies have examined the impacts of CD73 inhibition on tumor biology in depth. CD73 blockade, by inhibitor APCP or mAbs effectively abrogates tumor growth and metastasis and is associated with increased survival of tumor-bearing mice [165, 234, 291, 322-325]. Multiple underlying molecular mechanisms have been suggested: i) enhanced tumor antigen-specific T-cell homing to the tumors; ii) decreased apoptosis of and increased expansion of tumor-specific T cells; iii) enhanced intratumor Th1 and Th17 cell-associated cytokine release and; iv) reduced intratumor VEGF levels and impaired tumor angiogenesis. In addition, in animal models bearing subcutaneous MC38-OVA colon and RM-1 prostate cancers, antibody blockade of CD73 enhances the therapeutic efficiency of immunotherapies targeting immune checkpoint regulators programmed death (PD)-1 and cytotoxic T-lymphocyte antigen 4 (CTLA-4) [326].

Stagg and Smyth have further exploited the benefit of co-targeting the CD39-CD73-adenosine pathway in cancer therapy [21]. Concurrent blockade of CD39 and CD73 *via* mAbs (A1 clone for CD39 and 7G2 clone for CD73) substantially boosts the anticancer activity towards ovarian cancer (OvCA), principally by mitigating adenosine-mediated immune evasion mechanisms [320].

More recently, Hausler *et al.,* showed, in human primary ovarian cancer cells and cell lines, that inhibition of CD39 and/or CD73 using siRNAs or small-molecule inhibitors drives $CD4^{+}$ T cell proliferation and augments lytic activities of NK cells and cytotoxic T lymphocytes [327]. These preclinical studies have established the proof-of-concept for anticancer therapeutic strategies targeting CD39 and/or CD73.

In summary, CD39 and/or CD73 are novel therapeutic targets in several cancer types. Such adjunctive therapies have the potential to augment treatment efficacy of other (conventional and/or emerging) therapies. We believe that targeting CD39 holds greater promise in so far as this ectonucleotidase: i) tightly governs the first step of extracellular ATP metabolism; ii) is a master control node for ATP signaling transduction and; iii) is an upstream regulator of CD73 function; thereby dictating the fate of cells exposed to extracellular ATP. Altering the tumor microenvironment to maintain high levels of ATP while preventing phosphohydrolysis to immune-suppressive adenosine would augment antitumor activity. Specifically, blockade of CD39 on the host immune compartment and in the bulk of the tumor would effectively hinder growth of metastatic tumors by ultimately conferring an optimal antitumor microenvironment. Collectively, the molecular underpinnings of the primary anticancer role of CD39 blockade thus far include: i) inhibiting tumor angiogenesis and motility; ii) limiting local immunosuppressant adenosine generation by $CD39^{+}$ cells (*e.g.* immune suppressor and tumor cells and tumor-associated vasculatures); 3) monitoring high ATP levels that could directly kill tumor cells and impact associated ECs, induce Treg apoptosis, enhance cytotoxicity of DC-primed tumor specific CD8 CTLs, increase phagocytosis by functioning as a 'find me" signal, as well as skew Th cells towards the antitumor lineages Th1 and Th17.

Challenges with Clinical Applications of Purinergic Modulation in Cancer Therapy

Cancer is a very complex disease. Like any anticancer therapeutic approaches, purine-based drugs, inclusive of molecular compounds and monoclonal blockade antibodies, would encounter many hurdles that need to be circumvented to achieve optimal beneficial effects and to be successfully translated into the clinic.

Drug Selectivity and Specificity

Conventional therapeutic agents for cancer treatments, albeit valuable, have faced many problems, which include unsatisfactory specificity and efficacy, intrinsic toxicity, and development of resistance to drugs (intrinsic and acquired). Specificity and efficacy are key factors in cancer therapy. Non-selectivity and non-specificity result in severe adverse effects and are associated with morbidities, which largely limit cancer treatment outcomes. The activity of virtually all clinical chemotherapeutic agents is circumscribed by non-selective cytotoxicity towards both proliferating cells (inclusive of cancer and activated antitumor immune cells) and normal cells.

Cancer-killing compounds with distinct mechanisms of action have been developed for widespread clinical use, *e.g.* paclitaxel, trastuzumab, and taxane. However, majority of these drugs are associated with unacceptable off-target effects.

As to synthetic purine-based drugs, selectivity and specificity are also problematic, limiting potential clinical applications. As an example, ARL67156, a synthesized ATP analogue that is considered to selectively inhibit ecto-ATPase, has been shown to have weaker antagonism for P2X and P2Y12 receptors.

POM-1, the most selective CD39 inhibitor up to date, also exhibits inhibitory activity towards ENTPD2 and 3 (with an IC50 at 30 μM and 3.3 μM, respectively). Moreover, elevated cytotoxicity has been observed with long-term usage of these inhibitory compounds, limiting their clinical utility.

Furthermore, due to the important roles of purinergic signals in physiological processes such as maintenance of homeostasis, systemic blockade of purinergic signaling may disrupt multiple biological processes to cause further pathologic alterations in the body. For example, short-term blockade of CD39 might efficiently inhibit metastatic tumor growth *via* elicitation of a series of antitumor mechanisms, as alluded to above. However, long-term loss of CD39 function could lead to spontaneous formation of liver cancer in mice [97]. Therefore, targeted delivery of purine-based drugs for defined time periods is needed to circumvent these off-target effects, thereby achieving optimal anticancer outcomes.

Several novel and attractive targeted delivery strategies have been developed, *e.g.* direct intratumor injection of peptides for antigen-specific cancer immunotherapy [328]. This type of therapy only enhances tumor specific adaptive immune reactions but autoimmunity. Radiosensitizing chemotherapy is another novel approach that has been shown to improve the outcomes in comparison to radiation alone. The delivery of radiation therapy with yttrium90 (90Y) radioembolization, in combination with a radiosensitizing chemotherapeutic agent, provides the opportunity to enhance radiation effects on hepatic malignancies [329]. ATP administration has been shown to act synergistically with radiotherapy. Cotreatment of ATP with radiotherapy increases cell death of human glioma cells, when compared to ATP or radiotherapy treatment alone [129].

Nanostructures, including magnetic nanoparticles, liposomes, and polymers, have been shown to improve drug efficiency by specifically targeting cancer cells [330, 331]. Moreover, multiple surface markers provide a more efficient way to selectively detect cancer cells. Such cancer cell-specific strategies might be anticipated to have enhanced selectivity against tumor cells [332].

Innovative mAbs that bind specific tumor cell surface markers might exhibit less toxicity in cancer therapy. Over the past decade, the utility of mAbs targeting tumor antigens as an alternative anticancer approach has been actively exploited, entailing great promise, *i.e.* mAbs targeting EGFR, HER2/Neu, VEGF, CTLA-4, CD20, CD30, and CD52 [333]. Recently, potent anticancer effect of immunomodulatory antibodies or antibody-conjugated drugs has been noted in cancer clinic. Preclinical assessments of blocking mAbs against CD39 have shown promising immunotherapeutic activity against cancer. However, difficulties with production of CD39 blocking mAbs have been noted. The possible explanations for this may be the following: i) CD39 activity is critical for B cell expansion and function; ii) extracellular domains of CD39 are highly conserved and are not immunogenic and; iii) optimal CD39 activity/function is conferred by formation of dimers or tetramers through the transmembrane regions [334], which is such a dynamic process making CD39 polymers as moving objects that are extremely difficult to target. An alternative strategy would be to generate mAbs that could effectively clear CD39 from the cell surface, as shown by Terp *et al.,* that mAbs bind CD73 can result in internalization of the proteins [87].

Another concern regarding clinical applications would be how to specifically block tumor-associated CD39 without off-target endothelial effects, given the ubiquitous expression on normal vasculatures. Theoretically, disruption of vascular CD39 might be possibly linked to clotting defects, cardiac vasculature dysfunction, and fibrosis. Whether any unforeseen toxicity is associated with saturating dose of CD39 mAbs remains to be evaluated using preclinical cancer models.

To date, preclinical anticancer immunotherapeutic evaluations of CD39 and CD73 mAbs have mostly been carried out in cancer cell lines and in small animal models. Precise delineation of the mechanisms of action and cautious assessments of safety for any given purine-based drugs using clinically relevant animal models are absolute requisites before any clinical translation. This would also greatly benefit from further optimization and personalization of treatment strategies that are largely dependent upon tumor stages *e.g.* early (with local tumors) *vs* advanced (with metastases) and tumor types.

Drug Resistance

Cancer cells often develop insensitivity/resistance to targeted therapies. Drug insensitivity/resistance, either *de novo* or acquired, often leads to recurrence and relapse of treated cancer patients and is another major concern in the treatment of metastatic cancers. A better understanding of the underlying mechanisms prior to clinical trials is the key to improve drugs to overcome drug resistance. Intratumoral heterogeneity is a general trait of most tumors. Intrinsic resistance may activate a subpopulation of tumor cells *e.g.* cancer stem cells (CSCs), leading to recurrence after treatment [335]. The underpinnings for acquired resistance include genetic and epigenetic alternations of crucial genes in cancer cells, induction of immune suppressor cell expression/function, as well as activation of compensatory oncogenic signaling pathways due to disruption of the negative feedback mechanisms [336]. These are underscored by the findings that high dose IL-2 therapy in melanoma patients induces expansion and expression of CD39, CD73, and TGF-β of the inducible T cell costimulator $(ICOS)^+$ Tregs, causing rapid disease progression in non-responders [337]; and that metastases quickly develop in breast cancer patients lacking a P2X7 function allele, following anthracycline treatment [17, 338].

Though combination therapies have been actively pursued and used in oncology clinics to enhance antitumor activity and prevent resistance, the clinical outcomes are still disappointing. The ideal would be achieving drug efficacy of any targeted cancer therapy while obviating emergence of resistance, by integrating major antitumor mechanisms. A good proof-of-principle study in this regard has recently been conducted by Dr. Yu's laboratory [339]. In trastuzumab-resistant breast cancer, maximal therapeutic activity is noted with multi-targeted combinational therapies: inhibiting tumor cells by an AKT inhibitor, and concomitantly augmenting antitumor T cell responses *via* mAb blockade of HER2/Neu and CTLA-4. With regard to purinergic modulation, theoretically, upon induction of ATP release (as by chemotherapy and/or radiotherapy), solo blockade of CD39 would achieve maximal antitumor efficacy: elicitation of antitumor immunity, enhancement of direct tumor-killing activity, and inhibition of tumor angiogenesis, *via* actions on distinct cell types including immune cells, tumor cells, and tumor-associated ECs.

Another new therapeutic avenue against cancer while overcoming drug resistance is targeting cancer stemness. As an intrinsic mechanism for development of resistance, these highly tumorigenic CSCs have been shown to play an essential role in cancer growth, metastasis, and resistance. CSCs are a unique subpopulation of tumor cells that can generate all types of cells in the tumor mass through the self-renewal process. CSCs are generally refractory to conventional cancer drugs that directly disrupt tumor cell growth. Targeting CSC pathways have the potential to kill not only CSCs but also the bulk of the tumor. Several CSC pathway inhibitors, developed by Boston Biomedical (www.bostonbiomedical.com), that target both CSCs and non-stem cancer cells have shown potent antitumor and anti-metastatic activity in a wide range of cancer types in preclinical studies. Multiple ongoing clinical trials testing these drugs in treating patients with solid tumors, alone or in combination with standard-of-care therapies, have entered different phases. CD39 is recently identified as a novel marker for hematopoietic stem cells (HSCs) in both mice and humans [340]. Expression and enzymatic activity of CD39 confer HSC mobility and functionality, *e.g.* limiting inflammation and promoting regeneration after liver resection.

Lack of Clinical Relevant Animal Models and Robust Preclinical Translational Approaches

Animal models incompletely recapitulate the full-spectrum of pathogenesis of human cancer. Hence, owing to the complexity of carcinogenesis, ideal animal models for any given type of cancer are not available. Therapeutic evaluations of purine-based drugs have mostly been based on cancer cell lines and xenograft models. It has increasingly been acknowledged that most cancer drugs developed on the basis of such xenograft studies have not translated well into the clinic. Alternatively, genetically engineered mouse (GEM) models might provide better options. Well-conducted cancer research studies using the global CD39 null mice have unraveled multiple critical purinergic mechanisms underpinning pathogenesis of malignancy, which are seminal contributions to the cancer drug discovery field. Our recent generation of floxed CD39 mice would be valuable tools to dissect the discrete roles of CD39 and related purinergic signaling in distinct types of cell responses during multi-event tumorigenesis (unpublished data in Robson lab).

Another key element that has delayed cancer drug discovery is the lack of a robust platform for preclinical translational screening and testing. Recently, Jaffe *et al.*, has demonstrated that global chromatin profiling using a high-information-content mass spectrometry approach is efficacious in identifying novel therapeutic target for acute lymphoblastic leukemia [341]. In addition, system biology utilizing computational models might also provide useful clues to the dynamics of a given oncogenic pathway component in response to cancer drugs [342].

We have also established a mathematical model to simulate how cells respond to various stimuli and/or pharmacological inhibitors. We note that this modeling system accurately and robustly predicts the final biological consequences of different treatments, alone or in combination, on a given cell type (manuscript in preparation by Robson lab). None of the conventional *in vitro* culture systems has such powerful capacity. Moreover, with recent advances in next-generation sequencing and computer technology, multi-omics analyses (inclusive of genomics, transcriptomics, proteomics, and metabolomics) have been substantiated as useful tools for stratification and diagnosis and prognosis of cancer patients [343]. The magnitude of multi-omics science in personalized cancer medicine is further highlighted by the findings that genetic variations exist that control expression levels of CD39 [344] and P2X7 [345].

Taken together, most studies with regard to purinergic modulation have hitherto focused on tumor-associated immune responses. Nevertheless, nucleotides and nucleosides have exhibited strong direct effects on tumor cells per se, which implies another valuable approach in cancer therapy. The potentials of P2 and P1 receptor agonists/antagonists as anticancer drugs have opened favorable perspectives for the development of innovative purine-based therapeutics to treat cancer. Similarly, these therapeutic compounds targeting purinergic receptors also face many problems, as alluded for CD39 and CD73 above, *e.g.* lacking tumor specificity. The effectiveness of purine-based therapeutic approaches targeting activity/function of ectonucleotidases, P2, or P1 receptors, alone or in combination with immune-stimulatory cytokines, immune cell therapies, cancer vaccines, or traditional or state-of-art chemotherapy and/or radiotherapy, remain to be extensively evaluated.

CONCLUSION AND FUTURE DIRECTIONS

The identification and characterization of extracellular nucleotides and nucleosides in the tumor microenvironment has been important in advancing knowledge of cancer. Understanding unique purinergic mechanisms underlying

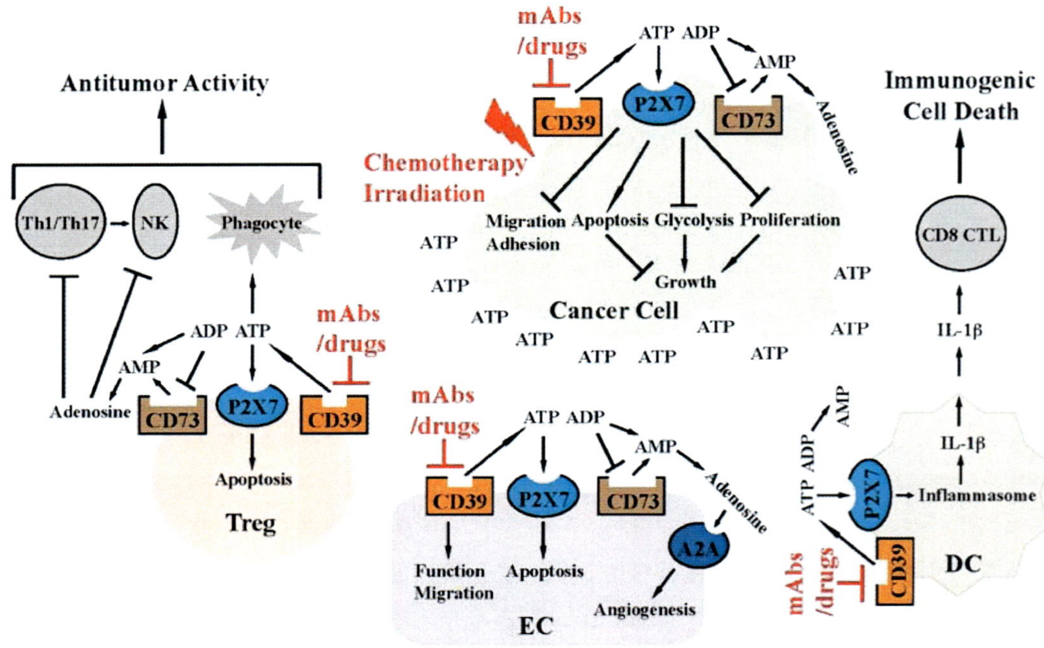

Fig. (1). Proposed impact of CD39 blockade in combination with chemotherapy and/or radiotherapy. Chemotherapy and/or radiotherapy will induce ATP release by cancer cells. Concurrent blockade of CD39 (*via* monoclonal antibodies (mAbs)) or pharmacological inhibitors) will alter the tumor microenvironment by boosting ATP levels and precluding subsequent phosphohydrolysis to tumor-promoting adenosine. Theoretically, this combinational therapeutic approach addresses several distinct aspects of tumor biology, *viz.*, limiting angiogenesis, augmenting antitumor immune responses, and directly killing cancer cells per se, thereby achieving maximal anticancer activity. Pathway key: →: Stimulation; ⊥: Inhibition.

the pathogenesis of malignancy would be fundamental for the discovery and development of effective drugs to treat cancer. The molecular bases of inflammation and immunity are of paramount importance. Approaches that limit or resolve chronic inflammation and augment antitumor immune responses might provide potent anticancer therapeutics limiting cancer development and progression.

Pivotal roles of ectoenzyme-modulated purinerigic signaling have been established in virtually all aspects of tumor biology, notably tumor growth and metabolism, angiogenesis, inflammation, immunity, and metastasis. Our efforts are devoted at developing agents targeting ectoenzymes (specifically CD39) and altering purinergic mechanisms. Together with chemotherapy and/or radiotherapy, this innovative therapeutic strategy has the capacity to target distinct elements of tumor biology, *viz.*, inhibition of angiogenesis, augmentation of antitumor immunity, and direct cytotoxicity towards tumor cells. This might be achieved in such a way that confers an immune-friendly tumor microenvironment, thereby achieving maximal anticancer activity (as illustrated in Fig. **1**).

Purinergic signaling plays distinct roles in tumor biology that is chiefly dependent upon context, *i.e.*, transplanted *vs* autochthonous tumors; acute *vs* chronic inflammation, and is dictated by the balance between pericellular nucleotides and nucleosides. It is noteworthy that, akin to several other key regulators of inflammation and angiogenesis *e.g.* NF-κB and DNA-binding protein inhibitor ID-1 [346, 347], purinergic modulation also has divergent impacts according to the nature of the tumor biology targeted and the kinetics of responses observed. Hence, accurate cancer patient stratification and well-tailored individualized treatment strategy will be required for clinical applications of purine-based drugs.

ACKNOWLEDGEMENTS

This study was supported by the grants from National Institutes of Health (RO1-HL094400 and NHLBI PO1-HL076540) of the United States and Promotive Research Fund for Excellent Young and Middle-aged Scientists of Shandong Province (No. BS2013YY003) of China.

CONFLICT OF INTEREST

The authors confirm that they have no conflict of interest in generating this work.

REFERENCES

[1] Trautmann A. Extracellular ATP in the immune system: more than just a "danger signal". Sci Signal 2009; 2: pe6.

[2] Burnstock G, Campbell G, Satchell D, Smythe A. Evidence that adenosine triphosphate or a related nucleotide is the transmitter substance released by non-adrenergic inhibitory nerves in the gut. Br J Pharmacol 1970; 40: 668-88.

[3] Ralevic V, Burnstock G. Receptors for purines and pyrimidines. Pharmacol Rev 1998; 50: 413-92.

[4] Eltzschig H K, Sitkovsky M V, Robson S C. Purinergic signaling during inflammation. N Engl J Med 2012; 367: 2322-33.

[5] Save S, Persson K. Extracellular ATP and P2Y receptor activation induce a proinflammatory host response in the human urinary tract. Infect Immun 2010; 78: 3609-15.
[6] MacDonald P E, Braun M, Galvanovskis J, Rorsman P. Release of small transmitters through kiss-and-run fusion pores in rat pancreatic beta cells. Cell Metab 2006; 4: 283-90.
[7] Zhang Z, Chen G, Zhou W, *et al*. Regulated ATP release from astrocytes through lysosome exocytosis. Nat Cell Biol 2007; 9: 945-53.
[8] Burnstock G. Physiology and pathophysiology of purinergic neurotransmission. Physiol Rev 2007; 87: 659-797.
[9] Gatof D, Kilic G, Fitz J G. Vesicular exocytosis contributes to volume-sensitive ATP release in biliary cells. Am J Physiol Gastrointest Liver Physiol 2004; 286: G538-46.
[10] Kang J, Kang N, Lovatt D, *et al*. Connexin 43 hemichannels are permeable to ATP. J Neurosci 2008; 28: 4702-11.
[11] Huang Y J, Maruyama Y, Dvoryanchikov G, Pereira E, Chaudhari N, Roper S D. The role of pannexin 1 hemichannels in ATP release and cell-cell communication in mouse taste buds. Proc Natl Acad Sci U S A 2007; 104: 6436-41.
[12] Liu H T, Toychiev AH, Takahashi N, Sabirov R ZOkada Y. Maxi-anion channel as a candidate pathway for osmosensitive ATP release from mouse astrocytes in primary culture. Cell Res 2008; 18: 558-65.
[13] Koyama T, Kimura C, Hayashi M, Watanabe M, Karashima Y, Oike M. Hypergravity induces ATP release and actin reorganization *via* tyrosine phosphorylation and RhoA activation in bovine endothelial cells. Pflugers Arch 2009; 457: 711-9.
[14] Suadicani SO, Brosnan CF, Scemes E. P2X7 receptors mediate ATP release and amplification of astrocytic intercellular Ca2+ signaling. J Neurosci 2006; 26: 1378-85.
[15] Eltzschig H K. Adenosine: an old drug newly discovered. Anesthesiology 2009; 111: 904-15.
[16] Selzner N, Selzner M, Graf R, Ungethuem U, Fitz J G, Clavien P A. Water induces autocrine stimulation of tumor cell killing through ATP release and P2 receptor binding. Cell Death Differ 2004; 11 Suppl 2: S172-80.
[17] Ghiringhelli F, Apetoh L, Tesniere A, *et al*. Activation of the NLRP3 inflammasome in dendritic cells induces IL-1beta-dependent adaptive immunity against tumors. Nat Med 2009; 15: 1170-8.
[18] Seminario-Vidal L, Lazarowski E R, Okada S F. Assessment of extracellular ATP concentrations. Methods Mol Biol 2009; 574: 25-36.
[19] Burnstock G. Historical review: ATP as a neurotransmitter. Trends Pharmacol Sci 2006; 27: 166-76.
[20] Burnstock G, Kennedy C. Is there a basis for distinguishing two types of P2-purinoceptor? Gen Pharmacol 1985; 16: 433-40.
[21] Stagg J, Smyth M J. Extracellular adenosine triphosphate and adenosine in ca7ncer. Oncogene 2010; 29: 5346-58.
[22] Volonte C, Amadio S, D'Ambrosi N, Colpi M, Burnstock G. P2 receptor web: complexity and fine-tuning. Pharmacol Ther 2006; 112: 264-80.
[23] Khakh B S, North R A. P2X receptors as cell-surface ATP sensors in health and disease. Nature 2006; 442: 527-32.
[24] Vaughn B P, Robson S C, Burnstock G. Pathological roles of purinergic signaling in the liver. J Hepatol 2012; 57: 916-20.

[25] Mulryan K, Gitterman D P, Lewis C J, *et al.* Reduced vas deferens contraction and male infertility in mice lacking P2X1 receptors. Nature 2000; 403: 86-9.
[26] North R A. Molecular physiology of P2X receptors. Physiol Rev 2002; 82: 1013-67.
[27] Bleehen T, Keele C A. Observations on the algogenic actions of adenosine compounds on the human blister base preparation. Pain 1977; 3: 367-77.
[28] Hamilton S G, Warburton J, Bhattacharjee A, Ward J, McMahon S B. ATP in human skin elicits a dose-related pain response which is potentiated under conditions of hyperalgesia. Brain 2000; 123 (Pt 6): 1238-46.
[29] Lewis C, Neidhart S, Holy C, North R A, Buell G, Surprenant A. Coexpression of P2X2 and P2X3 receptor subunits can account for ATP-gated currents in sensory neurons. Nature 1995; 377: 432-5.
[30] Allsopp R C, Lalo U, Evans R J. Lipid raft association and cholesterol sensitivity of P2X1-4 receptors for ATP: chimeras and point mutants identify intracellular amino-terminal residues involved in lipid regulation of P2X1 receptors. J Biol Chem 2010; 285: 32770-7.
[31] Garcia-Marcos M, Perez-Andres E, Tandel S, *et al.* Coupling of two pools of P2X7 receptors to distinct intracellular signaling pathways in rat submandibular gland. J Lipid Res 2006; 47: 705-14.
[32] Barth K, Weinhold K, Guenther A, Linge A, Gereke M, Kasper M. Characterization of the molecular interaction between caveolin-1 and the P2X receptors 4 and 7 in E10 mouse lung alveolar epithelial cells. Int J Biochem Cell Biol 2008; 40: 2230-9.
[33] Gonnord P, Delarasse C, Auger R, *et al.* Palmitoylation of the P2X7 receptor, an ATP-gated channel, controls its expression and association with lipid rafts. FASEB J 2009; 23: 795-805.
[34] Deaglio S, Robson S C. Ectonucleotidases as regulators of purinergic signaling in thrombosis, inflammation, and immunity. Adv Pharmacol 2011; 61: 301-32.
[35] Abbracchio M P, Burnstock G, Verkhratsky A, Zimmermann H. Purinergic signalling in the nervous system: an overview. Trends Neurosci 2009; 32: 19-29.
[36] Hollopeter G, Jantzen H M, Vincent D, *et al.* Identification of the platelet ADP receptor targeted by antithrombotic drugs. Nature 2001; 409: 202-7.
[37] Marteau F, Le Poul E, Communi D, *et al.* Pharmacological characterization of the human P2Y13 receptor. Mol Pharmacol 2003; 64: 104-12.
[38] Rayah A, Kanellopoulos J M, Di Virgilio F. P2 receptors and immunity. Microbes Infect 2012; 14: 1254-62.
[39] Lammer A B, Beck A, Grummich B, *et al.* The P2 receptor antagonist PPADS supports recovery from experimental stroke *in vivo*. PLoS One 2011; 6: e19983.
[40] Jacobson K A, Boeynaems J M. P2Y nucleotide receptors: promise of therapeutic applications. Drug Discov Today 2010; 15: 570-8.
[41] Klinger M, Freissmuth M, Nanoff C. Adenosine receptors: G protein-mediated signalling and the role of accessory proteins. Cell Signal 2002; 14: 99-108.
[42] Fishman P, Bar-Yehuda S, Synowitz M, *et al.* Adenosine receptors and cancer. Handb Exp Pharmacol 2009; 399-441.
[43] Ohana G, Bar-Yehuda S, Barer F, Fishman P. Differential effect of adenosine on tumor and normal cell growth: focus on the A3 adenosine receptor. J Cell Physiol 2001; 186: 19-23.
[44] Hoskin D W, Mader J S, Furlong S J, Conrad D M, Blay J. Inhibition of T cell and natural killer cell function by adenosine and its contribution to immune evasion by tumor cells (Review). Int J Oncol 2008; 32: 527-35.

[45] Chen J F, Eltzschig H K, Fredholm B B. Adenosine receptors as drug targets--what are the challenges? Nat Rev Drug Discov 2013; 12: 265-86.

[46] Banz Y, Beldi G, Wu Y, Atkinson B, Usheva A, Robson S C. CD39 is incorporated into plasma microparticles where it maintains functional properties and impacts endothelial activation. Br J Haematol 2008; 142: 627-37.

[47] Robson S C, Wu Y, Sun X, Knosalla C, Dwyer K, Enjyoji K. Ectonucleotidases of CD39 family modulate vascular inflammation and thrombosis in transplantation. Semin Thromb Hemost 2005; 31: 217-33.

[48] Wu Y, Sun X, Kaczmarek E, *et al.* RanBPM associates with CD39 and modulates ecto-nucleotidase activity. Biochem J 2006; 396: 23-30.

[49] Heine P, Braun N, Sevigny J, Robson S C, Servos J, Zimmermann H. The C-terminal cysteine-rich region dictates specific catalytic properties in chimeras of the ectonucleotidases NTPDasel and NTPDase2. Eur J Biochem 2001; 268: 364-73.

[50] Grinthal A, Guidotti G. Dynamic motions of CD39 transmembrane domains regulate and are regulated by the enzymatic active site. Biochemistry 2004; 43: 13849-58.

[51] Kukulski F, Levesque S A, Lavoie E G, *et al.* Comparative hydrolysis of P2 receptor agonists by NTPDases 1, 2, 3 and 8. Purinergic Signal 2005; 1: 193-204.

[52] Bigonnesse F, Levesque S A, Kukulski F, *et al.* Cloning and characterization of mouse nucleoside triphosphate diphosphohydrolase-8. Biochemistry 2004; 43: 5511-9.

[53] Lavoie E G, Kukulski F, Levesque S A, Lecka J, Sevigny J. Cloning and characterization of mouse nucleoside triphosphate diphosphohydrolase-3. Biochem Pharmacol 2004; 67: 1917-26.

[54] Vorhoff T, Zimmermann H, Pelletier J, Sevigny J, Braun N. Cloning and characterization of the ecto-nucleotidase NTPDase3 from rat brain: Predicted secondary structure and relation to other members of the E-NTPDase family and actin. Purinergic Signal 2005; 1: 259-70.

[55] Robson S C, Sevigny J, Zimmermann H. The E-NTPDase family of ectonucleotidases: Structure function relationships and pathophysiological significance. Purinergic Signal 2006; 2: 409-30.

[56] Bastid J, Cottalorda-Regairaz A, Alberici G, Bonnefoy N, Eliaou J F, Bensussan A. ENTPD1/CD39 is a promising therapeutic target in oncology. Oncogene 2013; 32: 1743-51.

[57] Ghiringhelli F, Bruchard M, Chalmin F, Rebe C. Production of adenosine by ectonucleotidases: a key factor in tumor immunoescape. J Biomed Biotechnol 2012; 2012: 473712.

[58] Camici M, Fini C, Ipata P L. Isolation and kinetic properties of 5'-nucleotidase from guinea-pig skeletal muscle. Biochim Biophys Acta 1985; 840: 6-12.

[59] Zimmermann H. 5'-Nucleotidase: molecular structure and functional aspects. Biochem J 1992; 285 (Pt 2): 345-65.

[60] Gordon E L, Pearson J D, Slakey L L. The hydrolysis of extracellular adenine nucleotides by cultured endothelial cells from pig aorta. Feed-forward inhibition of adenosine production at the cell surface. J Biol Chem 1986; 261: 15496-507.

[61] Robson S C. Role of CD73 and extracellular adenosine in disease : Presented by Maria P. Abbracchio. Purinergic Signal 2011; 7: 367-72.

[62] Visovatti S H, Hyman M C, Bouis D, Neubig R, McLaughlin V V, Pinsky D J. Increased CD39 nucleotidase activity on microparticles from patients with idiopathic pulmonary arterial hypertension. PLoS One 2012; 7: e40829.

[63] Sauer A V, Brigida I, Carriglio N, *et al.* Alterations in the adenosine metabolism and CD39/CD73 adenosinergic machinery cause loss of Treg cell function and autoimmunity in ADA-deficient SCID. Blood 2012; 119: 1428-39.

[64] Colgan S P, Eltzschig H K, Eckle T, Thompson L F. Physiological roles for ecto-5'-nucleotidase (CD73). Purinergic Signal 2006; 2: 351-60.

[65] Feng L, Sun X, Csizmadia E, *et al.* Vascular CD39/ENTPD1 directly promotes tumor cell growth by scavenging extracellular adenosine triphosphate. Neoplasia 2011; 13: 206-16.

[66] Niemela J, Ifergan I, Yegutkin G G, Jalkanen S, Prat A, Airas L. IFN-beta regulates CD73 and adenosine expression at the blood-brain barrier. Eur J Immunol 2008; 38: 2718-26.

[67] Algars A, Karikoski M, Yegutkin G G, Stoitzner P, Niemela J, Salmi M, Jalkanen S. Different role of CD73 in leukocyte trafficking *via* blood and lymph vessels. Blood 2011; 117: 4387-93.

[68] Fausther M, Lecka J, Soliman E, *et al.* Coexpression of ecto-5'-nucleotidase/CD73 with specific NTPDases differentially regulates adenosine formation in the rat liver. Am J Physiol Gastrointest Liver Physiol 2012; 302: G447-59.

[69] Corriden R, Chen Y, Inoue Y, *et al.* Ecto-nucleoside triphosphate diphosphohydrolase 1 (E-NTPDase1/CD39) regulates neutrophil chemotaxis by hydrolyzing released ATP to adenosine. J Biol Chem 2008; 283: 28480-6.

[70] Doherty G A, Bai A, Hanidziar D, *et al.* CD73 is a phenotypic marker of effector memory Th17 cells in inflammatory bowel disease. Eur J Immunol 2012; 42: 3062-72.

[71] Dwyer K M, Deaglio S, Gao W, Friedman D, Strom T B, Robson S C. CD39 and control of cellular immune responses. Purinergic Signal 2007; 3: 171-80.

[72] Sun X, Wu Y, Gao W, *et al.* CD39/ENTPD1 expression by CD4+Foxp3+ regulatory T cells promotes hepatic metastatic tumor growth in mice. Gastroenterology 2010; 139: 1030-40.

[73] Deaglio S, Dwyer K M, Gao W, *et al.* Adenosine generation catalyzed by CD39 and CD73 expressed on regulatory T cells mediates immune suppression. J Exp Med 2007; 204: 1257-65.

[74] Borsellino G, Kleinewietfeld M, Di Mitri D, *et al.* Expression of ectonucleotidase CD39 by Foxp3+ Treg cells: hydrolysis of extracellular ATP and immune suppression. Blood 2007; 110: 1225-32.

[75] Zhou Q, Yan J, Putheti P, *et al.* Isolated CD39 expression on CD4+ T cells denotes both regulatory and memory populations. Am J Transplant 2009; 9: 2303-11.

[76] Beldi G, Wu Y, Banz Y, *et al.* Natural killer T cell dysfunction in CD39-null mice protects against concanavalin A-induced hepatitis. Hepatology 2008; 48: 841-52.

[77] Eltzschig H K, Kohler D, Eckle T, Kong T, Robson S C, Colgan S P. Central role of Sp1-regulated CD39 in hypoxia/ischemia protection. Blood 2009; 113: 224-32.

[78] Muller W A. Sorting the signals from the signals in the noisy environment of inflammation. Sci Signal 2011; 4: pe23.

[79] Zeh H J, 3rd, Lotze M T. Addicted to death: invasive cancer and the immune response to unscheduled cell death. J Immunother 2005; 28: 1-9.

[80] la Sala A, Sebastiani S, Ferrari D, Di Virgilio F, Idzko M, Norgauer J, Girolomoni G. Dendritic cells exposed to extracellular adenosine triphosphate acquire the migratory

properties of mature cells and show a reduced capacity to attract type 1 T lymphocytes. Blood 2002; 99: 1715-22.
[81] la Sala A, Ferrari D, Corinti S, Cavani A, Di Virgilio F, Girolomoni G. Extracellular ATP induces a distorted maturation of dendritic cells and inhibits their capacity to initiate Th1 responses. J Immunol 2001; 166: 1611-7.
[82] Hasko G, Kuhel D G, Salzman AL, Szabo C. ATP suppression of interleukin-12 and tumour necrosis factor-alpha release from macrophages. Br J Pharmacol 2000; 129: 909-14.
[83] Martin C, Leone M, Viviand X, Ayem ML, Guieu R. High adenosine plasma concentration as a prognostic index for outcome in patients with septic shock. Crit Care Med 2000; 28: 3198-202.
[84] Sperlagh B, Doda M, Baranyi M, Hasko G. Ischemic-like condition releases norepinephrine and purines from different sources in superfused rat spleen strips. J Neuroimmunol 2000; 111: 45-54.
[85] Aliagas E, Vidal A, Texido L, Ponce J, Condom E, Martin-Satue M. High Expression of Ecto-Nucleotidases CD39 and CD73 in Human Endometrial Tumors. Mediators Inflamm 2014; 2014: 509027.
[86] Resta R, Yamashita Y, Thompson LF. Ecto-enzyme and signaling functions of lymphocyte CD73. Immunol Rev 1998; 161: 95-109.
[87] Terp MG, Olesen KA, Arnspang EC, *et al.* Anti-human CD73 monoclonal antibody inhibits metastasis formation in human breast cancer by inducing clustering and internalization of CD73 expressed on the surface of cancer cells. J Immunol 2013; 191: 4165-73.
[88] Coussens LM, Werb Z. Inflammation and cancer. Nature 2002; 420: 860-7.
[89] Grivennikov S I, Greten F R, Karin M. Immunity, inflammation, and cancer. Cell 2010; 140: 883-99.
[90] Mantovani A, Allavena P, Sica A, Balkwill F. Cancer-related inflammation. Nature 2008; 454: 436-44.
[91] Zou W, Restifo NP. T(H)17 cells in tumour immunity and immunotherapy. Nat Rev Immunol 2010; 10: 248-56.
[92] Van Meir EG, Hadjipanayis CG, Norden AD, Shu HK, Wen PY, Olson J J. Exciting new advances in neuro-oncology: the avenue to a cure for malignant glioma. CA Cancer J Clin 2010; 60: 166-93.
[93] Vander Heiden MG, Cantley LC, Thompson CB. Understanding the Warburg effect: the metabolic requirements of cell proliferation. Science 2009; 324: 1029-33.
[94] Ellis BC, Graham LD, Molloy PL. CRNDE, a long non-coding RNA responsive to insulin/IGF signaling, regulates genes involved in central metabolism. Biochim Biophys Acta 2014; 1843: 372-86.
[95] Li M, Durbin KR, Sweet SM, Tipton JD, Zheng Y, Kelleher NL. Oncogene-induced cellular senescence elicits an anti-Warburg effect. Proteomics 2013; 13: 2585-96.
[96] Phan LM, Yeung SC, Lee MH. Cancer metabolic reprogramming: importance, main features, and potentials for precise targeted anti-cancer therapies. Cancer Biol Med 2014; 11: 1-19.
[97] Sun X, Han L, Seth P, *et al.* Disordered purinergic signaling and abnormal cellular metabolism are associated with development of liver cancer in Cd39/ENTPD1 null mice. Hepatology 2013; 57: 205-16.

[98] Baffy G, Derdak Z, Robson S C. Mitochondrial recoupling: a novel therapeutic strategy for cancer? Br J Cancer 2011; 105: 469-74.

[99] Li W, Nichols K, Nathan C A, Zhao Y. Mitochondrial uncoupling protein 2 is up-regulated in human head and neck, skin, pancreatic, and prostate tumors. Cancer Biomark 2013; 13: 377-83.

[100] Ayyasamy V, Owens K M, Desouki M M, *et al.* Cellular model of Warburg effect identifies tumor promoting function of UCP2 in breast cancer and its suppression by genipin. PLoS One 2011; 6: e24792.

[101] Derdak Z, Mark N M, Beldi G, Robson S C, Wands J R, Baffy G. The mitochondrial uncoupling protein-2 promotes chemoresistance in cancer cells. Cancer Res 2008; 68: 2813-9.

[102] Fang M, Shen Z, Huang S, *et al.* The ER UDPase ENTPD5 promotes protein N-glycosylation, the Warburg effect, and proliferation in the PTEN pathway. Cell 2010; 143: 711-24.

[103] Pines A, Perrone L, Bivi N, *et al.* Quadrifoglio F, Tell G. Activation of APE1/Ref-1 is dependent on reactive oxygen species generated after purinergic receptor stimulation by ATP. Nucleic Acids Res 2005; 33: 4379-94.

[104] White N, Burnstock G. P2 receptors and cancer. Trends Pharmacol Sci 2006; 27: 211-7.

[105] Shabbir M, Ryten M, Thompson C, Mikhailidis D, Burnstock G. Purinergic receptor-mediated effects of ATP in high-grade bladder cancer. BJU Int 2008; 101: 106-12.

[106] White N, Ryten M, Clayton E, Butler P, Burnstock G. P2Y purinergic receptors regulate the growth of human melanomas. Cancer Lett 2005; 224: 81-91.

[107] Greig A V, Linge C, Healy V, *et al.* Expression of purinergic receptors in non-melanoma skin cancers and their functional roles in A431 cells. J Invest Dermatol 2003; 121: 315-27.

[108] Dixon C J, Bowler W B, Fleetwood P, Ginty A F, Gallagher J A, Carron J A. Extracellular nucleotides stimulate proliferation in MCF-7 breast cancer cells *via* P2-purinoceptors. Br J Cancer 1997; 75: 34-9.

[109] Schafer R, Sedehizade F, Welte T, Reiser G. ATP- and UTP-activated P2Y receptors differently regulate proliferation of human lung epithelial tumor cells. Am J Physiol Lung Cell Mol Physiol 2003; 285: L376-85.

[110] Scodelaro Bilbao P, Boland R. Extracellular ATP regulates FoxO family of transcription factors and cell cycle progression through PI3K/Akt in MCF-7 cells. Biochim Biophys Acta 2013; 1830: 4456-69.

[111] Nishimaki N, Tsukimoto M, Kitami A, Kojima S. Autocrine regulation of gamma-irradiation-induced DNA damage response *via* extracellular nucleotides-mediated activation of P2Y6 and P2Y12 receptors. DNA Repair (Amst) 2012; 11: 657-65.

[112] Ide S, Nishimaki N, Tsukimoto M, Kojima S. Purine receptor P2Y6 mediates cellular response to gamma-ray-induced DNA damage. J Toxicol Sci 2014; 39: 15-23.

[113] Kim S G, Gao Z G, Soltysiak K A, Chang T S, Brodie C, Jacobson K A. P2Y6 nucleotide receptor activates PKC to protect 1321N1 astrocytoma cells against tumor necrosis factor-induced apoptosis. Cell Mol Neurobiol 2003; 23: 401-18.

[114] Burnstock G, Di Virgilio F. Purinergic signalling and cancer. Purinergic Signal 2013; 9: 491-540.

[115] Mediavilla-Varela M, Luddy K, Noyes D, Khalil F K, Neuger A M, Soliman H, Antonia S. Antagonism of adenosine A2A receptor expressed by lung adenocarcinoma tumor cells and cancer associated fibroblasts inhibits their growth. Cancer Biol Ther 2013; 14(9).

[116] Kalhan A, Gharibi B, Vazquez M, *et al.* Adenosine A2A and A2B receptor expression in neuroendocrine tumours: potential targets for therapy. Purinergic Signal 2012; 8: 265-74.

[117] Wei Q, Costanzi S, Balasubramanian R, Gao Z G, Jacobson K A. A2B adenosine receptor blockade inhibits growth of prostate cancer cells. Purinergic Signal 2013; 9: 271-80.

[118] Serra S, Horenstein A L, Vaisitti T, *et al.* CD73-generated extracellular adenosine in chronic lymphocytic leukemia creates local conditions counteracting drug-induced cell death. Blood 2011; 118: 6141-52.

[119] Mirza A, Basso A, Black S, *et al.* RNA interference targeting of A1 receptor-overexpressing breast carcinoma cells leads to diminished rates of cell proliferation and induction of apoptosis. Cancer Biol Ther 2005; 4: 1355-60.

[120] Lelievre V, Muller J M, Falcon J. Adenosine modulates cell proliferation in human colonic adenocarcinoma. I. Possible involvement of adenosine A1 receptor subtypes in HT29 cells. Eur J Pharmacol 1998; 341: 289-97.

[121] Rapaport E. Treatment of human tumor cells with ADP or ATP yields arrest of growth in the S phase of the cell cycle. J Cell Physiol 1983; 114: 279-83.

[122] Weber F C, Esser P R, Muller T, *et al.* Lack of the purinergic receptor P2X(7) results in resistance to contact hypersensitivity. J Exp Med 2010; 207: 2609-19.

[123] Wilhelm K, Ganesan J, Muller T, *et al.* Graft-*versus*-host disease is enhanced by extracellular ATP activating P2X7R. Nat Med 2010; 16: 1434-8.

[124] Pellegatti P, Raffaghello L, Bianchi G, Piccardi F, Pistoia V, Di Virgilio F. Increased level of extracellular ATP at tumor sites: *in vivo* imaging with plasma membrane luciferase. PLoS One 2008; 3: e2599.

[125] Michaud M, Martins I, Sukkurwala A Q, *et al.* Autophagy-dependent anticancer immune responses induced by chemotherapeutic agents in mice. Science 2011; 334: 1573-7.

[126] Shabbir M, Burnstock G. Purinergic receptor-mediated effects of adenosine 5'-triphosphate in urological malignant diseases. Int J Urol 2009; 16: 143-50.

[127] Bian S, Sun X, Bai A, *et al.* P2X7 integrates PI3K/AKT and AMPK-PRAS40-mTOR signaling pathways to mediate tumor cell death. PLoS One 2013; 8: e60184.

[128] Deli T, Csernoch L. Extracellular ATP and cancer: an overview with special reference to P2 purinergic receptors. Pathol Oncol Res 2008; 14: 219-31.

[129] Gehring M P, Pereira T C, Zanin R F, *et al.* P2X7 receptor activation leads to increased cell death in a radiosensitive human glioma cell line. Purinergic Signal 2012; 8: 729-39.

[130] Wang Q, Wang L, Feng Y H, Li X, Zeng R, Gorodeski G I. P2X7 receptor-mediated apoptosis of human cervical epithelial cells. Am J Physiol Cell Physiol 2004; 287: C1349-58.

[131] Li X, Zhou L, Feng Y H, Abdul-Karim F W, Gorodeski G I. The P2X7 receptor: a novel biomarker of uterine epithelial cancers. Cancer Epidemiol Biomarkers Prev 2006; 15: 1906-13.

[132] Huang S, Chen Y, Wu W, *et al.* miR-150 promotes human breast cancer growth and malignant behavior by targeting the pro-apoptotic purinergic P2X7 receptor. PLoS One 2013; 8: e80707.

[133] Zhang X J, Zheng G G, Ma X T, *et al.* Expression of P2X7 in human hematopoietic cell lines and leukemia patients. Leuk Res 2004; 28: 1313-22.

[134] Gorodeski G I. P2X7-mediated chemoprevention of epithelial cancers. Expert Opin Ther Targets 2009; 13: 1313-32.

[135] Fang J, Chen X, Zhang L, *et al.* P2X7R suppression promotes glioma growth through epidermal growth factor receptor signal pathway. Int J Biochem Cell Biol 2013; 45: 1109-20.

[136] Mistafa O, Stenius U. Statins inhibit Akt/PKB signaling *via* P2X7 receptor in pancreatic cancer cells. Biochem Pharmacol 2009; 78: 1115-26.

[137] Mistafa O, Hogberg J, Stenius U. Statins and ATP regulate nuclear pAkt *via* the P2X7 purinergic receptor in epithelial cells. Biochem Biophys Res Commun 2008; 365: 131-6.

[138] Mistafa O, Ghalali A, Kadekar S, Hogberg J, Stenius U. Purinergic receptor-mediated rapid depletion of nuclear phosphorylated Akt depends on pleckstrin homology domain leucine-rich repeat phosphatase, calcineurin, protein phosphatase 2A, and PTEN phosphatases. J Biol Chem 2010; 285: 27900-10.

[139] Fang W G, Pirnia F, Bang Y J, Myers C E, Trepel J B. P2-purinergic receptor agonists inhibit the growth of androgen-independent prostate carcinoma cells. J Clin Invest 1992; 89: 191-6.

[140] Calvert R C, Shabbir M, Thompson C S, Mikhailidis D P, Morgan R J, Burnstock G. Immunocytochemical and pharmacological characterisation of P2-purinoceptor-mediated cell growth and death in PC-3 hormone refractory prostate cancer cells. Anticancer Res 2004; 24: 2853-9.

[141] White N, Butler P E, Burnstock G. Human melanomas express functional P2 X(7) receptors. Cell Tissue Res 2005; 321: 411-8.

[142] Coutinho-Silva R, Stahl L, Cheung K K, *et al.* P2X and P2Y purinergic receptors on human intestinal epithelial carcinoma cells: effects of extracellular nucleotides on apoptosis and cell proliferation. Am J Physiol Gastrointest Liver Physiol 2005; 288: G1024-35.

[143] Hopfner M, Lemmer K, Jansen A, *et al.* Expression of functional P2-purinergic receptors in primary cultures of human colorectal carcinoma cells. Biochem Biophys Res Commun 1998; 251: 811-7.

[144] Maaser K, Hopfner M, Kap H, *et al.* Extracellular nucleotides inhibit growth of human oesophageal cancer cells *via* P2Y(2)-receptors. Br J Cancer 2002; 86: 636-44.

[145] Yasuda Y, Saito M, Yamamura T, Yaguchi T, Nishizaki T. Extracellular adenosine induces apoptosis in Caco-2 human colonic cancer cells by activating caspase-9/-3 *via* A(2a) adenosine receptors. J Gastroenterol 2009; 44: 56-65.

[146] Rickles R J, Tam W F, Giordano T P, *et al.* Adenosine A2A and beta-2 adrenergic receptor agonists: novel selective and synergistic multiple myeloma targets discovered through systematic combination screening. Mol Cancer Ther 2012; 11: 1432-42.

[147] Antonioli L, Blandizzi C, Pacher P, Hasko G. Immunity, inflammation and cancer: a leading role for adenosine. Nat Rev Cancer 2013; 13: 842-57.

[148] Saito M, Yaguchi T, Yasuda Y, Nakano T, Nishizaki T. Adenosine suppresses CW2 human colonic cancer growth by inducing apoptosis *via* A(1) adenosine receptors. Cancer Lett 2010; 290: 211-5.

[149] Synowitz M, Glass R, Farber K, *et al.* A1 adenosine receptors in microglia control glioblastoma-host interaction. Cancer Res 2006; 66: 8550-7.

[150] Fishman P, Bar-Yehuda S, Ohana G, *et al.* Adenosine acts as an inhibitor of lymphoma cell growth: a major role for the A3 adenosine receptor. Eur J Cancer 2000; 36: 1452-8.

[151] Merighi S, Mirandola P, Milani D, *et al.* Adenosine receptors as mediators of both cell proliferation and cell death of cultured human melanoma cells. J Invest Dermatol 2002; 119: 923-33.

[152] Aghaei M, Panjehpour M, Karami-Tehrani F, Salami S. Molecular mechanisms of A3 adenosine receptor-induced G1 cell cycle arrest and apoptosis in androgen-dependent and independent prostate cancer cell lines: involvement of intrinsic pathway. J Cancer Res Clin Oncol 2011; 137: 1511-23.

[153] Bar-Yehuda S, Barer F, Volfsson L, Fishman P. Resistance of muscle to tumor metastases: a role for a3 adenosine receptor agonists. Neoplasia 2001; 3: 125-31.

[154] Bar-Yehuda S, Stemmer S M, Madi L, *et al.* The A3 adenosine receptor agonist CF102 induces apoptosis of hepatocellular carcinoma *via* de-regulation of the Wnt and NF-kappaB signal transduction pathways. Int J Oncol 2008; 33: 287-95.

[155] Otsuki T, Kanno T, Fujita Y, *et al.* A3 adenosine receptor-mediated p53-dependent apoptosis in Lu-65 human lung cancer cells. Cell Physiol Biochem 2012; 30: 210-20.

[156] Aghaei M, Karami-Tehrani F, Panjehpour M, Salami S, Fallahian F. Adenosine induces cell-cycle arrest and apoptosis in androgen-dependent and -independent prostate cancer cell lines, LNcap-FGC-10, DU-145, and PC3. Prostate 2012; 72: 361-75.

[157] Vincenzi F, Targa M, Corciulo C, *et al.* The anti-tumor effect of A3 adenosine receptors is potentiated by pulsed electromagnetic fields in cultured neural cancer cells. PLoS One 2012; 7: e39317.

[158] Madi L, Bar-Yehuda S, Barer F, Ardon E, Ochaion A, Fishman P. A3 adenosine receptor activation in melanoma cells: association between receptor fate and tumor growth inhibition. J Biol Chem 2003; 278: 42121-30.

[159] Fishman P, Bar-Yehuda S, Ohana G, *et al.* An agonist to the A3 adenosine receptor inhibits colon carcinoma growth in mice *via* modulation of GSK-3 beta and NF-kappa B. Oncogene 2004; 23: 2465-71.

[160] Fishman P, Madi L, Bar-Yehuda S, Barer F, Del Valle L, Khalili K. Evidence for involvement of Wnt signaling pathway in IB-MECA mediated suppression of melanoma cells. Oncogene 2002; 21: 4060-4.

[161] Dzhandzhugazyan K N, Kirkin A F, thor Straten P, Zeuthen J. Ecto-ATP diphosphohydrolase/CD39 is overexpressed in differentiated human melanomas. FEBS Lett 1998; 430: 227-30.

[162] Matsuo Y, Drexler H G, Harashima A, *et al.* A novel ALL-L3 cell line, BALM-25, expressing both immunoglobulin light chains. Leuk Lymphoma 2004; 45: 575-81.

[163] Moller P, Bruderlein S, Strater J, *et al.* MedB-1, a human tumor cell line derived from a primary mediastinal large B-cell lymphoma. Int J Cancer 2001; 92: 348-53.

[164] Bennett F, Rawstron A, Plummer M, de Tute R, Moreton P, Jack A, Hillmen P. B-cell chronic lymphocytic leukaemia cells show specific changes in membrane protein expression during different stages of cell cycle. Br J Haematol 2007; 139: 600-4.

[165] Jin D, Fan J, Wang L, *et al.* CD73 on tumor cells impairs antitumor T-cell responses: a novel mechanism of tumor-induced immune suppression. Cancer Res 2010; 70: 2245-55.

[166] Stella J, Bavaresco L, Braganhol E, *et al.* Differential ectonucleotidase expression in human bladder cancer cell lines. Urol Oncol 2010; 28: 260-7.

[167] Mikhailov A, Sokolovskaya A, Yegutkin G G, *et al.* CD73 participates in cellular multiresistance program and protects against TRAIL-induced apoptosis. J Immunol 2008; 181: 464-75.

[168] Bavaresco L, Bernardi A, Braganhol E, *et al.* The role of ecto-5'-nucleotidase/CD73 in glioma cell line proliferation. Mol Cell Biochem 2008; 319: 61-8.

[169] Ludwig H C, Rausch S, Schallock K, Markakis E. Expression of CD 73 (ecto-5'-nucleotidase) in 165 glioblastomas by immunohistochemistry and electronmicroscopic histochemistry. Anticancer Res 1999; 19: 1747-52.

[170] Sadej R, Spychala J, Skladanowski A C. Expression of ecto-5'-nucleotidase (eN, CD73) in cell lines from various stages of human melanoma. Melanoma Res 2006; 16: 213-22.

[171] Kondo T, Nakazawa T, Murata S I, Katoh R. Expression of CD73 and its ecto-5'-nucleotidase activity are elevated in papillary thyroid carcinomas. Histopathology 2006; 48: 612-4.

[172] Fukuda K, Sakakura C, Miyagawa K, *et al.* Differential gene expression profiles of radioresistant oesophageal cancer cell lines established by continuous fractionated irradiation. Br J Cancer 2004; 91: 1543-50.

[173] Durak I, Cetin R, Canbolat O, Cetin D, Yurtarslani Z, Unal A. Adenosine deaminase, 5'-nucleotidase, guanase and cytidine deaminase activities in gastric tissues from patients with gastric cancer. Cancer Lett 1994; 84: 199-202.

[174] Eroglu A, Canbolat O, Demirci S, Kocaoglu H, Eryavuz Y, Akgul H. Activities of adenosine deaminase and 5'-nucleotidase in cancerous and noncancerous human colorectal tissues. Med Oncol 2000; 17: 319-24.

[175] Spychala J, Lazarowski E, Ostapkowicz A, Ayscue L H, Jin A, Mitchell B S. Role of estrogen receptor in the regulation of ecto-5'-nucleotidase and adenosine in breast cancer. Clin Cancer Res 2004; 10: 708-17.

[176] Clayton A, Al-Taei S, Webber J, Mason M D, Tabi Z. Cancer exosomes express CD39 and CD73, which suppress T cells through adenosine production. J Immunol 2011; 187: 676-83.

[177] Bautch V L, Ambler C A. Assembly and patterning of vertebrate blood vessels. Trends Cardiovasc Med 2004; 14: 138-43.

[178] Ferrara N. Vascular endothelial growth factor: basic science and clinical progress. Endocr Rev 2004; 25: 581-611.

[179] Jain R K. Molecular regulation of vessel maturation. Nat Med 2003; 9: 685-93.

[180] Hicklin D J, Ellis L M. Role of the vascular endothelial growth factor pathway in tumor growth and angiogenesis. J Clin Oncol 2005; 23: 1011-27.

[181] Folkman J. Tumor angiogenesis: therapeutic implications. N Engl J Med 1971; 285: 1182-6.

[182] Holmgren L, O'Reilly M S, Folkman J. Dormancy of micrometastases: balanced proliferation and apoptosis in the presence of angiogenesis suppression. Nat Med 1995; 1: 149-53.

[183] Bergers G, Benjamin L E. Tumorigenesis and the angiogenic switch. Nat Rev Cancer 2003; 3: 401-10.

[184] Kesisis G, Broxterman H, Giaccone G. Angiogenesis inhibitors. Drug selectivity and target specificity. Curr Pharm Des 2007; 13: 2795-809.

[185] Jain R K, Duda D G, Clark J W, Loeffler J S. Lessons from phase III clinical trials on anti-VEGF therapy for cancer. Nat Clin Pract Oncol 2006; 3: 24-40.

[186] Sunderkotter C, Steinbrink K, Goebeler M, Bhardwaj RSorg C. Macrophages and angiogenesis. J Leukoc Biol 1994; 55: 410-22.

[187] Carmeliet P. Mechanisms of angiogenesis and arteriogenesis. Nat Med 2000; 6: 389-95.

[188] Buxton I L, Yokdang N, Matz R M. Purinergic mechanisms in breast cancer support intravasation, extravasation and angiogenesis. Cancer Lett 2010; 291: 131-41.

[189] Wang L, Karlsson L, Moses S, *et al.* P2 receptor expression profiles in human vascular smooth muscle and endothelial cells. J Cardiovasc Pharmacol 2002; 40: 841-53.

[190] Takagi H, King G L, Robinson G S, Ferrara N, Aiello L P. Adenosine mediates hypoxic induction of vascular endothelial growth factor in retinal pericytes and endothelial cells. Invest Ophthalmol Vis Sci 1996; 37: 2165-76.

[191] Grant M B, Tarnuzzer R W, Caballero S, *et al.* Adenosine receptor activation induces vascular endothelial growth factor in human retinal endothelial cells. Circ Res 1999; 85: 699-706.

[192] Feoktistov I, Goldstein A E, Ryzhov S, Zeng D, Belardinelli L, Voyno-Yasenetskaya T, Biaggioni I. Differential expression of adenosine receptors in human endothelial cells: role of A2B receptors in angiogenic factor regulation. Circ Res 2002; 90: 531-8.

[193] Dorsam R T, Kunapuli S P. Central role of the P2Y12 receptor in platelet activation. J Clin Invest 2004; 113: 340-5.

[194] Kaiser R A, Buxton I L. Nucleotide-mediated relaxation in guinea-pig aorta: selective inhibition by MRS2179. Br J Pharmacol 2002; 135: 537-45.

[195] Kaiser R A, Oxhorn B C, Andrews G, Buxton I L. Functional compartmentation of endothelial P2Y receptor signaling. Circ Res 2002; 91: 292-9.

[196] Kaczmarek E, Erb L, Koziak K, *et al.* Modulation of endothelial cell migration by extracellular nucleotides: involvement of focal adhesion kinase and phosphatidylinositol 3-kinase-mediated pathways. Thromb Haemost 2005; 93: 735-42.

[197] Satterwhite C M, Farrelly A M, Bradley M E. Chemotactic, mitogenic, and angiogenic actions of UTP on vascular endothelial cells. Am J Physiol 1999; 276: H1091-7.

[198] Tanaka N, Nejime N, Kagota S, *et al.* ATP participates in the regulation of microvessel permeability. J Pharm Pharmacol 2006; 58: 481-7.

[199] Yang S, Cheek D J, Westfall D P, Buxton I L. Purinergic axis in cardiac blood vessels. Agonist-mediated release of ATP from cardiac endothelial cells. Circ Res 1994; 74: 401-7.

[200] Buxton I L, Kaiser R A, Oxhorn B C, Cheek D J. Evidence supporting the Nucleotide Axis Hypothesis: ATP release and metabolism by coronary endothelium. Am J Physiol Heart Circ Physiol 2001; 281: H1657-66.

[201] Burnstock G. Pathophysiology and therapeutic potential of purinergic signaling. Pharmacol Rev 2006; 58: 58-86.

[202] Kashiwagi S, Izumi Y, Gohongi T, *et al.* NO mediates mural cell recruitment and vessel morphogenesis in murine melanomas and tissue-engineered blood vessels. J Clin Invest 2005; 115: 1816-27.

[203] Erb L, Liu J, Ockerhausen J, *et al.* An RGD sequence in the P2Y(2) receptor interacts with alpha(V)beta(3) integrins and is required for G(o)-mediated signal transduction. J Cell Biol 2001; 153: 491-501.

[204] Seye C I, Yu N, Gonzalez F A, Erb L, Weisman G A. The P2Y2 nucleotide receptor mediates vascular cell adhesion molecule-1 expression through interaction with VEGF receptor-2 (KDR/Flk-1). J Biol Chem 2004; 279: 35679-86.

[205] Buvinic S, Bravo-Zehnder M, Boyer J L, Huidobro-Toro J P, Gonzalez A. Nucleotide P2Y1 receptor regulates EGF receptor mitogenic signaling and expression in epithelial cells. J Cell Sci 2007; 120: 4289-301.

[206] Rumjahn S M, Yokdang N, Baldwin K A, Thai J, Buxton I L. Purinergic regulation of vascular endothelial growth factor signaling in angiogenesis. Br J Cancer 2009; 100: 1465-70.

[207] Cho C H, Lee C S, Chang M, *et al.* Localization of VEGFR-2 and PLD2 in endothelial caveolae is involved in VEGF-induced phosphorylation of MEK and ERK. Am J Physiol Heart Circ Physiol 2004; 286: H1881-8.

[208] Labrecque L, Royal I, Surprenant D S, Patterson C, Gingras D, Beliveau R. Regulation of vascular endothelial growth factor receptor-2 activity by caveolin-1 and plasma membrane cholesterol. Mol Biol Cell 2003; 14: 334-47.

[209] Ikeda S, Ushio-Fukai M, Zuo L, *et al.* Novel role of ARF6 in vascular endothelial growth factor-induced signaling and angiogenesis. Circ Res 2005; 96: 467-75.

[210] Massimino M L, Griffoni C, Spisni E, Toni M, Tomasi V. Involvement of caveolae and caveolae-like domains in signalling, cell survival and angiogenesis. Cell Signal 2002; 14: 93-8.

[211] Yamamoto K, Sokabe T, Matsumoto T, *et al.* Impaired flow-dependent control of vascular tone and remodeling in P2X4-deficient mice. Nat Med 2006; 12: 133-7.

[212] Freeman K W, Bowman B R, Zetter B R. Regenerative protein thymosin beta-4 is a novel regulator of purinergic signaling. FASEB J 2011; 25: 907-15.

[213] Hill L M, Gavala M L, Lenertz L Y, Bertics P J. Extracellular ATP may contribute to tissue repair by rapidly stimulating purinergic receptor X7-dependent vascular endothelial growth factor release from primary human monocytes. J Immunol 2010; 185: 3028-34.

[214] Baroja-Mazo A, Barbera-Cremades M, Pelegrin P. The participation of plasma membrane hemichannels to purinergic signaling. Biochim Biophys Acta 2013; 1828: 79-93.

[215] Weinhold K, Krause-Buchholz U, Rodel G, Kasper M, Barth K. Interaction and interrelation of P2X7 and P2X4 receptor complexes in mouse lung epithelial cells. Cell Mol Life Sci 2010; 67: 2631-42.

[216] Vergani A, Tezza S, D'Addio F, *et al.* Long-term heart transplant survival by targeting the ionotropic purinergic receptor P2X7. Circulation 2013; 127: 463-75.

[217] Moldovan N I. Role of monocytes and macrophages in adult angiogenesis: a light at the tunnel's end. J Hematother Stem Cell Res 2002; 11: 179-94.

[218] Aga M, Johnson C J, Hart A P, *et al.* Modulation of monocyte signaling and pore formation in response to agonists of the nucleotide receptor P2X(7). J Leukoc Biol 2002; 72: 222-32.

[219] Guha A, Bach R, Konigsberg W, Nemerson Y. Affinity purification of human tissue factor: interaction of factor VII and tissue factor in detergent micelles. Proc Natl Acad Sci U S A 1986; 83: 299-302.

[220] Clark A N, Youkey R, Liu X, *et al.* A1 adenosine receptor activation promotes angiogenesis and release of VEGF from monocytes. Circ Res 2007; 101: 1130-8.

[221] Erlinge D, Burnstock G. P2 receptors in cardiovascular regulation and disease. Purinergic Signal 2008; 4: 1-20.

[222] Schuchardt M, Tolle M, van der Giet M. P2Y purinoceptors as potential emerging therapeutical target in vascular disease. Curr Pharm Des 2012; 18: 6169-80.

[223] Hinze A V, Mayer P, Harst A, von Kugelgen I. P2X1 receptor-mediated inhibition of the proliferation of human coronary smooth muscle cells involving the transcription factor NR4A1. Purinergic Signal 2013; 9: 677-86.

[224] Leibovich S J, Chen J F, Pinhal-Enfield G, *et al.* Synergistic up-regulation of vascular endothelial growth factor expression in murine macrophages by adenosine A(2A) receptor agonists and endotoxin. Am J Pathol 2002; 160: 2231-44.

[225] Feoktistov I, Ryzhov S, Goldstein A E, Biaggioni I. Mast cell-mediated stimulation of angiogenesis: cooperative interaction between A2B and A3 adenosine receptors. Circ Res 2003; 92: 485-92.

[226] Jackson E K, Ren J, Gillespie D G, Dubey R K. Extracellular 2',3'-cyclic adenosine 5'-monophosphate is a potent inhibitor of preglomerular vascular smooth muscle cell and mesangial cell growth. Hypertension 2010; 56: 151-8.

[227] Beldi G, Wu Y, Sun X, *et al.* Regulated catalysis of extracellular nucleotides by vascular CD39/ENTPD1 is required for liver regeneration. Gastroenterology 2008; 135: 1751-60.

[228] Sheth S, Bleibel W, Thukral C, *et al.* Heightened NTPDase-1/CD39 expression and angiogenesis in radiation proctitis. Purinergic Signal 2009; 5: 321-6.

[229] Jackson S W, Hoshi T, Wu Y, *et al.* Disordered purinergic signaling inhibits pathological angiogenesis in cd39/Entpd1-null mice. Am J Pathol 2007; 171: 1395-404.

[230] Levesque S A, Kukulski F, Enjyoji K, Robson S C, Sevigny J. NTPDase1 governs P2X7-dependent functions in murine macrophages. Eur J Immunol 2010; 40: 1473-85.

[231] Goepfert C, Imai M, Brouard S, Csizmadia E, Kaczmarek E, Robson S C. CD39 modulates endothelial cell activation and apoptosis. Mol Med 2000; 6: 591-603.

[232] Goepfert C, Sundberg C, Sevigny J, *et al.* Disordered cellular migration and angiogenesis in cd39-null mice. Circulation 2001; 104: 3109-15.

[233] Behdad A, Sun X, Khalpey Z, *et al.* Vascular smooth muscle cell expression of ectonucleotidase CD39 (ENTPD1) is required for neointimal formation in mice. Purinergic Signal 2009; 5: 335-42.

[234] Allard B, Turcotte M, Spring K, Pommey S, Royal I, Stagg J. Anti-CD73 therapy impairs tumor angiogenesis. Int J Cancer 2014; 134: 1466-73.

[235] Braganhol E, Morrone F B, Bernardi A, *et al.* Selective NTPDase2 expression modulates *in vivo* rat glioma growth. Cancer Sci 2009; 100: 1434-42.

[236] Kunzli B M, Berberat P O, Giese T, *et al.* Upregulation of CD39/NTPDases and P2 receptors in human pancreatic disease. Am J Physiol Gastrointest Liver Physiol 2007; 292: G223-30.

[237] Di Virgilio F, Robson S C. Identification of novel immunosuppressive pathways paves the way for drug discovery. Curr Opin Pharmacol 2009; 9: 445-6.

[238] Janeway C A, Jr. How the immune system works to protect the host from infection: a personal view. Proc Natl Acad Sci U S A 2001; 98: 7461-8.

[239] Martins I, Tesniere A, Kepp O, *et al.* Chemotherapy induces ATP release from tumor cells. Cell Cycle 2009; 8: 3723-8.

[240] Aymeric L, Apetoh L, Ghiringhelli F, *et al.* Tumor cell death and ATP release prime dendritic cells and efficient anticancer immunity. Cancer Res 2010; 70: 855-8.

[241] Mattarollo S R, Loi S, Duret H, Ma Y, Zitvogel L, Smyth M J. Pivotal role of innate and adaptive immunity in anthracycline chemotherapy of established tumors. Cancer Res 2011; 71: 4809-20.

[242] Elliott M R, Chekeni F B, Trampont P C, *et al.* Nucleotides released by apoptotic cells act as a find-me signal to promote phagocytic clearance. Nature 2009; 461: 282-6.

[243] Huang T T, Ojcius D M, Young J D, *et al.* The anti-tumorigenic mushroom Agaricus blazei Murill enhances IL-1beta production and activates the NLRP3 inflammasome in human macrophages. PLoS One 2012; 7: e41383.

[244] Idzko M, Dichmann S, Ferrari D, *et al.* Nucleotides induce chemotaxis and actin polymerization in immature but not mature human dendritic cells *via* activation of pertussis toxin-sensitive P2y receptors. Blood 2002; 100: 925-32.

[245] Yip L, Woehrle T, Corriden R, *et al.* Autocrine regulation of T-cell activation by ATP release and P2X7 receptors. FASEB J 2009; 23: 1685-93.

[246] Schenk U, Westendorf A M, Radaelli E, *et al.* Purinergic control of T cell activation by ATP released through pannexin-1 hemichannels. Sci Signal 2008; 1: ra6.

[247] Bours M J, Swennen E L, Di Virgilio F, Cronstein B N, Dagnelie P C. Adenosine 5'-triphosphate and adenosine as endogenous signaling molecules in immunity and inflammation. Pharmacol Ther 2006; 112: 358-404.

[248] Wang S, Miyazaki Y, Shinozaki Y, Yoshida H. Augmentation of antigen-presenting and Th1-promoting functions of dendritic cells by WSX-1(IL-27R) deficiency. J Immunol 2007; 179: 6421-8.

[249] Mascanfroni I D, Yeste A, Vieira S M, *et al.* IL-27 acts on DCs to suppress the T cell response and autoimmunity by inducing expression of the immunoregulatory molecule CD39. Nat Immunol 2013; 14: 1054-63.

[250] Sekar D, Hahn C, Brune B, Roberts E, Weigert A. Apoptotic tumor cells induce IL-27 release from human DCs to activate Treg cells that express CD69 and attenuate cytotoxicity. Eur J Immunol 2012; 42: 1585-98.

[251] Longhi M S, Moss A, Bai A, *et al.* Characterization of Human CD39(+) Th17 Cells with Suppressor Activity and Modulation in Inflammatory Bowel Disease. PLoS One 2014; 9: e87956.

[252] Aswad F, Kawamura H, Dennert G. High sensitivity of CD4+CD25+ regulatory T cells to extracellular metabolites nicotinamide adenine dinucleotide and ATP: a role for P2X7 receptors. J Immunol 2005; 175: 3075-83.

[253] Schenk U, Frascoli M, Proietti M, *et al.* ATP inhibits the generation and function of regulatory T cells through the activation of purinergic P2X receptors. Sci Signal 2011; 4: ra12.

[254] Beavis P A, Stagg J, Darcy P K, Smyth M J. CD73: a potent suppressor of antitumor immune responses. Trends Immunol 2012; 33: 231-7.

[255] Sitkovsky M, Lukashev D. Regulation of immune cells by local-tissue oxygen tension: HIF1 alpha and adenosine receptors. Nat Rev Immunol 2005; 5: 712-21.

[256] Synnestvedt K, Furuta G T, Comerford K M, *et al.* Ecto-5'-nucleotidase (CD73) regulation by hypoxia-inducible factor-1 mediates permeability changes in intestinal epithelia. J Clin Invest 2002; 110: 993-1002.

[257] Morote-Garcia J C, Rosenberger P, Kuhlicke J, Eltzschig H K. HIF-1-dependent repression of adenosine kinase attenuates hypoxia-induced vascular leak. Blood 2008; 111: 5571-80.

[258] Di Virgilio F, Boeynaems J M, Robson S C. Extracellular nucleotides as negative modulators of immunity. Curr Opin Pharmacol 2009; 9: 507-13.

[259] Sitkovsky M, Lukashev D, Deaglio S, Dwyer K, Robson S C, Ohta A. Adenosine A2A receptor antagonists: blockade of adenosinergic effects and T regulatory cells. Br J Pharmacol 2008; 153 Suppl 1: S457-64.

[260] Raskovalova T, Huang X, Sitkovsky M, Zacharia L C, Jackson E K, Gorelik E. Gs protein-coupled adenosine receptor signaling and lytic function of activated NK cells. J Immunol 2005; 175: 4383-91.

[261] Novitskiy S V, Ryzhov S, Zaynagetdinov R, *et al.* Adenosine receptors in regulation of dendritic cell differentiation and function. Blood 2008; 112: 1822-31.

[262] Hilchey S P, Kobie J J, Cochran M R, *et al.* Human follicular lymphoma CD39+-infiltrating T cells contribute to adenosine-mediated T cell hyporesponsiveness. J Immunol 2009; 183: 6157-66.

[263] Kobie J J, Shah P R, Yang L, Rebhahn J A, Fowell D J, Mosmann T R. T regulatory and primed uncommitted CD4 T cells express CD73, which suppresses effector CD4 T cells by converting 5'-adenosine monophosphate to adenosine. J Immunol 2006; 177: 6780-6.

[264] Mandapathil M, Hilldorfer B, Szczepanski M J, *et al.* Generation and accumulation of immunosuppressive adenosine by human CD4+CD25highFOXP3+ regulatory T cells. J Biol Chem 2010; 285: 7176-86.

[265] Ohta A, Gorelik E, Prasad S J, *et al.* A2A adenosine receptor protects tumors from antitumor T cells. Proc Natl Acad Sci U S A 2006; 103: 13132-7.

[266] Sitkovsky M V, Lukashev D, Apasov S, *et al.* Physiological control of immune response and inflammatory tissue damage by hypoxia-inducible factors and adenosine A2A receptors. Annu Rev Immunol 2004; 22: 657-82.

[267] Scheibner K A, Boodoo S, Collins S, *et al.* The adenosine a2a receptor inhibits matrix-induced inflammation in a novel fashion. Am J Respir Cell Mol Biol 2009; 40: 251-9.

[268] Stagg J, Divisekera U, Duret H, *et al.* CD73-deficient mice have increased antitumor immunity and are resistant to experimental metastasis. Cancer Res 2011; 71: 2892-900.

[269] Smyth M J, Teng M W, Swann J, Kyparissoudis K, Godfrey D I, Hayakawa Y. CD4+CD25+ T regulatory cells suppress NK cell-mediated immunotherapy of cancer. J Immunol 2006; 176: 1582-7.

[270] Kunzli B M, Bernlochner M I, Rath S, *et al.* Impact of CD39 and purinergic signalling on the growth and metastasis of colorectal cancer. Purinergic Signal 2011; 7: 231-41.

[271] Rumjahn S M, Javed M A, Wong N, Law W E, Buxton I L. Purinergic regulation of angiogenesis by human breast carcinoma-secreted nucleoside diphosphate kinase. Br J Cancer 2007; 97: 1372-80.

[272] Anzinger J, Malmquist N A, Gould J, Buxton I L. Secretion of a nucleoside diphosphate kinase (Nm23-H2) by cells from human breast, colon, pancreas and lung tumors. Proc West Pharmacol Soc 2001; 44: 61-3.

[273] Rumjahn S M, Baldwin K A, Buxton I L. P2y receptor-mediated angiogenesis *via* vascular endothelial growth factor receptor 2 signaling. Proc West Pharmacol Soc 2007; 50: 58-60.

[274] Chadet S, Jelassi B, Wannous R, *et al.* The activation of P2Y2 receptors increases MCF-7 breast cancer cells migration through the MEK-ERK1/2 signalling pathway. Carcinogenesis 2014; 35(6): 1238-47.

[275] Li W H, Qiu Y, Zhang H Q, *et al.* P2Y2 receptor promotes cell invasion and metastasis in prostate cancer cells. Br J Cancer 2013; 109: 1666-75.

[276] Chen L, He H Y, Li H M, *et al.* ERK1/2 and p38 pathways are required for P2Y receptor-mediated prostate cancer invasion. Cancer Lett 2004; 215: 239-47.

[277] Reymond N, d'Agua B B, Ridley A J. Crossing the endothelial barrier during metastasis. Nat Rev Cancer 2013; 13: 858-70.

[278] Schumacher D, Strilic B, Sivaraj K K, Wettschureck N, Offermanns S. Platelet-derived nucleotides promote tumor-cell transendothelial migration and metastasis *via* P2Y2 receptor. Cancer Cell 2013; 24: 130-7.

[279] Jantaratnotai N, McLarnon J G. Calcium dependence of purinergic subtype P2Y(1) receptor modulation of C6 glioma cell migration. Neurosci Lett 2011; 497: 80-4.

[280] Slater M, Danieletto S, Pooley M, Cheng Teh L, Gidley-Baird A, Barden J A. Differentiation between cancerous and normal hyperplastic lobules in breast lesions. Breast Cancer Res Treat 2004; 83: 1-10.

[281] Jelassi B, Chantome A, Alcaraz-Perez F, *et al.* P2X(7) receptor activation enhances SK3 channels- and cystein cathepsin-dependent cancer cells invasiveness. Oncogene 2011; 30: 2108-22.

[282] Gu L Q, Li F Y, Zhao L, *et al.* Association of XIAP and P2X7 receptor expression with lymph node metastasis in papillary thyroid carcinoma. Endocrine 2010; 38: 276-82.

[283] Takai E, Tsukimoto M, Harada H, Kojima S. Autocrine signaling *via* release of ATP and activation of P2X7 receptor influences motile activity of human lung cancer cells. Purinergic Signal 2014 March 14.

[284] Sadej R, Spychala J, Skladanowski A C. Ecto-5'-nucleotidase (eN, CD73) is coexpressed with metastasis promoting antigens in human melanoma cells. Nucleosides Nucleotides Nucleic Acids 2006; 25: 1119-23.

[285] Wang L, Zhou X, Zhou T, *et al.* Ecto-5'-nucleotidase promotes invasion, migration and adhesion of human breast cancer cells. J Cancer Res Clin Oncol 2008; 134: 365-72.

[286] Leth-Larsen R, Lund R, Hansen H V, *et al.* Metastasis-related plasma membrane proteins of human breast cancer cells identified by comparative quantitative mass spectrometry. Mol Cell Proteomics 2009; 8: 1436-49.

[287] Mandapathil M, Szczepanski M J, Szajnik M, *et al.* Increased ectonucleotidase expression and activity in regulatory T cells of patients with head and neck cancer. Clin Cancer Res 2009; 15: 6348-57.

[288] Linden J. Adenosine promotes tumor metastasis. Sci Signal 2013; 6: pe20.

[289] Denti S, Sirri A, Cheli A, *et al.* RanBPM is a phosphoprotein that associates with the plasma membrane and interacts with the integrin LFA-1. J Biol Chem 2004; 279: 13027-34.

[290] Wang L, Fan J, Thompson L F, *et al.* CD73 has distinct roles in nonhematopoietic and hematopoietic cells to promote tumor growth in mice. J Clin Invest 2011; 121: 2371-82.

[291] Stagg J, Divisekera U, McLaughlin N, *et al.* Anti-CD73 antibody therapy inhibits breast tumor growth and metastasis. Proc Natl Acad Sci U S A 2010; 107: 1547-52.

[292] Allard B, Turcotte M, Stagg J. CD73-generated adenosine: orchestrating the tumor-stroma interplay to promote cancer growth. J Biomed Biotechnol 2012; 2012: 485156.

[293] Whiteside T L, Mandapathil M, Schuler P. The role of the adenosinergic pathway in immunosuppression mediated by human regulatory T cells (Treg). Curr Med Chem 2011; 18: 5217-23.

[294] Surprenant A, North R A. Signaling at purinergic P2X receptors. Annu Rev Physiol 2009; 71: 333-59.

[295] Hasko G, Linden J, Cronstein B, Pacher P. Adenosine receptors: therapeutic aspects for inflammatory and immune diseases. Nat Rev Drug Discov 2008; 7: 759-70.

[296] Arias J I, Aller M A, Arias J. Cancer cell: using inflammation to invade the host. Mol Cancer 2007; 6: 29.

[297] Rakoff-Nahoum S. Why cancer and inflammation? Yale J Biol Med 2006; 79: 123-30.

[298] Adinolfi E, Raffaghello L, Giuliani A L, *et al.* Expression of P2X7 receptor increases *in vivo* tumor growth. Cancer Res 2012; 72: 2957-69.

[299] Adinolfi E, Amoroso F, Giuliani A L. P2X7 Receptor Function in Bone-Related Cancer. J Osteoporos 2012; 2012: 637863.

[300] Agteresch H J, Burgers S A, van der Gaast A, Wilson J H, Dagnelie P C. Randomized clinical trial of adenosine 5'-triphosphate on tumor growth and survival in advanced lung cancer patients. Anticancer Drugs 2003; 14: 639-44.

[301] Agteresch H J, Dagnelie P C, Rietveld T, van den Berg J W, Danser A H, Wilson J H. Pharmacokinetics of intravenous ATP in cancer patients. Eur J Clin Pharmacol 2000; 56: 49-55.

[302] Agteresch H J, Rietveld T, Kerkhofs L G, van den Berg J W, Wilson J H, Dagnelie P C. Beneficial effects of adenosine triphosphate on nutritional status in advanced lung cancer patients: a randomized clinical trial. J Clin Oncol 2002; 20: 371-8.

[303] Falzoni S, Donvito G, Di Virgilio F. Detecting adenosine triphosphate in the pericellular space. Interface Focus 2013; 3: 20120101.

[304] Jelassi B, Anchelin M, Chamouton J, *et al.* Anthraquinone emodin inhibits human cancer cell invasiveness by antagonizing P2X7 receptors. Carcinogenesis 2013; 34: 1487-96.

[305] Ghalali A, Wiklund F, Zheng H, Stenius U, Hogberg J. Atorvastatin prevents ATP-driven invasiveness *via* P2X7 and EHBP1 signaling in PTEN-expressing prostate cancer cells. Carcinogenesis Feb 17, 2014.

[306] Ren S, Zhang Y, Wang Y, *et al.* Targeting P2X(7) receptor inhibits the metastasis of murine P388D1 lymphoid neoplasm cells to lymph nodes. Cell Biol Int 2010; 34: 1205-11.

[307] Wei Q, Costanzi S, Liu Q Z, Gao Z G, Jacobson K A. Activation of the P2Y1 receptor induces apoptosis and inhibits proliferation of prostate cancer cells. Biochem Pharmacol 2011; 82: 418-25.

[308] Sarangi S, Pandey A, Papa A L, *et al.* P2Y12 receptor inhibition augments cytotoxic effects of cisplatin in breast cancer. Med Oncol 2013; 30: 567.

[309] Beavis P A, Divisekera U, Paget C, *et al.* Blockade of A2A receptors potently suppresses the metastasis of CD73+ tumors. Proc Natl Acad Sci U S A 2013; 110: 14711-6.

[310] Beavis P A, Milenkovski N, Stagg J, Smyth M J, Darcy P K. A blockade enhances anti-metastatic immune responses. Oncoimmunology 2013; 2: e26705.

[311] Cekic C, Sag D, Li Y, Theodorescu D, Strieter R M, Linden J. Adenosine A2B receptor blockade slows growth of bladder and breast tumors. J Immunol 2012; 188: 198-205.

[312] Merighi S, Benini A, Mirandola P, *et al.* Caffeine inhibits adenosine-induced accumulation of hypoxia-inducible factor-1alpha, vascular endothelial growth factor, and interleukin-8 expression in hypoxic human colon cancer cells. Mol Pharmacol 2007; 72: 395-406.

[313] Lukashev D, Sitkovsky M, Ohta A. From "Hellstrom Paradox" to anti-adenosinergic cancer immunotherapy. Purinergic Signal 2007; 3: 129-34.

[314] Ma D F, Kondo T, Nakazawa T, *et al.* Hypoxia-inducible adenosine A2B receptor modulates proliferation of colon carcinoma cells. Hum Pathol 2010; 41: 1550-7.

[315] Ohana G, Bar-Yehuda S, Arich A, *et al.* Inhibition of primary colon carcinoma growth and liver metastasis by the A3 adenosine receptor agonist CF101. Br J Cancer 2003; 89: 1552-8.

[316] Fishman P, Bar-Yehuda S, Barer F, Madi L, Multani A S, Pathak S. The A3 adenosine receptor as a new target for cancer therapy and chemoprotection. Exp Cell Res 2001; 269: 230-6.

[317] Cohen S, Stemmer S M, Zozulya G, *et al.* CF102 an A3 adenosine receptor agonist mediates anti-tumor and anti-inflammatory effects in the liver. J Cell Physiol 2011; 226: 2438-47.
[318] Kim H, Kang J W, Lee S, *et al.* A3 adenosine receptor antagonist, truncated Thio-Cl-IB-MECA, induces apoptosis in T24 human bladder cancer cells. Anticancer Res 2010; 30: 2823-30.
[319] Kim S J, Min H Y, Chung H J, *et al.* Inhibition of cell proliferation through cell cycle arrest and apoptosis by thio-Cl-IB-MECA, a novel A3 adenosine receptor agonist, in human lung cancer cells. Cancer Lett 2008; 264: 309-15.
[320] Hausler S F, Del Barrio I M, Diessner J, *et al.* Anti-CD39 and anti-CD73 antibodies A1 and 7G2 improve targeted therapy in ovarian cancer by blocking adenosine-dependent immune evasion. Am J Transl Res 2014; 6: 129-39.
[321] Muller C E, Iqbal J, Baqi Y, Zimmermann H, Rollich A, Stephan H. Polyoxometalates--a new class of potent ecto-nucleoside triphosphate diphosphohydrolase (NTPDase) inhibitors. Bioorg Med Chem Lett 2006; 16: 5943-7.
[322] Zhang B. Opportunities and challenges for anti-CD73 cancer therapy. Immunotherapy 2012; 4: 861-5.
[323] Forte G, Sorrentino R, Montinaro A, *et al.* Inhibition of CD73 improves B cell-mediated anti-tumor immunity in a mouse model of melanoma. J Immunol 2012; 189: 2226-33.
[324] Stagg J, Beavis P A, Divisekera U, *et al.* CD73-deficient mice are resistant to carcinogenesis. Cancer Res 2012; 72: 2190-6.
[325] Zhang B. CD73 promotes tumor growth and metastasis. Oncoimmunology 2012; 1: 67-70.
[326] Allard B, Pommey S, Smyth M J, Stagg J. Targeting CD73 enhances the antitumor activity of anti-PD-1 and anti-CTLA-4 mAbs. Clin Cancer Res 2013; 19: 5626-35.
[327] Hausler S F, Montalban del Barrio I, Strohschein J, *et al.* Ectonucleotidases CD39 and CD73 on OvCA cells are potent adenosine-generating enzymes responsible for adenosine receptor 2A-dependent suppression of T cell function and NK cell cytotoxicity. Cancer Immunol Immunother 2011; 60: 1405-18.
[328] Nobuoka D, Yoshikawa T, Fujiwara T, Nakatsura T. Peptide intra-tumor injection for cancer immunotherapy: enhancement of tumor cell antigenicity is a novel and attractive strategy. Hum Vaccin Immunother 2013; 9: 1234-6.
[329] Hickey R, Mulcahy M F, Lewandowski R J, *et al.* Chemoradiation of hepatic malignancies: prospective, phase 1 study of full-dose capecitabine with escalating doses of yttrium-90 radioembolization. Int J Radiat Oncol Biol Phys 2014; 88: 1025-31.
[330] Wilczewska A Z, Niemirowicz K, Markiewicz K H, Car H. Nanoparticles as drug delivery systems. Pharmacol Rep 2012; 64: 1020-37.
[331] Sofou S. Surface-active liposomes for targeted cancer therapy. Nanomedicine (Lond) 2007; 2: 711-24.
[332] Bae Y H, Park K. Targeted drug delivery to tumors: myths, reality and possibility. J Control Release 2011; 153: 198-205.
[333] Scott A M, Wolchok J D, Old L J. Antibody therapy of cancer. Nat Rev Cancer 2012; 12: 278-87.
[334] Wang T F, Ou Y, Guidotti G. The transmembrane domains of ectoapyrase (CD39) affect its enzymatic activity and quaternary structure. J Biol Chem 1998; 273: 24814-21.
[335] Abdullah L N, Chow E K. Mechanisms of chemoresistance in cancer stem cells. Clin Transl Med 2013;2: 3.

[336] Szakacs G, Paterson J K, Ludwig J A, Booth-Genthe C, Gottesman M M. Targeting multidrug resistance in cancer. Nat Rev Drug Discov 2006; 5: 219-34.

[337] Sim G C, Martin-Orozco N, Jin L, *et al.* IL-2 therapy promotes suppressive ICOS+ Treg expansion in melanoma patients. J Clin Invest 2014; 124: 99-110.

[338] Sluyter R, Stokes L. Significance of P2X7 receptor variants to human health and disease. Recent Pat DNA Gene Seq 2011; 5: 41-54.

[339] Wang Q, Li S H, Wang H, *et al.* Concomitant targeting of tumor cells and induction of T-cell response synergizes to effectively inhibit trastuzumab-resistant breast cancer. Cancer Res 2012; 72: 4417-28.

[340] Schmelzle M, Duhme C, Junger W, *et al.* CD39 modulates hematopoietic stem cell recruitment and promotes liver regeneration in mice and humans after partial hepatectomy. Ann Surg 2013; 257: 693-701.

[341] Jaffe J D, Wang Y, Chan H M, *et al.* Global chromatin profiling reveals NSD2 mutations in pediatric acute lymphoblastic leukemia. Nat Genet 2013; 45: 1386-91.

[342] Purvis J E, Karhohs K W, Mock C, Batchelor E, Loewer A, Lahav G. p53 dynamics control cell fate. Science 2012; 336: 1440-4.

[343] Miao R, Luo H, Zhou H, *et al.* Identification of prognostic biomarkers in hepatitis B virus-related hepatocellular carcinoma and stratification by integrative multi-omics analysis. J Hepatol May 22, 2014.

[344] Friedman D J, Kunzli B M, YI A R, *et al.* From the Cover: CD39 deletion exacerbates experimental murine colitis and human polymorphisms increase susceptibility to inflammatory bowel disease. Proc Natl Acad Sci U S A 2009; 106: 16788-93.

[345] Mitsiades C S, Mitsiades N. P2X7 polymorphism and chronic lymphocytic leukaemia. Lancet 2003; 361: 1478; author reply 1478-9.

[346] Pikarsky E, Ben-Neriah Y. NF-kappaB inhibition: a double-edged sword in cancer? Eur J Cancer 2006; 42: 779-84.

[347] Sikder H, Huso D L, Zhang H, *et al.* Disruption of Id1 reveals major differences in angiogenesis between transplanted and autochthonous tumors. Cancer Cell 2003; 4: 291-9.

CHAPTER 6

HER2 Targeted Monoclonal Antibodies and Tyrosine Kinase Inhibitors

Neil A. O'Brien[1], Alexandra Canonici[2], Karen Howe[2], Martina S.J. McDermott[3], Denis M. Collins[2], Brigid C. Browne[4], John Crown[2,5] and Norma O'Donovan[*,2]

[1]Department of Medicine, Division of Hematology/Oncology, Geffen School of Medicine at UCLA, Los Angeles, CA, USA; [2]National Institute for Cellular Biotechnology, Dublin City University, Ireland; [3]Department of Drug Discovery and Biomedical Sciences, South Carolina College of Pharmacy, University of South Carolina, Columbia; [4]The Kinghorn Cancer Centre, Garvan Institute of Medical Research, Sydney, Australia; and [5]St. Vincent's University Hospital, Dublin, Ireland

Abstract: HER2 is overexpressed in approximately 20-25% of breast cancers and defines an aggressive sub-type of the disease. Fortunately for patients with HER2 positive breast cancer, the prognosis has improved in the last 10 years due to the development of HER2 targeted therapies, in particular trastuzumab, the HER2-directed monoclonal antibody. Recent data show that approximately 9.5% of patients with HER2 positive metastatic breast cancer achieve a durable complete response (> 5 years) following trastuzumab-based therapy. However, 90% of these patients still continue to develop progressive disease. These data highlight the need to develop novel therapeutic strategies to overcome both innate and acquired resistance to HER2 directed therapeutics.

Lapatinib, a small molecule tyrosine kinase inhibitor of HER2 and EGFR, has efficacy in trastuzumab resistant breast cancer and is approved for the treatment of patients with trastuzumab-refractory HER2 positive metastatic breast cancer. However, in metastatic disease, therapeutic action is often short-lived with most patients developing progressive disease. Thus, HER2 positive tumors can be innately resistant, or acquire resistance, to both trastuzumab and lapatinib.

Over the past 2 years, two new HER2 targeted therapies, pertuzumab and T-DM1 have received approval for the treatment of HER2 positive metastatic breast cancer. The pertuzumab monoclonal antibody blocks dimerization of HER2 with other members of the HER family and clinically has been shown to improve overall survival when used in combination with trastuzumab and docetaxel. The novel antibody drug conjugate,

***Corresponding Author Norma O'Donovan:** National Institute for Cellular Biotechnology, Dublin City University, Glasnevin, Dublin 9, Ireland; Tel: 00353-1-7007497; Fax: 00353-1-7005484;
E-mail: norma.odonovan@dcu.ie

Atta-ur-Rahman / M. Iqbal Choudhary (Eds.)

T-DM1, which links trastuzumab to the cytotoxic agent emtansine, improves the response of patients with trastuzumab-refractory metastatic breast cancer, compared to the standard of care lapatinib plus capecitabine regimen. A number of second generation irreversible pan-HER tyrosine kinase inhibitors are currently in clinical development, including neratinib, afatinib and dacomitinib.

More recently, the utility of HER2-directly therapeutics has been expanded into non-breast tumors such as gastric cancers that carry the HER2-alteration. Data from ongoing clinical trials will determine if targeting HER2 can also improve the prognosis of these cancer patients.

Keywords: Afatinib, antibody-drug conjugate, dacomitinib, lapatinib, neratinib, pertuzumab, T-DMI, trastuzumab, tyrosine kinase inhibitor.

INTRODUCTION

Human epidermal growth factor receptor 2 (HER2/*neu*/c-ErbB-2) is a member of the epidermal growth factor receptor (EGFR) family, along with EGFR (HER-1 or erbB1), HER-3 (erbB3), and HER-4 (erbB4). The HER2 proto-oncogene encodes a 185 kDa transmembrane receptor tyrosine kinase (RTK), which is composed of an extracellular domain (ECD), a transmembrane domain, and a cytoplasmic tyrosine kinase domain. Alterations in HER2, specifically gene amplification and protein expression have been implicated in breast cancer progression in approximately 20-25% of breast cancers [1]. The discovery of HER2 overexpression and its association with tumor aggressiveness and poor outcome in breast cancer, made HER2 an attractive target for the development of new therapies for this sub-group of breast cancer patients. The HER2 targeted monoclonal antibodies and tyrosine kinase inhibitors, approved for clinical use or currently in pre-clinical/clinical development, for HER2 positive breast cancer are the focus of this review, but we will first, briefly, review the biology of HER2 with a focus on its role in cancer.

HER2 Signaling

In contrast to the other HER family members, HER2 does not bind any known ligands. However, ligand binding to other HER family members can induce homo-dimerization and/or hetero-dimerization with other family members. Studies of the crystal structure of the HER2 ectodomain revealed that HER2 is constitutively present in a conformation which facilitates formation of heterodimers with other HER receptors, without ligand binding [2, 3]. Receptor dimerization facilitates *trans*-phosphorylation of specific tyrosine residues in the intracellular domain, resulting in activation of the kinase function and activation of downstream signaling pathways, in particular the PI3K/AKT and MAPK pathways (Fig. **1**). The key downstream effects of HER2 activation of these pathways are promotion of cell cycle progression and inhibition of cellular apoptosis.

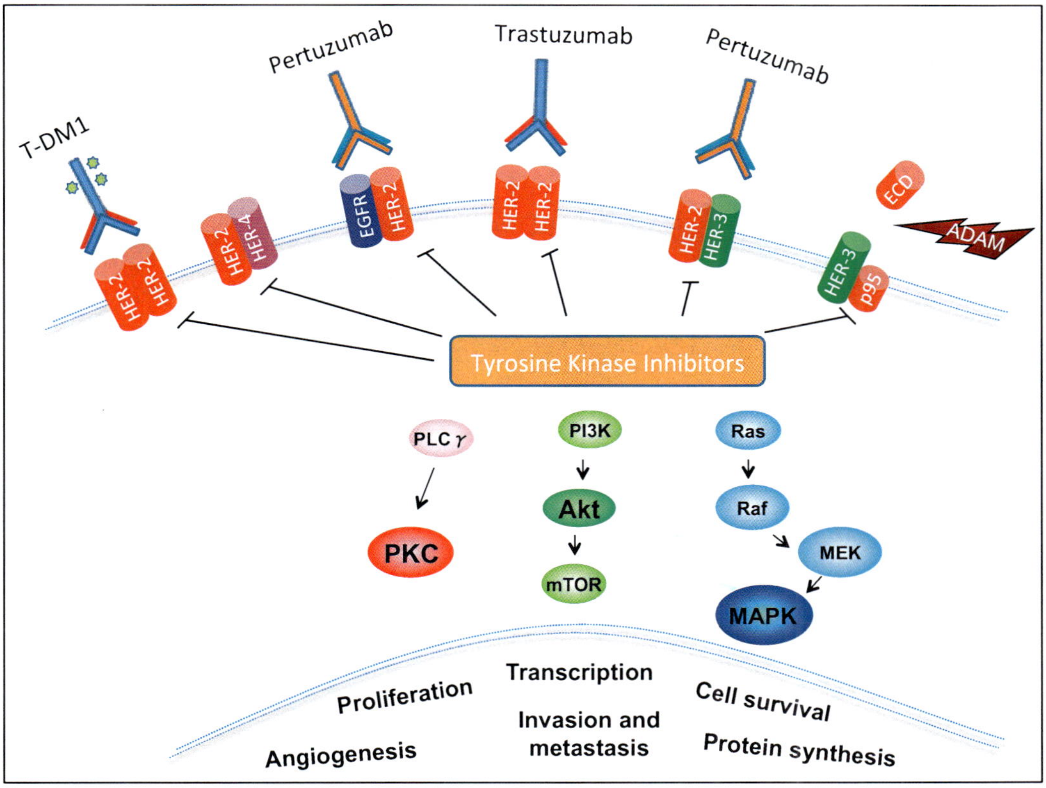

Fig. (1). Inhibition of HER-2 signaling: Trastuzumab binds the extracellular domain of HER2 and reduces HER2 signaling; pertuzumab also binds the extracellular domain and prevents HER2 homo- and hetero-dimerization; the tyrosine kinase inhibitors (TKIs) which bind to the intracellular domain and block kinase activation include; lapatinib which reversibly inhibits HER2 and EGFR; whereas neratinib, afatinib and dacomitinib are irreversible pan-HER inhibitors.

HER2 has been reported to be the preferred dimerization partner for other members of the HER family [4, 5], and dimers containing HER2 generate a stronger intracellular signal than other heterodimers [6]. HER2/HER3 dimers have been shown to be the most active and potent activators of the PI3K and MAPK pathways. In a recent study, Zhang *et al.* presented data which suggest a model of side-by-side HER2/HER3 dimers which promotes phosphorylation of the HER2 kinase domain [7]. The proposed tetrameric complex is believed to be responsible for activation of MAPK and PI3K signaling whereas the heterodimer causes activation of PI3K only [7, 8].

HER2 in Normal Cells

The HER receptors are expressed in multiple normal tissues and play important roles in normal cellular processes, particularly in development. HER2 plays a role in the development of the nervous system and the cardiac system. Mice with mutated HER2, HER3 or neuregulin-1 (NRG-1) proteins lack neural crest precursor cells [9], and loss of HER2, HER3, HER4, or NRGs, resulted in embryonic lethality due to cardiac abnormalities and brain defects [10-14].

Due to the fact that gene-targeting of HER family members is lethal *in utero*, it has been difficult to investigate the role of HER proteins in normal adult tissues. However, studies in mouse models suggest that they play an important in the initial stages of mammary gland development [15].

HER2 expression has been detected in a variety of epithelial cell types including gastro-intestinal, reproductive and urinary tract, skin, breast, placenta, ovaries and kidney [16-18]. In addition HER2 is expressed in adult cardiomyocytes, and mutated HER2 in cardiomyocytes causes cardiomyopathy in mice [19]. Thus, HER2 has important cardioprotective function [20, 21], which has important clinical implications for the HER2 monoclonal antibody trastuzumab, as will be discussed later.

HER2 IN CANCER

The rat homolog of HER2, *neu*, was originally identified in rat neuroblastoma cells [22] and overexpression of HER2 induced transformation of NIH/3T3 cells and NR6 mouse fibroblast cells [23-25]. Activation of HER2 in mammary acini, cultured in three-dimensional basement membrane gels, enhanced proliferation, inhibited apoptosis, and promoted formation of multiacinar structures, suggesting that HER2 can induce the early stages of mammary carcinogenesis *in vitro* [26]. Overexpression of HER2 in breast cancer cells caused increased PI3K signaling and enhanced tumorigenesis in nude mice [27]. HER2 has also been implicated in tumor cell invasion [28, 29] and angiogenesis [30].

HER2 in Breast Cancer

In 1987, Slamon *et al.* [1] reported that HER2 gene amplification, measured by Southern blotting, correlated significantly with prognosis in breast cancer. Patients with HER2 amplified lymph node positive breast cancer had a shorter time to relapse and overall survival (OS). HER2 overexpression correlates with several prognostic factors including tumor size, grade, lymph-node status, DNA aneuploidy, p53 mutation, proliferation index and urokinase-type plasminogen activator expression, and correlates inversely with estrogen receptor (ER) and progesterone receptor (PR) expression [31-34].

Clinically, HER2 amplification and/or overexpression is determined by *in situ* hybridization (ISH) and/or immunohistochemical (IHC) staining, respectively. The ASCO/CAP guidelines for HER2 testing state that the HER2 result is positive if: (i) IHC 3+ complete, intense circumferential membrane staining is observed in a homogeneous and contiguous population and within greater than 10% of the invasive tumor cells, or (ii) ISH positive using single probe or dual probe tests [35]. The ISH positive results are based on an average HER2 copy number $\geq$6.0 signals/cell for single probe or a HER2/CEP17 ratio of $\geq$2.0 or $<$2.0 but with an average HER2 copy number $\geq$6.0 signals/cell for dual-probe assays.

Cleavage of the ECD of HER2, by a disintegrin and metalloproteinase 10 (ADAM10) protease, generates a 95 kDa N-terminal truncated fragment of HER2 [36-38]. This truncated p95HER2 retains kinase activity [39]. The level of shed HER2 ECD detected in serum, also correlates with prognosis in breast cancer [40, 41]. Although measurement of p95HER2 in tumor samples by IHC is challenging due the lack of antibodies specific for this form of HER2, western blot analysis of breast tumors suggests that p95HER2 correlates with positive lymph node status and is detected more frequently in nodal metastasis than in primary tumors [36], and it also correlates with reduced 5-year disease free survival (DFS) [42].

HER2 TARGETED THERAPIES

HER2 targeted therapies can be divided into three main categories, namely monoclonal antibodies, tyrosine kinase inhibitors (TKIs) and more recently antibody-drug conjugates (ADCs). Two monoclonal antibodies, trastuzumab and pertuzumab, one ADC, T-DM1, and one TKI, lapatinib are currently approved for the treatment of patients with HER2 positive breast cancer, while several other TKIs are in preclinical/clinical development (Fig. **1**).

Trastuzumab (Herceptin™)

Trastuzumab: Discovery and Development

The discovery and development of trastuzumab spans many decades and is one of the most successful monoclonal antibody discoveries for the treatment of cancer. It originally stemmed from two pivotal discoveries in the 1980s; the identification of 185 kDa phosphoprotein called *neu* [22] and the discovery that *neu,* or HER2 as it is now referred to, was overexpressed in 20-25% of human primary breast cancers [1]. This molecular alteration represented an attractive target for the development of a new generation of targeted therapeutics. Several groups including researchers at Genentech developed murine monoclonal antibodies directed against the ECD of HER2, $p185^{HER2}$ [43, 44]. Shortly thereafter, screening panels of these antibodies revealed that some had anti-proliferative activity against HER2 overexpressing cell lines [43, 45]. Ultimately, Genentech Inc discovered a potent murine monoclonal antibody, muMAb 4D5 which significantly inhibited proliferation of HER2 overexpressing cells *in vitro* [46] and human breast cancer xenografts [47], with little effect on HER2 non-overexpressing cells. Due to these potent anti-tumor effects, the 4D5 murine monoclonal antibody was chosen for further clinical development.

The antibody was humanized to overcome the limiting factor of an anti-globulin response during therapy [48]. Utilizing gene conversion and site-directed mutagenesis, Carter *et al.*, subcloned the hypervariable region of the muMAb 4D5 into plasmids encoding the immunoglobulin G1 (IgG1) constant region and a human kappa light chain to generate eight chimeric antibodies [49]. One variant, humAb4d5-8 bound three times more tightly to the ECD of $p185^{HER2}$ than the muMAb 4D5 and had anti-proliferative effects on the HER2 overexpressing cell line, SKBR3 [49]. Interestingly, humAb4D5-8 also mediated an antibody dependent cellular cytoxicity (ADCC) response against SKBR3 cells in the presence of human effector cells whereas the murine variant does not [49]. This vector was then transduced into Chinese hamster ovary (CHO) cells that are used in large scale production and was further purified [45]. This humanized monoclonal antibody, named trastuzumab (Herceptin^{TM}), is 95% human and 5% murine and is specific for HER2 [45]. Trastuzumab is a 148 kDa IgG_1 monoclonal antibody [50], containing two antigen specific sites derived from 4D5, the human variable region and an immunoglobin G_1 conserved Fc portion [49, 51]. In 1998, trastuzumab received US Food and Drug Administration (FDA) approval for the treatment of patients with metastatic breast cancer [52], and in 2006 was approved for treatment of early stage breast cancer [53].

Trastuzumab: Preclinical Evaluation

Preliminary preclinical testing in HER2 positive breast cancer demonstrated that trastuzumab treatment results in induction of p27, inhibition of proliferation, induction of cell cycle arrest, reduced vascular endothelial growth factor (VEGF) expression, enhanced sensitivity to chemotherapy and induction of ADCC [54, 55]. Further preclinical studies have extensively investigated the activity of trastuzumab and as a result a number of potential mechanisms of action have been postulated for trastuzumab. In brief, trastuzumab binds to the HER2 ECD and is capable of inhibiting downstream signaling pathways and inducing cell cycle arrest, blocking ECD shedding and inducing an ADCC response [56-62]. The exact contribution of each of these mechanisms to the anti-tumor effects of trastuzumab in patients is not fully understood.

It was initially proposed that trastuzumab caused downregulation of HER2 by enhancing the endocytic degradation of the receptor [63-65]. However, Austin *et al.* [66] showed that trastuzumab is internalized and passively recycled to the membrane with HER2, suggesting that downregulation of HER2 does not contribute to the mechanism of action of trastuzumab. Furthermore, no downregulation of HER2 was observed in tumor samples from patients who received neoadjuvant trastuzumab therapy [67].

Upon binding to HER2, trastuzumab reduces the phosphorylation of HER2 which results in inhibition of the MAPK and PI3K/AKT signaling pathways, and ultimately leads to growth inhibition and apoptosis sensitization [56-59]. One of the key mechanisms of action of trastuzumab is believed to be disruption of ligand independent interaction between HER2 and HER3 which activates the PI3K/AKT pathway. HER2 overexpression leads to ligand-independent activation of HER2/HER3 complexes and HER3 phosphorylation [60]. This in turn activates the downstream PI3K/AKT pathway. Junttila *et al.* found trastuzumab inhibits this ligand-independent HER2/HER3 dimerization and in turn downregulates the PI3K pathway [60].

Trastuzumabs treatment blocks ECD shedding of HER2 from breast cancer cell lines, and therefore inhibits production of p95HER2 [61]. Clinical studies have shown a correlation between the decrease in circulating HER2 ECD in patient serum during trastuzumab treatment and tumor response and progression free survival (PFS) [68, 69].

The Fc portion of trastuzumab is capable of binding to Fc gamma receptors on immune cells and inducing ADCC (Fig. **2**) [62]. Studies in Fc receptor knockout mice showed that the anti-tumor activity of trastuzumab was significantly impaired, indicating that the Fc/Fcγ receptor interaction is important for the trastuzumab mediated ADCC [70]. Trastuzumab induced ADCC has been attributed to natural killer (NK) cells and T cells [62, 71]. In HER2 positive tumors from patients who responded to trastuzumab treatment, significantly higher levels of NK cells and ADCC were detected [71, 72]. A correlation between PFS and NK cells was also observed [72].

Finally, trastuzumab has been implicated in inhibition of angiogenesis. Izumi *et al.* showed that trastuzumab suppressed angiogenesis *via* reduction in pro-angiogenic factors *e.g.*: VEGF and promotion of anti-angiogenic factors *e.g.*:

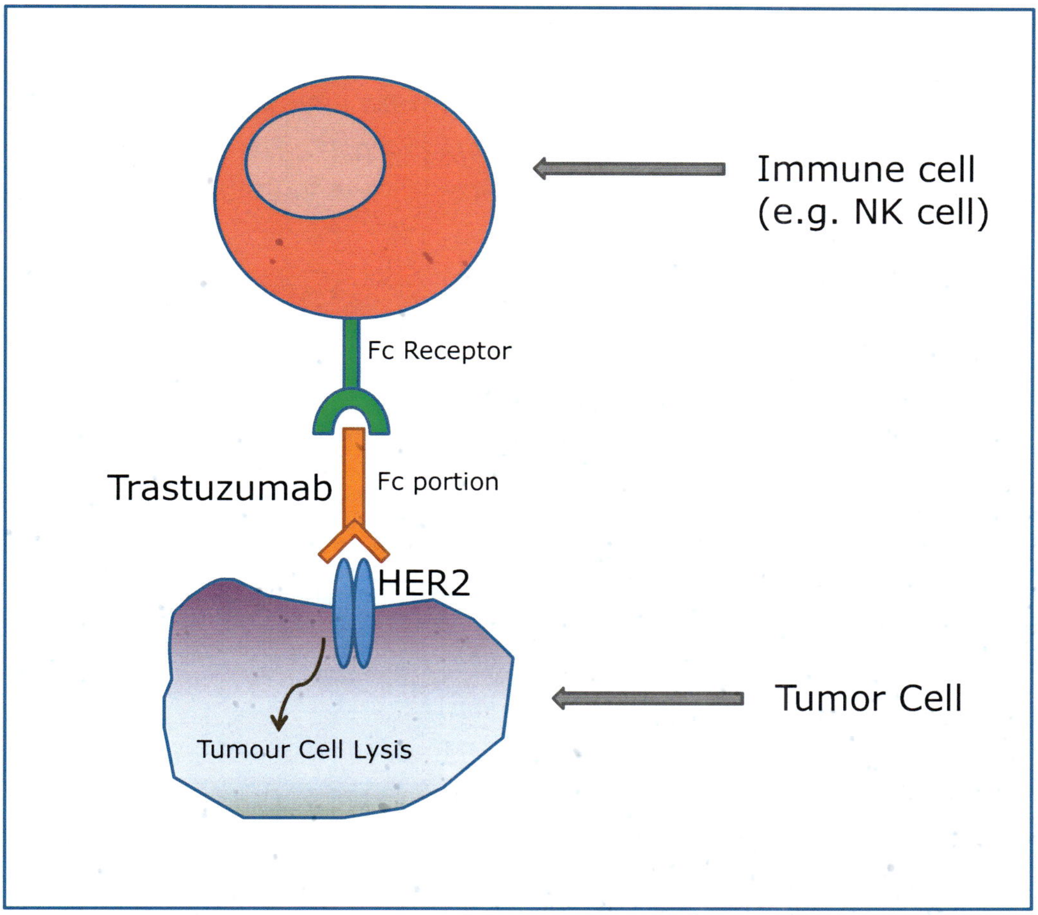

Fig. (2). Activation of ADCC upon trastuzumab binding. NK cells which express the Fc gamma receptors in turn bind to the Fc domain of trastuzumab which leads to tumor cell lysis or apoptosis.

thrombospondin-1 (TSP-1) only *in vivo* [73]. HER2 over-expressing cell lines were found to have increased VEGF mRNA and protein expression [74]. Klos *et al.,* showed that inhibition of angiogenesis was greater in xenografts treated with trastuzumab and paclitaxel compared to trastuzumab alone [75]. Another important finding from their study was that the PI3K/AKT/mTOR signaling pathway was involved in regulation of trastuzumab controlled VEGF activity [75]. Wen *et al.* [76] showed that in addition to decreasing VEGF levels, treatment with trastuzumab resulted in a decrease in interleukin-8 (IL-8) expression (pro-angiogenic) and an increase in TSP-1 expression (anti-angiogenic) *in vitro* and in BT474 xenografts [76].

Trastuzumab: Clinical Evaluation

In 1992, three phase I clinical trials were performed to determine the safety and pharmacokinetics (PK) of trastuzumab, administered at single weekly doses ranging from 10 and 500 mg [77]. Following completion of the phase I studies, two phase II trials of fixed dose trastuzumab (100 mg) alone or in combination with cisplatin were initiated in patients with HER2 overexpressing metastatic breast cancer [78, 79]. These trials produced an overall response of 12% and 24%, respectively. An international phase II clinical trial was carried out on 222 patients with HER2 positive metastatic breast cancer who had relapsed following prior chemotherapy treatment [80]. Unlike the previous studies, the trastuzumab dose was calculated on body weight (4 mg/kg loading dose followed by 2 mg/kg weekly). The objective response rate (ORR) in this clinical trial, determined by the independent response evaluation committee, was 15% (4% complete response (CR) and 11% partial response (PR)). CR was defined as the disappearance of radiographically, palpable, and/or visually apparent tumor. PR was defined as a ≥ 50% decrease in the dimensions of all measurable lesions [80]. The results confirmed that single agent trastuzumab could be safely administered in pre-treated patients.

Early PK studies on trastuzumab suggested a terminal half-life of 8 days [81]. However, subsequent studies determined that trastuzumab has a half-life of approximately 28 days [19]. Based on the longer half-life, a 3-weekly schedule, consisting of a loading dose of 8 mg/kg followed by 6 mg/kg once every 3 weeks was investigated [82]. A phase II study in patients with HER2 positive metastatic breast cancer reported that the 3-weekly trastuzumab regimen achieved similar results to the weekly regimen, and there were no increased or unexpected toxicities [83]. In addition, the administration of trastuzumab every 3 weeks resulted in PK similar to the weekly regimen. Although the weekly *versus* 3-weekly dosing has not been evaluated in a phase III clinical trial, both regimens have been used in phase II and III trials and are routinely used in clinical practice [51].

Phase II trials of trastuzumab with various chemotherapy regimens demonstrated response rates ranging from 24-88% [51]. Results of the pivotal phase III randomized clinical trial evaluating trastuzumab in HER2 metastatic breast cancer patients who were previously untreated, were reported in 2001 [52]. Of the 469 patients enrolled, 234 were randomized to chemotherapy alone and 235 to chemotherapy plus trastuzumab. Patients who had not previously received an anthracycline were treated with anthracycline (doxorubicin or epirubicin) and cyclophosphamide with (n=143) or without (n=138) trastuzumab. Patients who had previously received an anthracycline were treated with paclitaxel with (n=96) or without (n=92) trastuzumab. Trastuzumab in combination with chemotherapy improved the ORR (CR or PR as previously defined [80]) (50% *versus* 32%), PFS (7.4 *versus* 4.6 months), OS (25.1 *versus* 20.3 months) and resulted in a 20% reduction in risk of death, compared to chemotherapy alone. Upon disease progression, patients receiving chemotherapy only were allowed to cross over to receive trastuzumab. In 1998, based on the results of the phase III trial, the FDA granted approval for the use of trastuzumab with chemotherapy for the treatment of patients with HER2 positive metastatic breast cancer.

Although trastuzumab is generally not associated with serious side effects, cardiomyopathy was observed in a small percentage of patients in the early clinical trials. Cardiotoxicity occurred most frequently in patients receiving concurrent administration of anthracyclines (27% in patients treated with an anthracycline, cyclophosphamide, and trastuzumab; 8% in patients treated with an anthracycline and cyclophosphamide alone; 13% in patients treated with paclitaxel and trastuzumab; and 1 % in patients treated with paclitaxel alone) [52]. Based on the cardiotoxicity findings, concurrent administration of trastuzumab with anthracyclines is not recommended. Anthracyclines are themselves cardiotoxic and HER2 signaling *via* interaction with NRG-activated HER4 plays a role in the protection of cardiomyocytes from anthracycline-induced cell death. Therefore inhibition of HER2 by trastuzumab is believed to augment the cardiotoxicity of anthracyclines by blocking this protective signaling [14, 84].

The most significant advance in HER2 positive breast cancer came from the introduction of trastuzumab to adjuvant treatment of early stage HER2 positive breast cancer. Five randomized trials have evaluated trastuzumab in the adjuvant setting. Two phase III North American studies, North Central Cancer Treatment Group (NCCTG) N-9831 trial and the National Surgical Adjuvant Breast and

Bowel Project (NSABP) B-31 trial investigated doxorubicin and cyclophosphamide treatment followed by paclitaxel alone or in combination with trastuzumab for one year [53, 85]. The N-9831 trial differed slightly in paclitaxel administration schedule as patients in the third arm received trastuzumab alone upon completion of the chemotherapy regimen. Joint analysis of these trials at 3.9 years of median follow-up, revealed that addition of trastuzumab to paclitaxel in the adjuvant setting significantly improved DFS (hazard ratio (HR): 0.51, 95% confidence interval (CI) 0.44-0.59) and OS (HR: 0.59, 95% CI 0.48-0.73) [85].

The HERA (Trastuzumab Adjuvant) trial assigned 5000 women who had previously completed adjuvant chemotherapy to either undergo observation or receive trastuzumab every third week for 1 or 2 years [86]. Trastuzumab treatment after adjuvant chemotherapy for 1 or 2 years resulted in a 36% or 34% reduction in the risk of recurrence. They also concluded that 2 years of adjuvant treatment is not more effective than 1 year of treatment, which provides significant DFS and OS benefit for patients [87]. In the FinHer adjuvant study the docetaxel, trastuzumab and FEC (fluorouracil, epirubicin and cyclophosphamide) regimen improved distant disease-free survival (DDFS) compared to docetaxel and FEC alone or vinorelbine, trastuzumab and FEC [88]. Patients who received trastuzumab with chemotherapy had better DDFS than those who received chemotherapy alone.

The BCIRG-006 phase III adjuvant trial compared doxorubicin and cyclophosphamide followed by docetaxel alone (AC-T), doxorubicin and cyclophosphamide followed by docetaxel and trastuzumab (AC-T + H) or docetaxel, carboplatin and trastuzumab (TCH) in approximately 3,200 HER2 positive breast cancer patients [89, 90]. At 5 years, the addition of 1 year of adjuvant trastuzumab significantly improved DFS (75% for AC-T, 84% for AC-T plus trastuzumab, 81% for TCH) and OS (87% for AC-T, 92% for AC-T plus trastuzumab, 91% for TCH). This study also suggested that the TCH regimen is superior to the AC-T plus trastuzumab with respect to the safety profile and demonstrates comparable efficacy [90]. A meta-analysis of the five trials, showed that addition of trastuzumab to adjuvant chemotherapy produced a significant decrease in mortality ($p < 0.00001$), recurrence ($p < 0.00001$) and rates of metastasis ($p < 0.00001$), for patients with early stage HER2 positive breast cancer [91]. In 2006, the FDA granted approval for the use of trastuzumab in combination with chemotherapy for the treatment of patients with early stage HER2-overexpressing breast cancer.

In three recent studies, the addition of trastuzumab to chemotherapy as neoadjuvant treatment for HER2 positive breast cancer has resulted in pathological complete response (pCR) rates of 32-39% [92-94], compared to 19% pCR reported for HER2 positive patients treated with neoadjuvant chemotherapy without trastuzumab [92] or 16% pCR reported in a reference group of HER2 negative patients treated with neoadjuvant chemotherapy alone [94].

In addition to combining trastuzumab with chemotherapy, trials of trastuzumab in combination with other HER2 targeted therapies have been completed or are ongoing and will be discussed in the following sections. Furthermore, trastuzumab is also being tested in combination with therapies targeting the signaling pathways downstream of HER2, in particular the PI3K/AKT/mTOR pathway.

IgG monoclonal antibodies are considered to be excluded from the central nervous system (CNS) but it has been shown that IgG are transported across the blood brain barrier from brain to blood [95]. Assessment of trastuzumab levels in cerebral spinal fluid (CSF) showed that only minimal amounts of trastuzumab penetrated the CSF [96]. This is also reflected by evidence of CNS metastases developing in patients who are undergoing trastuzumab therapy [97]. Intrathecal trastuzumab, that is, injection of the drug into the spinal canal, has been tested and has been shown to eliminate neoplastic cells from the CSF of one patient [98].

Recently, a new formulation of trastuzumab has been approved for subcutaneous administration [99]. This new subcutaneous form can be administered in 2-5 min compared to the 30-90 min administration of intravenous trastuzumab, and has a PK profile and efficacy non-inferior to intravenous trastuzumab [99]. This new formulation is now approved for both early and late stage HER2 positive breast cancer.

Trastuzumab: Mechanisms of Resistance and Biomarkers

Despite the overall success of trastuzumab in the clinic, *de novo* or acquired resistance is an emerging problem for patients. In a recent study of metastatic

HER2 breast cancer patients, Gullo *et al.* reported that 9.5% of patients treated with trastuzumab in combination with chemotherapy achieved a durable CR, defined as continuously free of metastatic cancer for greater than 5 years [100]. Although this is the first indication that HER2 positive metastatic breast may be curable, the majority of patients with metastases develop progressive disease and ultimately succumb to the disease. Several resistance mechanisms have been proposed [101-103].

PTEN (Phosphatase and Tensin Homolog) Loss & PI3K/AKT Activity

Loss of PTEN due to mutations and loss of heterozygosity (LOH) has been reported in 50% of breast cancers [104, 105]. Restoring PTEN expression in PTEN null cells inhibits PI3K/AKT signaling and tumor formation [106]. Trastuzumab treatment results in PTEN membrane localization and an increase in phosphatase activity due to a reduction in Src-mediated PTEN tyrosine phosphorylation [57]. Nagata *et al.,* also showed that PTEN antisense nucleotides conferred trastuzumab resistance *in vitro* and *in vivo*. In HER2 positive breast tumors, PTEN deficiency is associated with reduced response to trastuzumab therapy compared to tumors with normal PTEN levels. PTEN loss-induced trastuzumab resistance was overcome by PI3K inhibitors, suggesting PI3K-targeting therapies may overcome resistance [57]. In a large scale RNA-interference screen it was reported that measuring PTEN loss and activating mutations of PI3K in combination was a superior marker of trastuzumab response [107]. O'Brien *et al.* reported that loss of PTEN combined with PI3K mutation, predicting activation of the PI3K/AKT pathway, correlated with trastuzumab resistance *in vitro* [108]. A molecular study carried out on 63 relapsed HER2 positive tumors found that PTEN reduction and activating mutations in PIK3CA occurred in 71% of trastuzumab refractory tumors [109]. However, in 2013, Perez *et al.* reported findings from the NCCTG-N9831 clinical trial where correlations between tumor PTEN protein expression and DFS were investigated [110]. PTEN expression in tumors did not correlate with DFS and adjuvant trastuzumab was beneficial to HER2 positive breast cancer patients regardless of tumor PTEN status [110]. Thus measurement of PTEN alone does not appear to predict trastuzumab response/resistance. However, combining PTEN levels with PI3K mutation status may be predictive of trastuzumab response/resistance, by providing a better indicator of the activation status of the PI3K/AKT signaling pathway.

Activation of Alternative Signaling Pathways

The insulin-like growth factor 1 receptor (IGFIR) may play a role in resistance. IGFIR is a transmembrane tyrosine kinase receptor and this pathway is involved in breast cancer proliferation and metastasis [111]. SKBR-3 breast cancer cells genetically altered to over-express IGFIR were insensitive to growth inhibition by trastuzumab and inhibition of IGFIR signaling restored trastuzumab sensitivity [112]. A study by Browne *et al.,* showed that IGFIR levels were increased in a trastuzumab resistant cell line model (SKBR3-Tr) and in agreement with Lu *et al.,* upon silencing of IGFIR expression there was an increased response to trastuzumab [113]. In a recent study, Browne *et al.,* reported that neither IGFIR nor pIGFIR expression predicts response to trastuzumab treatment in patients with early stage HER2 positive breast cancer (n=96) [114]. A large study of 1,746 early stage HER2 positive breast cancer patients also reported no difference in response to trastuzumab between IGFIR-negative and -positive patients [115]. However, co-targeting HER2 and IGFIR produced enhanced anti-proliferative activity in a subset of HER2 positive breast cancer cell lines [114].

The RTK, MET may also play a role in trastuzumab resistance [116]. Inhibition of MET increases trastuzumab sensitivity and upon MET activation cells were protected from growth inhibition by trastuzumab. Shattuck *et al.,* also found that MET is co-expressed with HER2 in HER2 positive breast cancer cells and patient samples [116].

Activation of other HER family members has been implicated in resistance, in particular EGFR and HER3. Activation of HER3 and formation of HER2/HER3 heterodimers results in PI3K/AKT pathway activation [65]. EGFR overexpression has been associated with trastuzumab resistance in both *in vitro* and *in vivo* resistance models [117, 118]. Gijsen *et al.* found that HER2 phosphorylation can be sustained by ligand-dependent activation of EGFR, HER3 and HER4 resulting in heterodimers capable of signaling downstream pathways [119]. The ligand release is mediated by ADAM17 protease through an AKT negative feedback loop. Combined treatment with trastuzumab and ADAM inhibitors blocked this feedback loop and reduced HER2 phosphorylation in SKBR3 cells [119].

HER2 ECD Shedding and p95HER2

HER2 ECD shedding and p95HER2 have been implicated in trastuzumab resistance. The HER2 ECD was examined in patients, with metastatic breast cancer, after initiating trastuzumab treatment (n=307) and a failure to reach a decline in HER2 ECD levels correlated with reduced response to trastuzumab [120]. Circulating HER2 ECD may bind trastuzumab and trastuzumab does not bind to the cleaved p95HER2. Xenograft tumors established using T47D [121] and MCF7 [122] cells forced to overexpress p95HER2 are insensitive to trastuzumab treatment. Retrospective studies have found an association with p95HER2 expression and trastuzumab resistance [36, 42, 122, 123]. Interestingly, O'Brien *et al.* found no association between p95HER2 and trastuzumab response in a panel of HER2 positive breast cancer cell lines [124]. They observed that p95HER2 levels tracked consistently with high HER2 and phospho-HER2 levels, suggesting that p95HER2 may not be an independent marker of response.

Steric Hindrance of Receptor-Antibody Interaction: Overexpression of MUC4

Trastuzumab resistance has been associated with over-expression of the membrane associated glycoprotein mucin 4 (MUC4) [125]. It is has been shown to bind and sterically hinder trastuzumab binding to HER2 [126]. Furthermore, upon knock down of MUC4 there was increased binding of trastuzumab [126]. Upregulation of MUC4 was found to be associated with resistance to both endocrine and HER2 targeted therapies in MCF7 cells and HER2 positive xenograft tumors [127].

Molecular Chaperones

Molecular chaperones such as heat shock protein 90 (HSP90) may play a role in trastuzumab resistance. HSP90 is known to regulate the stability of HER2 which decreases receptor turnover and thereby strengthens HER2 signaling effects [128]. Interestingly, p95HER2 is also a client protein of HSP90 [129]. An *in vivo* tumor model overexpressing p95HER2 displayed resistance to trastuzumab. However, treatment with HSP90 inhibitors induced loss of HER2 and p95HER2, resulting in growth inhibition and apoptosis induction [129]. HSP90 may not directly confer resistance but HSP90 inhibitors maybe an effective therapeutic strategy for trastuzumab resistant patients.

Although multiple mechanisms of both innate and acquired resistance have been postulated, no predictive biomarkers of resistance have been successfully validated clinically. Amplification and/or overexpression of HER2 are the only clinically validated predictive biomarkers of response to trastuzumab.

Trastuzumab: Development of Biosimilars

As trastuzumab goes off patent this year, 2014, in Europe and in 2019 in the United States, a new wave of biosimilars is in the pipeline. Synthon has completed a phase I trial comparing their biosimilar to trastuzumab and the resulting pharmacokinetic data has allowed for phase III trial progression [130]. Celltrion presented phase III results of its trastuzumab biosimilar, CT-P6 at ASCO 2013 [131]. This study showed equivalent efficacy of CT-P6 to trastuzumab in ORR in combination with paclitaxel as a first line treatment administered every 3 weeks and had a comparable safety profile [131]. Pfizer also presented results of its phase I trial for a trastuzumab biosimilar, PF-05280014 [132]. The data showed equivalent properties and similar safety profiles to both a US and EU sourced trastuzumab.

HerTraz or CANMAb (Mylan and Biocon) received regulatory approval in India in 2013 [133, 134]. Mylan and Biocon have exclusive commercialization rights for this biosimilar in numerous countries and plan to launch HerTraz/CANMAb in 2014 [133].

It is anticipated that biosimilars will lower the cost of receiving a HER2 targeted therapy, thereby providing more patients with access to targeted treatments, as trastuzumab treatment costs approximately $4,500 per month in the United States.

Pertuzumab (2C4, previously Omnitarg™, now Perjeta®)

Pertuzumab: Discovery and Mechanism of Action

Pertuzumab is a full-length recombinant humanized IgG1 monoclonal antibody that specifically targets the ECD of the ErbB2 receptor [135] and represents a novel class of HER2 dimerization inhibitors. The original mouse monoclonal antibody variant of pertuzumab, 2C4, was identified by researchers at Genentech during a screen for murine monoclonal antibodies that would immunoprecipitate the 185 kDa full-length protein product of the HER2 gene without cross reacting with EGFR [44]. Each of the 10 antibodies that were raised against the ECD of the ErbB2 receptor were isolated and characterized for their potential development as receptor based tumor therapies [44]. Another of these murine monoclonal antibodies identified in the same screen, named 4D5, was later humanized to become trastuzumab [49]. These studies also showed that 4D5 and 2C4 bound to distinct epitopes on the ECD of the ErbB2 receptor which is ultimately responsible for the subtle but clinically important differences between the mechanism of action of these two molecules [44]. Subsequent studies of the HER2-pertuzumab and HER2-trastuzumab complexes confirmed that pertuzumab binds to domain II of the ECD whereas trastuzumab binds to domain IV [3, 136].

By interacting with the juxtamembrane portion of the HER2 ECD at domain IV, trastuzumab can prevent shedding of the receptor ECD [66], but has little activity in blocking interaction with ligand activated members of the HER family [49, 137]. In contrast, pertuzumab binds directly to the dimerization interface at domain II and inhibits ligand-activated dimerization of HER2 with its oncogenic partners, HER3 and EGFR [136]. Ligand binding to EGFR or HER3 causes a conformational change and rotation of the receptor that brings domains I and III into a closed conformation which exposes domain II, allowing for dimerization with domain II of other type I RTKs [138-140]. Due to a truncation in the ligand binding domain of the HER2 ECD, the receptor is permanently in the closed/ligand bound conformation, thus domain II is permanently exposed, allowing for homo- and heterodimerization in the absence of ligand [141, 142].

Thus although HER2 has no known ligand, it is the preferred dimerization partner for other members of the HER-family [143]. In HER2 amplified breast cancer, extremely high levels of the HER2 protein are produced on the cell surface. This allows HER2 to dimerize readily with HER3 in the absence of ligand activation [144]. Together these proteins form what is believed to be the major oncogenic subunit in HER2-amplified breast cancer [145]. In this instance, trastuzumab is thought mediate its effects on downstream AKT signaling by sequestering HER2 away from HER3 and thus limiting the access to HER3 [65, 146], as such trastuzumab is only effective in HER2-amplified tumors. Pertuzumab, on the other hand, is unable to block this ligand independent dimerization associated with HER2-amplification, however it is effective in blocking ligand mediated HER2 activation through HER3 and EGFR [44, 65, 137]. This opens the possibility of pertuzumab having activity outside of HER2-amplfied breast cancer in cells that express lower levels of HER2 where trastuzumab is ineffective [137].

Despite the complementary manner in which these two monoclonal antibodies interact with the HER2 protein, both will ultimately down regulate HER2 driven PI3K/mTOR signaling and induce G_1-S cell cycle arrest. In the presence of the HER3 ligand NRG-1β, pertuzumab treatment induces a loss of HER2 and HER3 phosphorylation [44, 65, 137], which results in a loss of AKT phosphorylation *via* inhibition of PI3K. At this point it appears the mechanisms of action of pertuzumab and trastuzumab converge and both induce an inhibition of cell proliferation through upregulation of the cyclin dependent kinase 2 (CDK2) inhibitor protein p27 [63, 147-149]. Inhibition of AKT signaling has the potential to inhibit DNA damage repair pathways, indicating the potential for pertuzumab treatment to induce apoptosis. Furthermore, pertuzumab has been shown to mediate a similar effect on ADCC as trastuzumab. Both molecules are IgG1 monoclonal antibodies, and when bound to cell surface HER2 can recruit activated NK cells through interaction of the Fcγ receptor of the NK cell with the Fc domains of the monoclonal antibodies [136, 150].

Pertuzumab: Preclinical Evaluation

Given that it does not strictly require HER2-amplification to have activity, pertuzumab preclinical efficacy as both a single agent and combination has been investigated in a range of cancer types, including breast, prostate, lung and ovarian.

Early studies showed that the mouse monoclonal antibody 2C4 had single agent activity in human cell line xenograft models of breast and prostate cancer independent of HER2-amplification status. *In vitro* activity was also observed in

HER2-normal cell lines when first stimulated with the HER3 ligand NRG-1β, proving that HER2 signaling could be blocked by targeting co-factor mediated activation [137]. These findings were confirmed *in vivo* by using a breast cancer cell line xenograft model that produces high levels of the HER3 ligand, NRG-1β, but does not carry the HER2-amplification [145]. In this model, pertuzumab activity was far superior to that of trastuzumab, indicating a role for pertuzumab in the treatment of HER2 cofactor driven tumors. These studies also confirm the previous findings that in breast cancer at least; HER3 is the major co-activator of HER2 and not EGFR [145, 151, 152]. HER3 levels have also been shown to be a biomarker of response to pertuzumab in ovarian cancer cell lines [153].

In addition to inhibiting HER2 co-activation, pertuzumab has also been investigated pre-clinically as a secondary HER2-targeting therapeutic that may provide benefit to patients that progress on trastuzumab-based therapy. The fact that trastuzumab and pertuzumab have independent and shared mechanisms of action makes them good candidates for combination. Preliminary *in vitro* studies showed that combined treatment of a HER2-amplified cell line resulted in greater decrease in HER2/PI3K/AKT signaling and a greater induction of apoptosis and ADCC than observed with either agent alone. Furthermore, these effects were more evident in HER2-amplified breast cell lines that co-expressed high levels of HER3 that those with high EGFR [154, 155]. *In vivo* studies using cell line xenografts of HER2-amplified cell lines showed that the trastuzumab/pertuzumab combination was well tolerated in mice and a marginal increase in efficacy in comparison to either single agent was observed [145, 156]. It is possible that the modest differences from single agent to combination can be attributed to the fact trastuzumab monotherapy was so active in these models. However, when this combination was tested in a HER2-amplifed xenograft model of trastuzumab resistance, significant benefit was observed when trastuzumab was combined with pertuzumab, indicating that pertuzumab may provide benefit in trastuzumab-refractory breast cancer [157]. Combined efficacy was also observed in a xenograft model of non-small cell lung cancer (NSCLC). Molecular characterization of these models revealed high levels of HER2 and HER3 protein in the breast cancer tumors but high levels of HER2 and EGFR protein in the NSCLC tumors, indicating that pertuzumab could have activity against both the

HER2-HER3 dimers in breast and HER2-EGFR dimers in lung cancer where EGFR alterations may be more prevalent [157]. The combination of pertuzumab with the trastuzumab-emtaninse ADC (T-DM1, Kadcyla®, Genentech) has also been evaluated in *in vitro* and *in vivo* preclinical studies [158]. The addition of pertuzumab increased the cytotoxicity observed with T-DM1 alone in HER2-amplified breast cancer cell lines. Combined anti-tumor efficacy was also observed in xenograft models of NSCLC and in models of HER2-amplifed and NRG-1β-driven breast cancer [158].

Pertuzumab: Clinical Evaluation

Even though originally identified in the same study, the paths of trastuzumab and pertuzumab to the clinic have been markedly distinct. Whereas the therapeutic benefit of trastuzumab has long been established [52, 80, 159], pertuzumab eventually received FDA approval for treatment of cancer patients in 2012 [160].

The dimerization inhibition properties of pertuzumab indicated that unlike trastuzumab, activity would not be restricted to HER2-amplified breast cancer [137]. The original phase I clinical trial reported that pertuzumab was well tolerated and showed indications of clinical activity [161]. This gave encouragement that a HER-dimerization inhibitor could be an effective anti-cancer strategy, possibly even in HER2-normal or in non-breast tumors. Single agent pertuzumab was investigated for safety and efficacy in two independent phase II clinical trials in prostate [162] and lung cancer (NSCLC) [163]. Although well tolerated as a monotherapy, very limited efficacy was observed in both studies. A marginal improvement on this clinical efficacy was observed in a phase II trial of ovarian cancer. Interestingly, PFS in patients with high HER2 levels was 20.9 weeks compared to 5.8 weeks in patients with low HER2 [164], indicating that the response biomarker for pertuzumab may indeed be HER2. Further evidence that HER2-amplification may be required for a clinical response was provided by data from a phase II clinical trial of single agent pertuzumab in patients with HER2-non-amplified (and low protein by IHC) advanced metastatic breast cancer [165]. The limited efficacy observed in this international multicenter clinical trial led the investigators to conclude that there was little benefit to further investigation of single agent pertuzumab in HER2-negative patients [165]. Thus, the pre-clinical evidence with pertuzumab did not meet the expectations of predicting clinical benefit outside of HER2-amplifed cancer, at least in the metastatic setting. However, there was still the possibility that the limited efficacies observed in these phase II studies could be improved upon by combining pertuzumab with cytotoxic chemotherapy or other targeted agents, such as trastuzumab.

A phase II single arm clinical study showed that the combination of trastuzumab and pertuzumab was well tolerated with an ORR of 24.2% (7.6% CR and 16.7% PR) in patients with advanced HER2-positive breast cancer that had previously progressed on trastuzumab therapy [166]. Another phase II trial directly compared the benefits of neoadjuvant trastuzumab or pertuzumab *versus* the combination in locally advanced, inflammatory, or early HER2-positive breast cancer (NeoSphere). Patients were randomized to four arms of A) trastuzumab plus docetaxel, B) pertuzumab plus docetaxel, C) trastuzumab plus pertuzumab plus docetaxel or D) trastuzumab plus pertuzumab without docetaxel [167]. A phase Ib study had already demonstrated the safety of combining pertuzumab with the antimicrotubule agent docetaxel [168]. Significantly improved pCRs were observed in the trastuzumab/pertuzumab plus docetaxel arm (45.8%) *vs* the trastuzumab plus docetaxel arm (29.0%). Although toxicities were less in the non-docetaxel containing combination arm, pCR rates were also lower (16.8%) [167]. Further analyses of these data highlighted the remarkable efficacy of the trastuzumab/pertuzumab docetaxel combination in the patients with HER2 positive and ER negative (63%) tumors relative to those with HER2 positive and ER positive (26%) tumors, suggesting that this may be the patient sub-type that would benefit most from this combination [167, 169]. The potential of pertuzumab to augment trastuzumab activity was confirmed in the CLEOPATRA phase III clinical trial of 808 patients that had not received prior trastuzumab therapy [160]. Patients with HER2 positive metastatic breast cancer were randomly assigned to receive trastuzumab and docetaxel plus pertuzumab or the control regimen of trastuzumab and docetaxel. Significantly improved PFS (18.7 *vs* 12.4 months) and OS (estimated median OS at 3 yrs: 65.8% *versus* 50.4%) was observed in the pertuzumab/trastuzumab plus docetaxel arm relative to the control arm [160, 170]. Given that these improved responses were not accompanied by significant increases in adverse events (including cardiac toxicities), the pertuzumab/trastuzumab plus docetaxel combination received FDA approval in June 2012 as first-line therapy for patients with HER2-amplified metastatic breast cancer. Furthermore, supporting efficacy and safety data from the NeoSphere and TRYPHAENA phase II clinical trials led to the combination of pertuzumab plus trastuzumab plus docetaxel receiving accelerated FDA approval in September 2013 as first-line treatment for patients at high risk of metastasis or death, *i.e.*, patients with locally advanced, inflammatory or early stage HER2-amplifed breast cancer [167, 171].

The pertuzumab/trastuzumab combination is currently being further investigated in HER2-amplifed early (non-metastatic) breast cancer in the APHINITY phase II clinical trial (NCT01358877) [172]. In addition, a series of clinical studies are also underway to find the best chemotherapeutic agents to combine with pertuzumab and trastuzumab. Pertuzumab is also being investigated for efficacy and tolerability in combination with T-DM1 in HER2-amplfied breast cancer in the MARIANNE clinical trial (NCT01120184) [173]. The findings from this phase III study, which will be the first to evaluate the combination of a HER2-dimerization inhibitor and a HER2-directed ADC, are eagerly awaited.

Pertuzumab: Biomarkers of Response and Resistance

The preclinical data with pertuzumab strongly suggested that there would be clinical efficacy outside of HER2-amplified tumors. However, after rigorously testing this hypothesis in the clinic, it appears, for the moment at least, that the optimal response phenotype pertuzumab is indeed HER2-amplified breast cancer. *In vitro* studies of cell lines supplemented with NRG-1β ligand stimulation indicated impressive anti-proliferative activity for pertuzumab in non HER2-amplified cells. However, outside of this artificially created environment, *i.e.*, the clinic, pertuzumab performs poorly in HER2-normal patients. It remains to be seen if a tumor sub-group exists that produces high levels of HER3 activating ligands that may achieve benefit from pertuzumab mono- or combination therapy.

Undoubtedly, the majority of the mechanisms of resistance to trastuzumab, described earlier, will apply to pertuzumab. Alterations in PI3K/PTEN/mTOR pathway signaling will surely affect pertuzumab response downstream of HER2-targeting. Steric hindrance or enzymatic cleavage of the HER2 ECD would also limit pertuzumab activity. However, given that the clinical indications for pertuzumab treatment are for combination with trastuzumab, it is imperative to identify additional biomarkers of response and resistance to combined therapy. Careful molecular analysis of patient tissues collected from clinical studies such as CLEOPATRA, NeoSphere and TRYPHAENA will help to further stratify patients most likely to respond to combined HER2-targeted therapy and identify the escape pathways that can be targeted alternatively or in combination.

T-DM1(Kadcyla™)

T-DM1: Discovery and Mechanism of Action

Ado-trastuzumab emtansine (T-DM1) (Kadcyla™, Genentech) is an ADC which is composed of the HER2 monoclonal antibody trastuzumab linked, *via* 4-(3-mercapto-2,5-dioxo-1-pyrrolidinylmethyl)-cyclohexanecarboxylic acid (MCC), to the cytotoxic chemotherapy drug mertansine (Fig. **3**). Mertansine is a maytansanoid, that is, a derivative of maytansine. Maytansine is an antibiotic which was originally isolated from an Ethiopian plant, *Maytenus serrate*. It binds to tubulin and inhibits microtubule assembly, thereby causing microtubule disassembly and perturbing mitosis. Maytansine is highly toxic for human cancer cells, *in vitro*, with IC_{50} values in the sub-nanomolar range. It was ineffective in clinical trials however, due to high systemic toxicity resulting in a low therapeutic index [174, 175]. In 1992, ImmunoGen Inc. described an ADC consisting of maytansine conjugated by a disulphide linker to an anti-HER2 antibody TA.1 [175]. Treatment of HER2 positive SKBR-3 cells with 0.1 nM TA.1(-SS-May)4 conjugate killed 99.9% of the tumor cells, with an IC_{50} value of 3 pM). The conjugate was 1000-fold less toxic to HER2 negative cells.

In 2008, Lewis-Phillips *et al.* first described T-DM1, which was co-developed by ImmunoGen and Genentech, by linking trastuzumab to mertansine (DM1) *via* a non-reducible linker [176]. The non-reducible thioether linker provided improved efficacy and PK and reduced toxicity compared to the reducible disulfide linkers. The disulfide-linked DM1-containing ADCs were rapidly cleared, whereas, PK studies in mice over 1 week showed that serum concentrations of T-DM1 were similar to total serum trastuzumab concentrations.

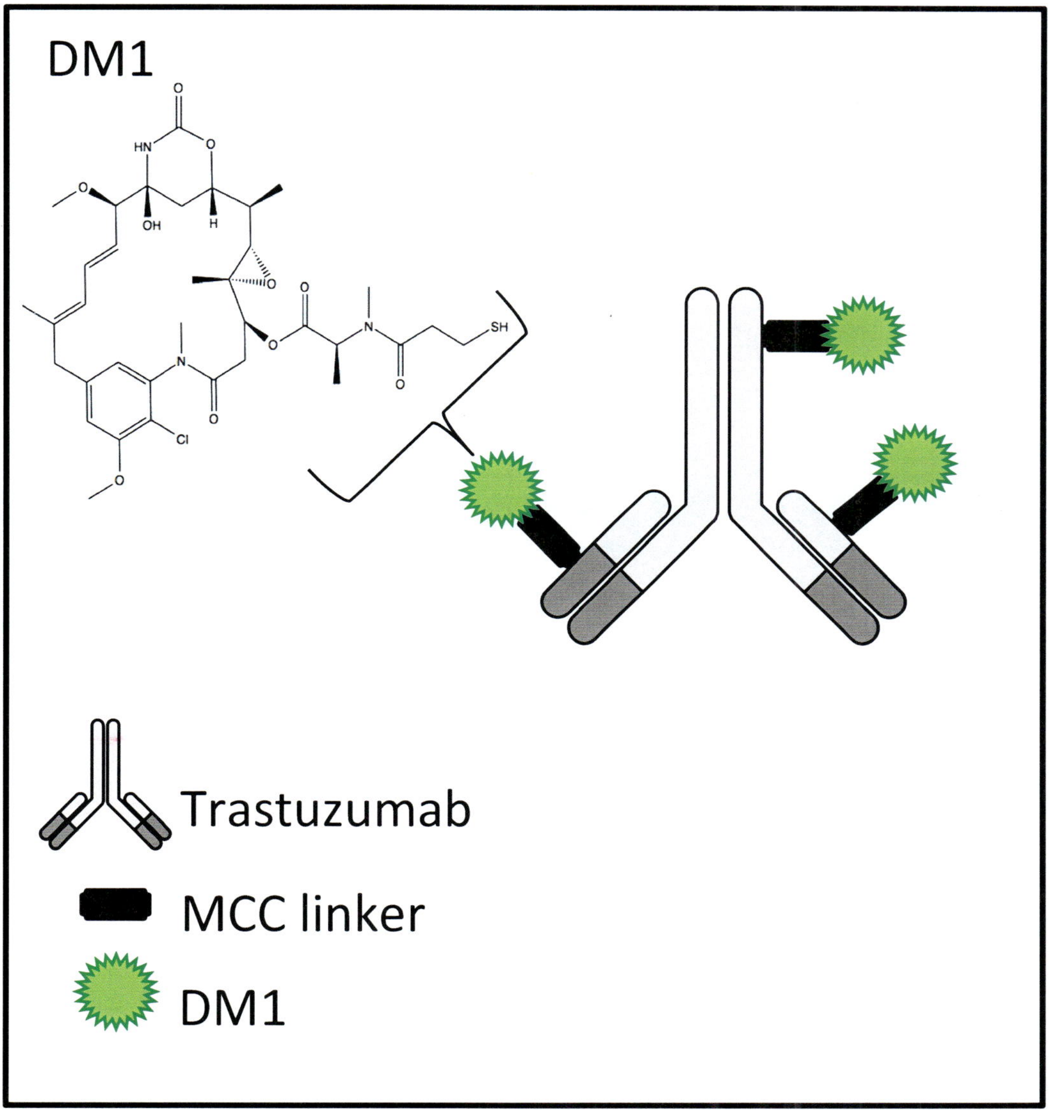

Fig. (3). Structure of T-DM1, consisting of an average of 3-4 DM1 molecules linked to trastuzumab *via* a nonreducible thioether linker (MCC).

The drug to antibody ratio in T-DM1 is approximately 3.5:1 [176, 177]. Upon binding to HER2-overexpressing tumor cells, T-DM1 is internalized along with HER2 and is postulated to undergo intracellular proteolytic degradation to release the active maytansinoid. Consistent with this, protease inhibitors block the activity of T-DM1, *in vitro* [176].

The rationale for developing the T-DM1 ADC included the suitability of HER2 as a clinically validated target and the potent cytotoxicity of the DM1, coupled with the favorable characteristics of the MCC linker [177].

T-DM1: Preclinical Evaluation

In vitro evaluation of T-DM1 confirmed selective activity in HER2 positive breast cancer cell lines, with minimal anti-proliferative activity in non-HER2 amplified cell lines, and increased potency compared to free trastuzumab or free DM1. In contrast, free DM1 shows similar potency in HER2 amplified and HER2 non-amplified cell lines [176].

While trastuzumab is cytostatic *in vitro*, T-DM1 induced caspase-dependent apoptosis and cell lysis in the HER2 positive breast cancer cell lines. Evaluation of *in vivo* efficacy showed that T-DM1 caused dose-dependent inhibition of tumor growth and regression in the 3 HER2 positive breast cancer models tested [176]. In addition to induction of apoptosis, Barok *et al.* [178] reported that T-DM1 induced mitotic catastrophe in HER2 positive (JIMT-1) xenograft tumors. The authors hypothesize that the induction of mitotic catastrophe might occur in cells that are not highly sensitive to T-DM1, possibly due to lower cytoplasmic concentrations of DM1 than would be achieved in sensitive cells where apoptosis induction occurs.

Junttila *et al.* compared the mechanisms of action of T-DM1 to unconjugated trastuzumab. In a trastuzumab-insensitive xenograft model of HER2 positive breast cancer, T-DM1 significantly inhibited tumor growth, whereas free DM1, at a dose equivalent to that conjugated to trastuzumab in T-DM1 showed minimal anti-tumor activity [179]. In addition, no significant therapeutic effect was observed when unconjugated trastuzumab was delivered in combination with DM1, ruling out the possibility of chemosensitization effects. *In vitro* binding assays confirmed that the affinity of T-DM1 for HER2 is similar to free trastuzumab (KD = 0.140 ± 0.02 nM *versus* 0.170 ± 0.003 nM). T-DM1 showed similar inhibition of AKT phosphorylation and inhibition of HER2 ectodomain shedding as unconjugated trastuzumab, in HER2 positive breast cancer cells *in vitro*. In contrast to trastuzumab response, PI3K mutation status did not impact on T-DM1 response *in vitro*.

In vitro ADCC assays performed with PBMCs confirmed that T-DM1 retains the ability to activate immune cell mediated ADCC, similar to trastuzumab. Barok *et al.* also confirmed that T-DM1 induces ADCC similar to trastuzumab in HER2 positive breast cancer cell lines, including JIMT1 cells which, although HER2 amplified, expresses moderate levels of HER2 [178].

In HER2 positive breast cancer cell lines which were innately resistant to lapatinib (MCF7-neo/HER2) or were conditioned to develop resistance to lapatinib (SKBR3), T-DM1 inhibited growth a low concentrations. T-DM1 is also active against trastuzumab resistant cell lines, including HER2 positive breast cancer cell lines and HER2 positive cell lines from a number of other tissues of origin (lung, gastric and ovarian carcinoma)[176].

In vivo studies with xenograft models of the trastuzumab and lapatinib resistant JIMT-1 cells, suggest that T-DM1 efficacy may be dependent on tumor burden [178]. In JIMT-1 xenografts with established tumors, T-DM1 partially but significantly inhibited tumor growth. Treatment with T-DM1 from the time of inoculation blocked the development of JIMT-1 xenograft tumors for up to 15 weeks. Interestingly, when the JIMT-1 xenografts were treated with trastuzumab for 40 days, then switched to T-DM1 treatment, T-DM1 was unable to inhibit tumor growth.

In depth *in vivo* modelling studies show that the anti-tumor effects of T-DM1 were schedule independent. The modelling suggested that T-DM1 can be dosed weekly or 3-weekly with no impact on efficacy, if the troughs between doses are greater than the tumoristatic concentration (TSC; the stationary drug concentration at which the growth rate equals the kill rate) [180].

Preclinical studies characterizing the antigen-dependent and non-antigen-dependent toxicity profiles of T-DM1 were performed in monkeys and rats, as T-

DM1 binds primate ErbB2 but not rodent c-neu [181]. T-DM1 was safely tolerated at doses up to 40 mg/kg in rats and 30 mg/kg in monkeys, whereas the maximum tolerated dose (MTD) of DM1 was 0.2 mg/kg. This tolerance of higher doses of DM1 in T-DM1, supports the principle that ADCs improve the therapeutic index. The safety profiles for T-DM1 and DM1 were similar, with bone marrow/hematologic, hepatic, and neuronal toxicities observed. The toxicity profile is consistent with the mode of action of DM1, *i.e.* inhibition of tubulin polymerization. T-DM1, similar to trastuzumab, did not cause acute changes in cardiac conduction or hemodynamic parameters. However, reduction in left ventricular ejection fraction, which occurs in a small percentage of patients treated with trastuzumab, was not assessed in these preclinical studies.

T-DM1: Clinical Evaluation

Single Agent Studies

A phase I first-in-human study of T-DM1 was conducted in patients with advanced HER2-positive breast cancer, who had progressed on trastuzumab-based therapy [177]. Two drug administration schedules were evaluated in separate cohorts within the phase I study: every 3 weeks and weekly. Dose-limiting grade 4 thrombocytopenia was experienced by two patients receiving 4.8-mg/kg. No dose limiting toxicities were reported in the cohort of patients treated with 3.6 mg/kg and that was declared the MTD. A total of 15 patients were treated with the MTD. The half-life of T-DM1 at this dose was 3.5 days, with peak plasma levels of DM1 less than 10 ng/mL. Systemic clearance of T-DM1 was more rapid than the clearance rate reported for unconjugated trastuzumab [83]. Integrated population based pharmcokinetic modelling of T-DM1 conjugate and total trastuzumab clearance data suggests that the 2/3 times faster T-DM1 conjugate clearance is due to a deconjugation process, in addition to proteolytic cleavage, which occurs for trastuzumab [182].

Thrombocytopenia emerged as the most common adverse event and key dose limiting toxicity associated with T-DM1 [177]. Thrombocytopenia is a common occurrence with cytotoxic chemotherapy and is believed to be caused by antimitotic effects on megakaryocyte precursors. To investigate the mechanism of

T-DM1-induced thrombocytopenia, Thon *et al.,* used a novel high-content quantitative live-cell imaging assay, and showed that T-DM1 is taken up by mouse megakaryocytes and it then inhibits megakaryocyte differentiation and decreases proplatelet production by disrupting the microtubule cytoskeleton [183].

The clinical benefit rate (PR plus stable disease (SD) at 6 months, defined by RECIST) in the 15 patients treated with the MTD in the phase I study was 73%, and the confirmed response rate among patients with measurable disease in this group (n=9) was 44% [177].

The phase I study of weekly T-DM1 established a MTD of 2.4 mg/kg [184]. Objective PRs, determined using RECIST, were observed in 46.4 % of patients and the 6-month clinical benefit rate (PR plus SD) was 57.1%. The adverse events experienced by patients receiving the weekly T-DM1 regimen were similar to those experienced by patients receiving the 3-weekly regimen.

In the phase I studies, only 1 of the 47 patients had an anti-therapeutic antibody (ATA) response [177, 184]. Across four studies of single agent T-DM1 at 3.6 mg/kg every 3 weeks, ATA was detected in approximately 4.5 % of patients (13/286) [185]. The PK profiling across the four studies also showed that T-DM1 exposure does not correlate with clinical responses or adverse events.

In two phase II single arm clinical trials, T-DM1 was evaluated in (i) patients with progressive HER2 positive metastatic breast cancer following prior anti-HER2 targeted therapy and prior chemotherapy and (ii) patients who have previously received all standard anti-HER2 therapies [186, 187]. In both studies, T-DM1 was administered 3 weekly at 3.6 mg/kg. The ORRs (CR or PR) were 25.9 % and 34.5 %, respectively. In both studies the response rates were higher in patients with HER2 positivity confirmed by central laboratory testing. In a phase II randomized trial, first line treatment with T-DM1 provided a significant improvement in PFS, with a favorable safety profile, compared to trastuzumab plus docetaxel, for HER2 positive metastatic breast cancer (14.2 *versus* 9.2 months; HR, 0.59; 95% CI, 0.36 to 0.97) [188]. OS rates were similar between treatment arms.

The randomized phase III EMILIA trial reported that T-DM1 significantly prolonged PFS (9.6 *versus* 6.4 months; HR, 0.65; 95% CI, 055 to 0.77; p<0.001) and OS (30.9 *versus* 25.1 months; HR, 0.68; 95% CI, 0.55 to 0.85; p<0.001) compared to lapatinib plus capecitabine in patients with HER2 positive advanced breast cancer previously treated with trastuzumab and a taxane [189]. Adverse events of grade 3 or higher were less frequent in patients receiving T-DM1 than for patients receiving lapatinib plus capecitabine (40.8 *versus* 57.0%). For patients who experienced T-DM1 related thrombocytopenia, the first occurrence of grade 3/4 thrombocytopenia was reported within the first two cycles of treatment and with dose modifications, the majority of these patients continued treatment.

On the basis of the EMILIA phase III results, in February 2013, the US FDA granted approval for T-DM1 for the treatment of patients with HER2 positive metastatic breast cancer following progression on trastuzumab and a taxane.

In a retrospective exploratory analysis of data from EMILIA, in the subset of patients with brain metastases at baseline, T-DM1 was associated with significantly improved OS compared with lapatinib plus capecitabine [190].

A phase II single arm study evaluated the cardiac safety of T-DM1 administered to patients with early stage HER2 positive breast cancer following (neo)-adjuvant anthracycline-based chemotherapy [191]. No symptomatic left ventricular dysfunction was observed. Of the 50 patients who received neo-adjuvant T-DM1, the pCR rate was 56.0% (*95% CI, 41.3%–69.6%*).

A phase III, randomized, open-label trial comparing T-DM1 and trastuzumab as adjuvant therapy for HER2-positive primary breast cancer (KATHERINE) is currently recruiting patients.

Combination Studies

Based on preclinical data showing that T-DM1 combined with docetaxel or pertuzumab enhanced antitumor activity [192, 193], a number of phase I/II trials have examined T-DM1 in combination with pertuzumab and/or chemotherapy (taxanes). The PK, safety and efficacy of T-DM1 combined with pertuzumab were studied in a phase Ib/II trial in 67 patients with HER2 positive, locally advanced or metastatic breast cancer [182]. Based on the PK and pharmacodynamic data the risk of therapeutic protein-drug interaction is low when T-DM1 and pertuzumab are administered together. Among the 64 patients in the dose expansion phase, who received T-DM1 (3.6 mg/kg) and pertuzumab (420 mg), the ORR (CR or PR) was 40.6 % (95% CI: 28.5 to 53.6%), with a median PFS of 6.6 months (95% CI: 4.21 to 9.46 months).

A phase Ib study examined the combination of T-DM1 (weekly and 3-weekly), paclitaxel and pertuzumab in patients with HER2 positive metastatic breast cancer previously treated with trastuzumab [194]. The MTD for the 3-weekly dosing was 3.6 mg/kg T-DM1 and this dose was further evaluated in a phase IIa trial of the T-DM1, paclitaxel and pertuzumab combination in patients with locally advanced or metastatic breast cancer [195]. Adding pertuzumab to the T-DM1 plus paclitaxel combination did not increase the incidence of grade 3/4 adverse events. However, the paclitaxel dose intensity was low and peripheral neuropathy leading to paclitaxel discontinuation was common. The ORR (CR or PR defined by RECIST) for patients with measurable disease was 50% (21/42), 47.6% for patients who received T-DM1 plus paclitaxel and 52.4% for patients who received T-DM1, paclitaxel and pertuzumab.

A phase Ib/II neoadjuvant trial of T-DM1 and docetaxel with or without pertuzumab, reported a pCR of 58.6% (41/70), 56.8% in the T-DM1 plus docetaxel arm and 60.6% in the T-DM1, docetaxel and pertuzumab arm [196]. No definitive conclusion could be made about the relative efficacy of the doublet and triplet combinations due to the non-randomized and non-stratified nature of the trial and the small sample size.

The efficacy of the T-DM1 plus pertuzumab combination is currently being investigated in the three arm MARIANNE trial, comparing T-DM1 plus pertuzumab or T-DM1 plus pertuzumab-placebo, *versus* the combination of trastuzumab plus taxane in patients with HER2-positive locally advanced or metastatic breast cancer (NCT01120184).

In the adjuvant setting, a phase III trial is ongoing to evaluate T-DM1 in combination with pertuzumab *versus* trastuzumab in combination with pertuzumab and a taxane in patients with HER2-positive primary invasive breast cancer (NCT01966471).

In addition, T-DM1 is undergoing testing in combination with hormone therapy and a number of other targeted therapies as outlined in Table **1**.

Table 1. Ongoing Clinical Trials Evaluating T-DM1 in Combination with Chemotherapeutic Agents and Targeted Therapies (*Source: www.clinicaltrials.gov, Accessed 18/03/2014*)

Regimen	Phase	Patients	NCT Number
T-DM1 + Capecitabine	II	HER2-positive metastatic breast cancer or locally advanced or metastatic gastric cancer	NCT01702558
T-DM1 + ABT-737 (BCL-2 inhibitor)	I/II	HER2 positive breast cancer	NCT02070094
T-DM1 + BYL719 (PI3K inhibitor)	I	HER2 positive metastatic breast cancer pts who progress on prior trastuzumab & taxane treatment	NCT02038010
T-DM1 with/without standard endocrine therapy *versus* trastuzumab with standard endocrine therapy	II	Operable HER2 positive/hormone receptor positive breast cancer	NCT01745965
T-DM1 + pertuzumab *versus* trastuzumab + pertuzumab + taxane	III	Following anthracyclines as adjuvant therapy in operable HER2 positive breast cancer	NCT01966471
T-DM1 + ONT-380 (reversible, selective HER2 TKI)	Ib	HER2 positive breast cancer	NCT01983501
Trastuzumab + pertuzumab followed by T-DM1	II	HER2 positive metastatic breast cancer	NCT01835236
Neoadjuvant T-DM1 with lapatinib and abraxane *versus* trastuzumab with lapatinib and paclitaxel	II	HER2 positive breast cancer	NCT02073487
T-DM1 with abraxane and lapatinib	I	Metastatic HER2 positive breast cancer	NCT02073916

T-DM1: Mechanisms of Resistance and Biomarkers

T-DM1 has produced significant improvements in clinical response in patients with HER2 positive breast cancer, including patients with trastuzumab refractory disease. However, as with all existing HER2 targeted therapies, not all HER2 positive tumors respond. While little has been published on mechanisms of resistance to T-DM1, it is plausible to speculate that there may be some overlap with proposed mechanisms of resistance to trastuzumab, such as loss of expression of HER2, HER2 epitope masking or increased cleavage of the HER2 ECD.

In vivo studies using the JIMT-1 model showed that xenograft tumors treated with T-DM1 from the time of inoculation were almost completely growth inhibited by T-DM1, however tumors started to grow after approximately 15 weeks of treatment [178]. Furthermore, JIMT-1 xenograft tumors pretreated with trastuzumab did not respond to T-DM1. These studies suggest both acquired resistance to T-DM1 and overlapping resistance to trastuzumab and T-DM1. No obvious changes in HER2 expression were observed in the xenograft tumors following T-DM1 treatment. Furthermore, there was no evidence of increased HER2 ECD cleavage. In tumors treated with T-DM1 an apparent accumulation of HER2 stained intracellular granules, resembling enlarged lysosomes, was observed. The authors suggest that this may be indicative of a T-DM1-induced defect in intracellular trafficking of HER2 protein. Whether this potential defect plays a causative role in T-DM1 resistance remains to be determined.

A recent study showed that NRG-1 treatment reduced the cytotoxic activity of T-DM1 in 4 of 6 HER2 positive breast cancer cell lines [158]. This effect was blocked by treatment with pertuzumab, and the combination of T-DM1 and pertuzumab was synergistic *in vitro* and *in vivo*. The synergistic effect was not associated with enhanced ADCC, but instead is likely due to the combination effectively blocking HER2-HER3 and downstream AKT signaling.

In addition to mechanisms of resistance specific to HER2 targeting, resistance to DM1 may contribute to resistance to T-DM1, perhaps particularly in the context of acquired resistance. The multidrug resistance protein, P-glycoprotein (P-gp) has been implicated in resistance to the ADC, gemtuzumab ozogamicin, due to its ability to efflux the cytotoxic drug, calicheamicin, which is linked to the CD44 antibody [197, 198]. *In vitro* assays using P-gp overexpressing cells showed that DM1 is a substrate for P-gp [199, 200]. IHC studies of P-gp in breast cancer have shown that it is expressed in approximately 60% of invasive breast cancers [201, 202]. Thus, overexpression of P-gp could play a role in resistance to T-DM1 in breast cancer patients.

Based on the mechanism of action of T-DM1 it is not surprising that HER2 levels might predict response to treatment. In patients enrolled on a phase II study of

T-DM1, HER2 levels were retrospectively assessed by qRT-PCR. The ORR was found to be higher in patients with HER2 levels greater than the median (36%, 95% CI, 18.5-56.9%, n=25) compared to patients whose HER2 levels were lower than the median (28.0%, 95% CI, 12.1-47.5%, n=25) [186]. No other predictive biomarkers for response to T-DM1 have yet been identified.

Lapatinib (Tyverb®, Tykerb®)

Lapatinib: Mechanisms of Action

Lapatinib (Tyverb®, Tykerb®, GSK) is an orally administered, small molecule, selective, reversible inhibitor of EGFR and HER2 (Table **2**); it binds competitively to the ATP binding site of both receptors and thus prevents signal transduction through the MAPK and PI3K/AKT pathways, leading to increased apoptosis and decreased cell growth [203]. Lapatinib is a 4-anilinoquinazoline which inhibits HER2 with an IC_{50} of 9.2 nM, EGFR with an IC_{50} of 10.8 nM, HER4 with an IC_{50} of 0.367 μM and c-Src with an IC_{50} of 3.5 μM making lapatinib a highly selective HER2/EGFR inhibitor [204].

Inhibition of HER2 Signaling

Sensitivity to lapatinib is independent of the levels of EGFR protein expression in HER2 positive breast cancer cells. This suggests that the effects of lapatinib are as a result of inhibition of HER2 signaling rather than a combination of EGFR and HER2 inhibition. In patient samples, lapatinib responsiveness correlated with HER2 expression but not EGFR expression. Patients with HER2 positive breast cancer benefit from lapatinib treatment, regardless of the EGFR expression status of their tumor [203-206]. Xia *et al.* showed that lapatinib inhibits both MAPK and PI3K/AKT signaling in HER2 positive breast cancer cell lines, tumor xenografts and in clinical tumor biopsies obtained from HER2 positive breast cancer patients treated with lapatinib [203]. In a panel of breast cancer cell lines, lapatinib response correlated with inhibition of HER2, Raf, AKT and Erk phosphorylation [206].

Table 2. Tyrosine Kinase Inhibitors Targeting the HER Family which are Currently in Use or Being Tested in HER2 Positive Breast Cancer

Name	Chemical Name	Drug Class	Targets	IC_{50} (nM)	Current Status in HER2$^+$ Breast Cancer	Refs.
Lapatinib	N-{3-Chloro-4-[(3-fluorobenzyl)oxy] phenyl}-6-[5-({[2-(methylsulfonyl)ethyl]amino}methyl)-2-furyl]-4-quinazolinamine	Reversible HER2 and EGFR TKI	EGFR	11	Approved for metastatic HER2 positive breast cancer	[204]
			HER2	9		
			HER4	367		
Neratinib	2-butenamide, N-[4-[[3-chloro-4-(2-pyridinylmethoxy) phenyl] amino]-3-cyano-7-ethoxy-6-quinolinyl]-4-(dimethylamino)-, (2E)-, (2Z)-2-butenedioate (1:1)	Irreversible pan-HER TKI	EGFR	92	Phase III	[273]
			HER2	59		
			HER4	19		
			Phospho-EGFR	3		
			Phospho-HER2	5		
Afatinib	*N*-[4-[(3-chloro-4-fluorophenyl)amino]-7-[[(3*S*)-tetrahydro-3-furanyl]oxy]-6-quinazolinyl]-4-(dimethylamino)-2-butenamide	Irreversible pan-HER TKI	$EGFR^{WT}$	0.5	Phase III	[292]
			$EGFR^{L858R}$	0.2		
			$EGFR^{L858R/T790M}$	9		
			HER2	14		
			Phospho-$EGFR^{WT}$	8		
			Phospho-$EGFR^{L858R/T790M}$	49		
			Phospho-HER2	75		
			HER4	1		
Dacomitinib	2E)-N-16-4-(piperidin-1-yl)but-2-enamide	Irreversible pan-HER TKI	EGFR	6	Phase I	[306]
			HER2	46		
			HER4	74		

Cell Cycle Arrest and Apoptosis

Treatment of HER2 positive breast cancer cells with lapatinib results in cell cycle arrest, with cells accumulating in the G1 phase [204, 206]. In addition to induction of cell cycle arrest and in contrast to trastuzumab, lapatinib induces apoptosis in HER2 positive breast cancer cells. Lapatinib-induced apoptosis has been correlated with decreased expression of survivin [207]. Survivin is an inhibitor of apoptosis protein (IAP) which has been shown to protect breast cancer cells from apoptosis induction [208]. The down-regulation of survivin was also observed in HER2-overexpressing tumor samples from breast cancer patients who participated in a phase 1 pilot study of lapatinib [209]. Lapatinib-mediated apoptosis has also been associated with the upregulation of Bcl-2 interacting mediator of cell death (BIM), a pro-apoptotic member of the Bcl-2 family [210]. Lapatinib-mediated apoptosis can also be increased through inhibition of the anti-apoptotic protein, myeloid cell leukaemia 1 (MCL-1) [211].

Autophagy

Autophagy is a process involving the formation of membrane bound vacuoles containing lytic proteins which results in the degradation of cellular proteins and cytoplasmic organelles [212]. Lapatinib treatment, in combination with a Bcl-2 inhibitor, obatoclax, caused synergistic cell killing by inducing autophagic cell death indicating a non-protective role for lapatinib-induced autophagy [213]. Lapatinib treatment induced both autophagy and apoptosis in breast cancer cell lines and combined treatment with 3-methyladenine (3-MA), an autophagy inhibitor, attenuated the induction of apoptosis, and stimulated DNA synthesis and colony formation [214]. This suggests that the lapatinib simultaneously induces apoptosis and autophagy to facilitate cell death.

Induction of Stress Response Pathways

Although trastuzumab treatment is associated with cardiotoxicity, a study of 3,558 patients showed that lapatinib treatment is not frequently associated with cardiotoxicity (1.6%) [215]. GW2974, a lapatinib analogue, protects cardiac myocytes from apoptotic stimuli by activating AMP-regulated protein kinase (AMPK), which switches cells from an anabolic to a catabolic state of metabolism which suggests that activation of AMPK by lapatinib may be necessary to preferentially induce apoptosis in tumor cells while sparing cardiac cells [216]. AMPK activation also regulates tumor cell growth through the inhibition of the mTOR pathway, leading to inhibition of protein synthesis [217].

Pharmacokinetics

Following oral administration, lapatinib has a moderate rate of absorption with peak plasma concentrations achieved several hours post-treatment, and is assumed to have a low bioavailability. Lapatinib undergoes metabolism *via* hepatic and intestinal cytochrome P450 and is eliminated by biotransformation. The serum concentrations of lapatinib peak 4 hours after treatment, increase with increasing dose and achieve steady state in 6 to 7 days, suggesting an effective half-life of 24 hours. At the dose of 1,250 mg daily, the peak plasma concentration of lapatinib in patients was 2.4 μg/ml (2.5 μM), (ranging from 1.57 to 3.77 μg/ml), and the steady-state trough concentrations of lapatinib range from 0.3 to 0.6 μg/ml (0.318-0.636 μM) [205].

Lapatinib: Clinical Evaluation

Monotherapy

Phase I trials evaluating the safety and PK of lapatinib were conducted in patients with advanced malignancies exhibiting overexpression of EGFR and/or HER2 and provided evidence of lapatinib activity. These studies show that lapatinib is well tolerated at doses of up to 1,600 mg/day. The predominant drug-related adverse events reported were diarrhea and rash [205]. Lapatinib was then examined in phase II trials, with a focus on breast cancer as most of the patients who exhibited a PR to lapatinib in the phase I trials had breast cancer. Phase II trials of single agent lapatinib in patients with metastatic breast cancer, revealed that lapatinib showed limited clinical benefit as a monotherapy in HER2 positive breast cancer but showed no clinical benefit in HER2 negative breast cancer [218, 219]. Lapatinib monotherapy also showed clinical activity and manageable toxicity in HER2-overexpressing breast cancer patients who had progressed on trastuzumab [218, 220]. As first-line therapy, lapatinib monotherapy produced an ORR (CR or PR defined by RECIST) of 24% and clinical benefit rate (CR, PR, or SD for 24 weeks) of 43% in patients with HER2-amplified locally advanced or metastatic breast cancer [221].

Lapatinib and Capecitabine

Capecitabine (Xeloda®, Roche) is a pro-drug which is enzymatically converted to 5-fluorouracil in the tumor, where it inhibits DNA synthesis [222]. Preclinical studies of a lapatinib analogue (GW282974X) with the capecitabine metabolite 5'-deoxy-5-fluorouridine demonstrated synergistic activity in breast cancer cell lines [223]. The optimal tolerated regimen was determined in a phase I trial: 1,250 mg lapatinib daily and 2,000 mg/m2/day capecitabine on days 1 to 14 of a 21-day cycle [224]. Of the 45 patients enrolled, 1 had a CR and 3 had a PR. A randomized phase III trial compared capecitabine alone to lapatinib plus capecitabine, in patients with HER2 positive, locally advanced or metastatic breast cancer that had progressed following treatment with trastuzumab plus chemotherapy. The study was stopped at the interim analysis as the addition of lapatinib to capecitabine demonstrated a statistically significant improvement in median PFS (8.5 *versus* 4.5 months), with no increase in toxicity [225]. Updated results suggested a trend towards improved OS and a reduction in the risk for progression to CNS disease in the combination group [226]. The final analysis of the trial results suggest a 20 % decrease in the risk of death for patients treated with the combination *versus* capecitabine alone [227]. In March 2007, lapatinib in combination with capecitabine, was approved by the US FDA, for the treatment of patients with advanced or HER2-overexpressing metastatic breast cancer, previously treated with trastuzumab and an anthracycline, or taxane. Lapatinib in combination with capecitabine was the first therapy approved for the treatment of patients with trastuzumab-refractory HER2-positive metastatic breast cancer.

In the phase III trial, diarrhea was reported more frequently in patients receiving lapatinib plus capecitabine than capecitabine alone. However, a pooled analysis of diarrhea events in patients treated with lapatinib alone or in combination with capecitabine or taxanes, concluded that most diarrhea events were low grade and proactive management can prevent severe diarrhea [228].

Overexpression of HER2 has been correlated with an increased risk of developing CNS metastases [229]. In a preclinical mouse model of brain metastasis, lapatinib reduced the levels of phosphorylated HER2 and inhibited the formation of brain metastasis [230]. Lapatinib alone showed modest CNS activity in patients with brain metastasis from HER2 positive breast cancer, who had been previously treated with trastuzumab [231]. However, when lapatinib was combined with capecitabine in the LANDSCAPE trial an objective CNS response was reported in 66% of patients and 20% of patients had a volumetric reduction greater than 80%

suggesting that lapatinib and capecitabine has activity as a first-line treatment for brain metastases in HER2-positive breast cancer patients [232]. A recent study which measured the levels of lapatinib and capecitabine in brain metastases showed that clinically relevant concentrations were detected in some brain metastases providing further evidence that lapatinib and capecitabine can cross the blood-brain barrier [233].

Lapatinib and Letrozole

ER and HER2 are frequently co-expressed in breast cancer and data from pre-clinical *in vitro* studies suggests that combined inhibition of HER2 and ER was superior to either single agent [234]. Letrozole is an aromatase inhibitor which blocks the growth of ER positive tumors. An initial phase 1 trial indicated the feasibility of safely combining letrozole and lapatinib [235]. The efficacy of lapatinib and letrozole was evaluated in a double-blind, placebo-controlled trial whereby the addition of lapatinib to letrozole was well tolerated and led to a significantly increased PFS (8.2 v 3.0 months; HR = 0.71; 95% CI, 0.53-0.96; $p = 0.019$), and clinical benefit rate (CR or PR or SD for at least 6 months, defined by RECIST) (48% v 29%; odds ratio = 0.4; 95% CI, 0.2-0.8; $p = 0.003$) relative to letrozole alone in women with metastatic breast cancer who coexpress ER and HER2 [236, 237]. This led to the approval of lapatinib in combination with letrozole for the treatment of postmenopausal women with ER positive and HER2 positive advanced breast cancer, for whom hormonal therapy is indicated.

Lapatinib and Taxanes

Lapatinib in combination with paclitaxel, a microtubule interfering drug, has been evaluated as a first-line treatment for patients with metastatic breast cancer. Patients with HER2-negative metastatic breast cancer failed to benefit from the addition of lapatinib to paclitaxel while paclitaxel-lapatinib significantly improved clinical outcomes in HER2-positive patients [238]. Combination lapatinib and paclitaxel treatment was assessed in a phase III randomized trial in patients with newly diagnosed HER2 positive metastatic breast cancer. The addition of lapatinib to paclitaxel increased OS from 20.5 to 27.8 months [239]. These studies demonstrate that lapatinib in combination with paclitaxel provides a significant survival advantage compared to paclitaxel alone for patients with HER2 positive metastatic breast cancer.

A phase I study of lapatinib in combination with docetaxel indicated that the combination is well-tolerated [240]. A phase I/II study evaluating lapatinib in combination with docetaxel as first-line treatment is currently ongoing (NCT01044485). Preliminary safety data demonstrated that the optimal tolerated regimen (docetaxel 75 mg/m^2 once every 3 weeks and lapatinib 1,250 mg once daily) could be safely administered without systematic use of G-CSF in non-pretreated patients with locally advanced or metastatic HER2 breast cancer [241].

Lapatinib and Trastuzumab

Preclinical data suggests that lapatinib has synergistic effects in combination with trastuzumab [206, 207]. A phase III study evaluated the effects of lapatinib with/without trastuzumab in patients with HER2 postitve breast cancer who had progressed on trastuzumab and reported a significant increase in PFS (HR = 0.73; 95% CI, 0.57- 0.93; p = 0.008) in the combination group compared to lapatinib alone [242]. There was also a significant increase in median OS of 4.5 months with the lapatinib and trastuzumab combination treatment compared to lapatinib alone [243].

Preclinical studies also suggested that dual targeting with trastuzumab and lapatinib in combination with chemotherapy might improve response compared to either agent with chemotherapy [207]. A phase Ib study of trastuzumab, lapatinib and docetaxel reported an ORR (CR or PR defined by RECIST) of 31% in 45 patients with measurable disease [244].

The NeoALTTO randomized phase III study, evaluated the efficacy of lapatinib and/or trastuzumab plus paclitaxel, as neoadjuvant therapy in patients with HER2 positive breast cancer. pCR was significantly higher in the group given lapatinib and trastuzumab (51.3 %), compared to trastuzumab alone (29.5 %) or lapatinib alone (24.7 %), suggesting that dual HER2 inhibition is more effective than single agent inhibition in the neoadjuvant setting [245]. The most commonly reported adverse reactions reported by patients receiving lapatinib on the NeoALTTO trial were diarrhea, including grade 3 and grade 4 reactions, dermatological complaints including rashes and hepatotoxicity which in some cases was severe enough to result in death [246].

A phase II neoadjuvant study evaluated the combination of trastuzumab and/or lapatinib with carboplatin and docetaxel. In this study, the chemotherapy plus lapatinib arm (pCR 25%) was inferior to chemotherapy plus trastuzumab and lapatinib (pCR 52%) (p=0.021), but there was no significant difference between the trastuzumab arm (pCR 43%) and either the lapatinib or the trastuzumab plus lapatinib arm [247]. Preliminary data for another similar neoadjuvant study reported pCR rates of 48% for the carboplatin, docetaxel and trastuzumab regimen and 44% for the carboplatin, docetaxel, trastuzumab and lapatinib regimen. This study also reported that the addition of lapatinib to carboplatin, docetaxel and trastuzumab results in substantial gastrointestinal toxicity [248].

A large phase III study of lapatinib treatment for patients with early stage breast cancer, ALTTO (Adjuvant Lapatinib and/or Trastuzumab Treatment Optimization), was opened in April 2007, to compare lapatinib, trastuzumab, trastuzumab followed by lapatinib, and concomitant lapatinib and trastuzumab, combined with chemotherapy. At the planned interim analysis, the lapatinib-alone arm was discontinued, as it was deemed unlikely to meet the pre-specified criteria of non-inferiority to trastuzumab alone with respect to DFS [249]. Recently, the first results of the ALTTO trial, reported that trastuzumab combined with lapatinib failed to demonstrate a DFS advantage over trastuzumab alone at 4.5 years median follow-up [250].

Lapatinib is also currently being tested in phase I/II clinical trials in combination with a number of chemotherapeutic agents including, pemetrexed, topotecan, and gemcitabine, as well as other targeted therapies including the angiogenesis inhibitor pazopanib, the EGFR inhibitor cetuximab, the mTOR inhibitor rapamycin, the c-Met/VEGFR inhibitor forertinib and inhibitors of the PI3K/AKT pathway.

Lapatinib: Mechanisms of Resistance

Similar to trastuzumab, the primary target of lapatinib in HER2 positive breast cancer is HER2. However, both drugs target different parts of the HER2 protein and have both distinct and overlapping mechanisms of action. Furthermore, both preclinical [206] and clinical studies [225] have shown that lapatinib has anti-tumor activity in HER2 positive breast cancer cells that are resistant to trastuzumab. Thus it is not surprising that trastuzumab and lapatinib may have overlapping and non-overlapping mechanisms of resistance.

The mechanisms of innate lapatinib resistance remain poorly understood, at least in part due to the lack of sufficient preclinical models of innate resistance. Several mechanisms of innate trastuzumab resistance that do not seem to impact on sensitivity to lapatinib including; loss of PTEN, since lapatinib activity does not correlate with PTEN status [251], p95HER2 activity, p95HER2 retains the intracellular kinase domain which lapatinib targets [252] and IGFIR expression, since lapatinib treatment inhibited IGFIR signaling and induced apoptosis, even in the presence of IGF-1 [253].

Several groups have developed cell line models of acquired lapatinib resistance through continuous long-term exposure to lapatinib resulting in the emergence of a resistant cell population. Interrogation of these preclinical models of acquired lapatinib resistance has identified several proposed mechanisms of resistance:

Crosstalk with ER

ER signaling plays an essential role in breast cancer as over 60 % of breast cancers are ER positive. Several studies have found that comparing acquired lapatinib-resistant cells with sensitive cells revealed increased expression of ER itself [254] or genes relating to ER signaling including FOXO3a, suggesting a switch from HER2 "oncogene-addiction" to co-dependence on HER2 and ER [255]. Cells with acquired lapatinib-resistance were sensitive to a combination of lapatinib and the anti-estrogen fulvestrant [256]. Combining lapatinib with ER inhibition prevented the emergence of lapatinib-resistant BT474 cells [255]. Importantly, this study also reported increased ER signaling in tumor biopsies from lapatinib treated breast cancer patients.

AXL Overexpression

AXL is a membrane-bound RTK containing a kinase domain closely related to MET and an ECD resembling that of neural cell adhesion molecules [257].

Overexpression of AXL protein was detected in a cell line model of acquired lapatinib resistance and inhibition of AXL restored sensitivity to lapatinib in the lapatinib-resistant cells [256].

XIAP Overexpression

XIAP is an IAP that binds to and inhibits the activation of procaspase-9, procaspase-7 and procaspase-3 leading to inhibition of both intrinsic and extrinsic apoptotic pathways. Expression of XIAP correlates with shorter OS and may act as an independent prognostic biomarker for invasive ductal carcinoma [258, 259]. Acquired lapatinib resistant cells expressed 3-fold higher XIAP compared to sensitive cells, and the viability of these lapatinib-resistant cells was decreased by embelin treatment which down regulates XIAP. In addition, stable expression of XIAP, using a lentiviral system, was sufficient to induce resistance to lapatinib in sensitive cells [260].

Upregulation of SRC Family Kinases

Increased expression of several SRC family kinases was reported in multiple cell lines models of acquired lapatinib-resistance and treatment of the lapatinib-resistant cells with saracatinib (AZD0530) or dasatinib, both ATP competitive small molecule SRC inhibitors, resulted in inhibition of SRC phosphorylation and inhibition of cell growth. Combined treatment of lapatinib sensitive breast cancer cell lines with lapatinib and saracatinib prevented the emergence of lapatinib-resistant cells. Importantly this study also showed that the expression of several SRC family members were upregulated in a small cohort of primary HER2 positive tumors following lapatinib treatment [261]. Increased SRC kinase activity has also recently been reported in an additional model of acquired lapatinib resistance [262].

In addition to SRC, expression of focal adhesion kinase (FAK) was identified in models of acquired lapatinib resistance. SRC and FAK signaling are downstream of β1-integin-mediated signaling and inhibition of β1-integin significantly inhibited the growth of lapatinib-resistant cells but did not significantly affect sensitive cells, suggesting a role for β1-integrin in acquired resistance to lapatinib [263].

NFκB Signaling

Constitutive activation of NFκB (nuclear factor kappa-light-chain-enhancer of activated B cells) resulted in lapatinib resistance in lapatinib-sensitive cells. Acquired lapatinib-resistant cells exhibited upregulated NFκB and were resistant to either NFκB or HER2 inhibitors alone but sensitive to a combination of both inhibitors. In addition, a subset of NF-κB-responsive genes was overexpressed in HER2-positive patients and associated with a poor clinical outcome [264].

Lapatinib treatment also activates RelA, a subunit of NF-κB. Inhibition of RelA enhanced the apoptotic effects of lapatinib in lapatinib sensitive cells and could overcome acquired lapatinib resistance. There was also a small yet significant change in RelA expression between lapatinib responders and non-responders in lapatinib treated HER2-postive breast tumor samples [265].

Activation of PI3K

Two studies have shown that activating mutations in PI3K play a role in lapatinib resistance [266, 267]. Knockdown of p110α inhibited proliferation of lapatinib-resistant cells, both *in vitro* and *in vivo* when lapatinib was combined with a p110α-selective PI3K inhibitor BYL719 [266].

Lapatinib: Biomarkers

To date the only predictive biomarker for lapatinib response is amplification of HER2, however not all HER2 positive breast tumors respond to lapatinib, thus the lack of more stringent, robust predictive biomarkers of lapatinib response is a major clinical issue. However, a recent study performed a retrospective analysis of trastuzumab resistant patients treated with lapatinib plus capecitabine and identified Ki67 and liver metastases are significant prognostic factors for predicting PFS of subsequent lapatinib therapy [268]. High Ki67 index (marker of proliferation), liver metastases and number of liver metastases predicted shorter PFS. O'Brien *et al.* examined biomarkers of trastuzumab and lapatinib response in 18 HER2 positive breast cancer cell lines and showed that high levels of phospho-EGFR, phospho-HER2, phospho-HER3 and phospho-IGFIR predicted response to lapatinib, suggesting that tumors dependent on RTK signaling may be more sensitive to lapatinib [124]. Finn *et al.,* recently showed that in patients with HER2 positive ER positive breast cancer, with low levels of ER, the addition of lapatinib to letrozole significantly improved PFS (13.6 *versus* 6.7 months; p = 0.01), whereas no benefit was observed in patients with high levels of ER expression [269]. These data suggest that tumors with a clear dependence on HER2 signaling are most likely to respond to TKI such as lapatinib. O'Neill *et al.* identified a panel of five potential early pharmacodynamic biomarkers of response to lapatinib in HER2 positive breast cancer cell lines (RB1CC1, FOXO3A, NR3C1, ERBB3 and CCND1). These markers also predicted response to other HER2 targeted TKIs, trastuzumab and the combination of lapatinib with capecitabine *in vitro* [270, 271]. Biomarker driven clinical studies, such as the TRIO-B07 (NCT00769470) and TCHL (NCT01485926) neoadjuvant trials, will be key to identifying clinically relevant biomarkers of response and resistance to HER2-targeted therapies such as lapatinib [247, 248].

IRREVERSIBLE TYROSINE KINASE INHIBITORS

While the introduction the reversible TKI, lapatinib, has improved the prognosis for patients with HER2 positive breast cancer, drug resistance remains an obstacle to improving cure rates, particularly in the metastatic setting. Therefore, there is still a need for new targeted therapies for HER2 positive breast cancer. Recently, second generation irreversible TKIs have produced promising results in HER2 positive breast cancer. The pharmacological properties and anti-cancer activities of neratinib, afatinib and dacomitinib are discussed below.

Neratinib (HKI-272)

Neratinib: Discovery and Mechanisms of Action

Neratinib (HKI-272; Puma Biotechnology Inc) is a cyanquinoline irreversible pan-HER TKI (Table **2**). Neratinib was designed based on a homology model of the kinase domain of HER2 [272]. Neratinib inhibits the function of the kinase domain of the HER family members by forming a covalent interaction with a conserved cysteine residue (Cys 773 in the case of EGFR and Cys 805 in the case of HER2) in the ATP-binding pocket of the receptor [272]. This leads to reduction in the autophosphorylation of the receptor and subsequent phosphorylation of downstream substrates [272, 273]. Inhibition of receptor autophosphorylation was also observed *in vivo* in xenograft models [272, 273]. Neratinib is equally effective at inhibiting the growth and receptor autophosphorylation of cell lines that overexpress HER2 and EGFR [272]. It retains activity in the presence of the known EGFR and HER2 mutations [272]. One study showed in cell lines that neratinib interferes with ligand-induced dimerization of HER receptors, disrupts previously formed receptor dimers and prevents down-regulation of HER2 receptors thus potentially enhancing the ADCC activity of trastuzumab [274]. Using a genome-wide RNAi screen, Seyhan *et al.,* identified synthetic lethal or enhancer genes that interact with neratinib in the HER2 overexpressing breast cancer cell line SKBR3 [275]. The screen identified genes whose inhibition led to neratinib resistance including genes involved oncogenesis, transcription factors, cellular ion transport, protein ubiquitination, cell cycle, and genes known to interact with breast cancer-associated genes [275]. The novel resistance-associated genes identified in this study may enable the development of strategies to overcome neratinib resistance.

Neratinib: Preclinical Evaluation

Neratinib showed strong anti-proliferative activity in HER2 positive breast cancer *in vitro* and in xenograft models *in vivo* [273, 276]. It decreased the activation of the HER receptor family members and inhibited the PI3K and MAPK downstream signaling pathways *in vitro* and *in vivo* [273, 276]. Neratinib combined with trastuzumab showed additive effects in trastuzumab sensitive and resistant HER2 positive breast cancer cells *in vitro* and *in vivo* [276]. The combination of neratinib with trastuzumab prevented the reactivation of pHER3 and pAKT observed following treatment with either of the drugs alone [276]. A number of recent studies have shown that NRG and HER3 play a role in resistance to trastuzumab, lapatinib and T-DM1, therefore the ability of neratinib to block HER3 mediated activation of pAKT may overcome this mechanism of resistance, and suggest a potential role for neratinib or other irreversible TKIs in combination with trastuzumab and/or T-DM1 [158, 277, 278].

Neratinib inhibited cell cycle regulatory pathways which led to arrest of the cell cycle at the G1-S phase transition and decreased cellular proliferation [273]. These effects were mediated through inhibition of MAPK and AKT phosphorylation, down-regulation of cyclin D1 and induction of p27 [273]. Neratinib showed a strong additive effect in combination with paclitaxel and a synergistic effect with cytarabine in SKBR3 cells [275].

Neratinib: Clinical Evaluation

Phase I Studies

In patients with solid tumors, the absorption of neratinib was relatively slow after treatment with single doses ranging from 40 to 500 mg [279]. The MTD was determined to be 320 mg and the recommended dose for subsequent phase II trials was 240 mg daily [279]. Following administration of 240 mg neratinib, the peak plasma concentration ranged from 55.3 to 75.9 ng/ml in healthy subjects and cancer patients [279-281]. Neratinib monotherapy is generally well-tolerated and showed an acceptable safety profile in phase I clinical trials. The most common adverse effect reported in neratinib trials was diarrhea, which was manageable with anti-diarrheal agents and dose reductions. Other frequent neratinib-related toxicities included nausea, vomiting, fatigue, anorexia and rash. No cardiotoxicity was observed in healthy adult subjects and patients [280, 282]. Although not a primary endpoint of phase I studies, promising antitumor activity was observed in HER2 positive breast cancer patients previously treated with anthracyclines and taxanes [279] or previously treated with other HER2 targeted therapies (trastuzumab, lapatinib, T-DM1), taxane and chemotherapy [283]. Combined treatment with neratinib and the mTOR inhibitor, temsirolimus, also demonstrated activity in patients with HER2 positive metastatic breast cancer who had progressed on trastuzumab, including patients with known HER-PI3K driven cancers [284].

Phase II Studies

Several phase II trials have evaluated neratinib in patients with advanced HER2 positive breast cancer. Neratinib showed clinical activity in trastuzumab-pretreated and trastuzumab-naïve patients (median PFS of 22.3 and 39.6 weeks respectively) [285]. A phase I/II study is currently investigating the efficacy of neratinib in combination with trastuzumab in advanced breast cancer (NCT00398567). The combination of neratinib and paclitaxel in HER2 positive metastatic breast cancer patients produced an ORR of 73% (95% CI: 62.9-81.2%), including 7 (7%) patients who achieved a CR and 65 (66%) who achieved a PR, based on modified RECIST guidelines [286]. The neratinib/paclitaxel combination was associated with higher toxicity than neratinib monotherapy, though this level of toxicity was manageable [286]. A phase II trial is currently investigating the effect of paclitaxel with either neratinib or trastuzumab in metastatic HER2 positive breast cancer (NCT00915018) and an ongoing neo-adjuvant trial is recruiting patients to assess the efficacy of neratinib in combination with trastuzumab and paclitaxel (NCT01008150).

Neratinib in combination with vinorelbine showed antitumor activity in HER2 positive metastatic breast cancer patients pretreated with or without lapatinib, with an ORR (CR or PR based on modified RECIST v1.0 guidelines) of 41% (no prior lapatinib) and 8% (prior lapatinib) and median PFS of 22.7 and 48.0 weeks respectively [287]. Neutropenia was observed following treatment with neratinib in combination with paclitaxel or vinorelbine [287].

The efficacy of neratinib in comparison to lapatinib and capecitabine was assessed in patients with HER2 positive locally advanced/metastatic breast cancer [288]. The ORR was lower for the neratinib arm and median PFS was 4.5 months for neratinib *versus* 6.8 months for lapatinib and capecitabine [288]. However, the results were considered inconclusive as neither inferiority nor non-inferiority of neratinib *versus* lapatinib plus capecitabine could be demonstrated [288]. A phase I/II is currently recruiting patients to assess the combination of neratinib and temsirolimus in HER2 amplified metastatic breast cancer (NCT01111825) (Table **3**).

Phase III Studies

A phase III trial is currently recruiting patients to compare neratinib in combination with capecitabine to lapatinib and capecitabine in patients with HER2 positive metastatic breast cancer previously treated with HER2 targeted therapies (NCT01808573). A phase III trial evaluating neratinib after adjuvant trastuzumab in patients with early stage breast cancer has recently completed enrolment (NCT00878709) (Table **3**).

Table 3. Ongoing Clinical Trials Evaluating Neratinib and Afatinib in Breast Cancer (*Source: www.clinicaltrials.gov, accessed 13/03/2014*)

Regimen	Phase	Patients	NCT Number
NERATINIB			
Paclitaxel with neratinib and trastuzumab	I	Metastatic HER2 positive breast cancer	NCT01423123
Neratinib and temsirolimus	I/II	Metastatic HER2 positive or triple negative breast cancer	NCT01111825
Neratinib with paclitaxel	I/II	Breast cancer	NCT00445458
Neratinib with trastuzumab	I/II	Advanced HER2 positive breast cancer	NCT00398567
Neratinib and capecitabine	I/II	Breast cancer	NCT00741260
Neratinib with vinorelbine	I/II	Solid tumors and metastatic breast cancer	NCT00706030
Neratinib *versus* lapatinib plus capecitabine	II	HER2 positive metastatic or locally advanced breast cancer	NCT00777101
Neratinib with paclitaxel +/- trastuzumab followed by doxorubicin + cyclophosphamide	II	HER2 positive locally advanced breast cancer	NCT01008150
Neratinib	II	Metastatic HER2 non-amplified but HER2 mutant breast cancer	NCT01670877
Neratinib	II	Advanced HER2 positive breast cancer	NCT00300781
Neratinib with paclitaxel *versus* trastuzumab with paclitaxel	II	HER2 positive locally recurrent or metastatic breast cancer	NCT00915018
Neratinib	II	HER2 positive breast cancer with brain metastases	NCT01494662
Neratinib plus capecitabine *versus* lapatinib plus capecitabine	III	HER2 positive metastatic breast cancer	NCT01808573
AFATINIB			
Afatinib in combination with 3-weekly trastuzumab	I	HER2 positive cancer	NCT01649271
Afatinib with/without vinorelbine	II	HER2 positive breast cancer pts with brain metastases	NCT01441596
Afatinib and trastuzumab as neoadjuvant treatment	II	Locally advanced or operable breast cancer receiving taxane-anthracycline chemo	NCT01594177
Afatinib with/without weekly paclitaxel or weekly vinorelbine	II	HER2 positive metastatic breast cancer who failed HER2-targeted treatment in the neoadjuvant or adjuvant setting	NCT01271725
Afatinib with/without weekly vinorelbine	II	HER2 positive locally advanced or metastatic inflammatory breast cancer	NCT01325428
Afatinib with vinorelbine	III	HER2 positive metastatic breast cancer that failed one prior trastuzumab treatment	NCT01125566

Afatinib (BIBW 2992)

Afatinib: Mechanisms of Action

Afatinib (BIBW 2992; Boehringer Ingelheim GmbH) is an irreversible pan-HER TKI (Table **2**). Afatinib is an anilino-quinalozine derivative harboring a reactive acrylamide group [289]. Afatinib covalently binds specific cysteine residues within the ATP-binding site in the kinase domain of the receptor (Cys 773 in the case of EGFR and Cys 805 in the case of HER2) [290]. By irreversibly binding, it inhibits the autophosphorylation of the ErbB receptor family members, including EGFR mutants [289, 290]. It also inhibits EGFR- and HER2- containing dimers [290] and the proliferation of cancer cell lines driven by HER receptor signaling [289].

Afatinib: Preclinical Evaluation

Afatinib inhibited the growth of HER2 positive breast cancer cell lines *in vitro*, including trastuzumab and/or lapatinib resistant cells [291]. The anti-proliferative activity of afatinib combined with trastuzumab was additive in trastuzumab-sensitive and acquired trastuzumab resistant cell lines, however in trastuzumab and/or lapatinib resistant cell lines, the combination did not enhance response compared to afatinib alone [291]. Afatinib potently inhibited EGFR and HER2 phosphorylation in HER2 positive breast cancer cells *in vitro* [290]. It also decreased the phosphorylation of the downstream signaling molecule Erk [291]. Afatinib has also been tested *in vivo* and induced tumor regression in HER2 overexpressing trastuzumab-sensitive and trastuzumab-resistant breast cancer xenograft models [292].

Afatinib: Clinical Evaluation

Phase I

The PK profile of afatinib revealed moderately fast absorption [293]. The MTD has been established to range between 40 mg and 70 mg per day [294-296] and the dose recommended for phase II studies was between 50 and 70 mg once daily [294, 297]. Following administration of 50 mg afatinib once daily, the peak plasma concentration was 27.0 ng/ml in patients with advanced solid tumors [297]. Several phase I studies have tested alternative schedules for administering afatinib monotherapy. Evaluation of a two-week on/two-week off schedule in patients with advanced solid tumors, resulted in no CRs or PRs (assessed using RECIST) [4]. Of the 38 patients enrolled, 7 showed SD while 8 showed minor tumor regressions [4]. In a three-week on/one-week off schedule study, no CRs or PRs (evaluated according to RECIST) were observed [5]. Continuous daily treatment with afatinib was safe and showed durable antitumor activity in patients with advanced solid tumors, including breast carcinoma patients [296, 297]. The daily treatment regimen was selected for evaluation in the ongoing phase III trials. In phase I/II studies afatinib had a good safety profile. The most common adverse effects were diarrhea, mucosal inflammation, nausea, vomiting, fatigue, dermatitis acneiform and rash. In phase I-II trials, cardiotoxicity was observed between 0-5.3% with afatinib treatment [282].

A phase Ib study tested afatinib combined with cisplatin plus paclitaxel or cisplatin plus 5-fluorouracil in patients with advanced solid tumors [298]. Both afatinib combination regimens showed anti-tumor activity. Disease control was observed in 54% in patients treated with afatinib plus cisplatin and paclitaxel and 29% in patients treated with afatinib plus cisplatin and 5- fluorouracil. However, increased diarrhea and haematological toxicities were reported with the afatinib chemotherapy regimens, which require proactive and timely management to improve tolerability and minimize patient discontinuation [298]. Afatinib in combination with docetaxel showed a manageable adverse-event profile and anti-tumor activity, in patients with advanced solid tumors [299, 300].

Two phase I studies are testing combinations of afatinib with weekly (NCT00950742) and 3-weekly trastuzumab (NCT01649271). With weekly trastuzumab the MTD for afatinib has been determined as 20 mg daily. The study with 3-weekly trastuzumab is currently recruiting patients (Table **3**).

Phase II

Afatinib showed promising activity in patients with HER2 positive metastatic breast cancer who progressed after trastuzumab or were intolerant to that treatment [301]. Of the 41 patients treated, 19 (46%) achieved clinical benefit (no CR, 4 had a PR, 15 had SD, defined by RECIST). Median PFS was 15.1 weeks (95% CI: 8.1-16.7); median OS was 61.0 weeks (95% CI: 56.7-not evaluable) [301]. Preliminary data from a neoadjuvant study comparing afatinib to trastuzumab or lapatinib in patients with HER2 positive treatment-naïve locally advanced breast cancer, showed that afatinib had the highest PR (by RECIST) rate (80%, 75%, and 36.4% in patients treated with afatinib, lapatinib, and trastuzumab, respectively) [302].

The LUX-Breast 2 trial is currently recruiting patients to investigate the effect of afatinib alone and in combination with paclitaxel or vinorelbine in patients with HER2 positive metastatic breast cancer following progression on prior trastuzumab and/or lapatinib (NCT01271725) (Table **3**). The LUX-Breast 3 trial is investigating the effect of afatinib alone or in combination with vinorelbine in HER2 positive breast cancer patients suffering from brain metastases (NCT01441596) (Table **3**).

Two neo-adjuvant studies are evaluating afatinib treatment; (i) in combination with trastuzumab for locally advanced or operable HER2 positive breast cancer (NCT01594177) and afatinib alone and (ii) in combination with vinorelbine in HER2 positive locally advanced or metastatic inflammatory breast cancer in trastuzumab-naïve and trastuzumab resistant patients (NCT01325428). In the vinorelbine study, deep exosome sequencing will be exploited for biomarker discovery to elucidate potential mechanisms leading to drug resistance [303].

Phase III

The LUX-Breast 1 trial which is investigating the efficacy of afatinib in combination with vinorelbine in patients with HER2 positive metastatic breast cancer, who failed one prior trastuzumab treatment, has recently completed accrual (NCT01125566).

Dacomitinib (PF-00299804)

Dacomitinib: Mechanisms of Action

Dacomitinib (PF-00299804; Pfizer Inc) is a quinazalone-based irreversible pan-HER TKI (Table **2**). Dacomitinib achieves irreversible inhibition *via* covalent bonding of the cysteine residues in the ATP domain of HER family members' kinase domain [304]. It inhibits the phosphorylation of HER2, EGFR and HER4 in HER2 positive breast cancer cell lines [305], and mutant EGFR and HER2 in lung cancer cell lines [306].

Dacomitinib: Preclinical Evaluation

Dacomitinib inhibited proliferation of HER2 positive breast cancer cell lines, including trastuzumab and lapatinib resistant cells, with IC_{50} values ranging from <0.005-2.0 μM [305]. In the panel of 44 breast cancer cell lines tested, HER2 mRNA and protein levels correlated with response to dacomitinib. Dacomitinib decreased the phosphorylation of HER2, EGFR, HER4 and downstream signaling molecules AKT and Erk. Its anti-proliferative effects were exerted through cell cycle inhibition and induction of apoptosis [305].

Dacomitinib: Clinical Evaluation

The MTD and the recommended dose for phase II studies have been defined at 45 mg daily [307, 308]. The peak plasma concentration following 45 mg of dacominitib was determined at 21.2 ng/ml in patients and between 16.8 and 17.0 ng/ml in healthy subjects [308-310]. Pharmacokinetic analyses revealed that dacomitinib has a long-half life and an extensive tissue penetration [307]. In phase I studies, dacomitinib showed anti-tumor activity in advanced solid tumors [307, 308]. Janne *et al.*, reported that 7.3% (8) patients showed clinical benefit, defined as CR, PR, or SD for at least 24 weeks [307]. In the Japanese study, of 13 evaluable patients, one patient had a PR and SD was observed in 9 patients, including 1 breast cancer patient. However, no patient showed a CR [308]. The most common adverse events of dacomitinib include skin toxicities, fatigue, stomatitis, diarrhea, nausea and vomiting. Dacomitinib is currently in phase III trials in NSCLC but is not currently being evaluated in breast cancer.

Irreversible TKIs: Mechanisms of Resistance

The mechanisms of potential cellular resistance to irreversible TKIs are as yet poorly understood.

Seyhan *et al.*, investigated neratinib resistance using an RNAi screening approach to identify target genes that when knocked down induce resistance [275]. They identified 128 genes, including transcription factors, genes involved in oncogenesis, cellular ion transport, protein ubiquitination, cell cycle and genes known to interact with breast cancer associated genes, whose inhibition led to neratinib resistance *in vitro* [275]. In cell line models of acquired neratinib resistance, Breslin *et al.*, observed cross-resistance to afatinib and lapatinib [311]. Furthermore, trastuzumab and/or lapatinib resistant cells responded to neratinib [276, 312]. These results suggest both overlapping and non-overlapping mechanisms of resistance to different HER2 inhibitors. Overexpression of IGFIR in neratinib-resistant cells suggests its potential involvement in the development of resistance to this drug [311].

HER2 positive trastuzumab and/or lapatinib resistant cells retain sensitivity to afatinib or dacomitinib suggesting potential non-overlapping mechanisms of resistance [291, 305].

In lung cancers, hepatocyte growth factor (HGF) secreted in the tumor microenvironment may confer resistance to afatinib by activation of the Met/PI3K/AKT and Met/MAPK/ERK signaling pathways [313]. Dacomitinib resistant lung cancer cells maintained PI3K/AKT signaling through activation of IGFIR which was in turn mediated by downregulation of IGF binding protein 3 [314].

Irreversible TKIs: Biomarkers

Levels of HER2 and phospho-HER2 directly correlated with sensitivity to neratinib *in vitro* [276]. The downregulation of pAKT and pErk in response to neratinib treatment was also correlated with sensitivity to neratinib. However, no correlation was observed between several other potential biomarkers, including EGFR, p-95 HER2, HER3, IGFIR, AKT, PTEN and PI3K status, and response to neratinib. In HER2 positive breast cancer cell lines, overexpression of the neuropeptide neuromedin U has been associated with resistance to neratinib [315]. In addition to predicting response to lapatinb, the panel of pharmacodynamic markers identified by O'Neill *et al.,* also predicts response to neratinib and afatinib [271].

Sensitivity of HER2 positive breast cancer cell lines to dacomitinib was correlated with levels of HER2 expression and inversely correlated with HER3 mRNA levels [305]. No correlation between response to dacomitinib and either EGFR or HER4 mRNA levels was observed [305]. In a phase I trial of dacomitinib, Ki67 and pMAPK were measured in skin biopsy samples following dacomitinib treatment and the levels of both were found to be significantly decreased [306], and thus may represent potential surrogate pharmacodynamic biomarkers.

HER2 TARGETED THERAPIES IN HER2-LOW BREAST CANCER

A standardized protocol for the determination of HER2 positive tumors has been developed to ensure all patients that may potentially benefit from HER2 targeted therapies are identified. The differentiation between HER2 positive and HER2 negative breast cancer is defined by the ASCO/CAP guidelines as detailed above [316]. Inconsistencies and variations in methods, procedures and interpretations relating to the determination of HER2 status between laboratories has led to a continuous refinement of the histopathological procedures and algorithms that determine HER2 positivity [317]. A consequence of the discordance in HER2 testing was the retrospective discovery of the inclusion of HER2-negative patients in the NSABP-B31 and N9831 trials of trastuzumab in combination with chemotherapy in patients with HER2 positive early stage breast cancer [53, 318]. Most interestingly, and indeed controversially, the HER2-negative patients that data was available for, in NSABP-B31 and N9831, showed benefit for the addition of trastuzumab to chemotherapy [319, 320]. The limited numbers meant that these results were not sufficiently powered to provide evidence of a definitive benefit for the use of trastuzumab in HER2-low patients in the adjuvant setting. A retrospective review of HER2 status and testing of the patients involved in NSABP-B31 confirmed the initial findings and a predictive model of degree of response to trastuzumab was developed from archived NSABP-B31 tumor blocks using gene expression profiling techniques that demonstrated that HER2-negative tumors belong to the moderate benefit group [321]. These results provided the initiative for a large scale, randomized clinical trial of trastuzumab in HER2-low patients in the adjuvant setting, NSABP-B47 (NCT01275677) which is currently underway to examine if a trastuzumab/chemotherapy combination does indeed provide benefit in patients with HER2-low disease (IHC 1+/2+, no HER2 gene-amplification). Another consequence of these clinical observations has been an increased interest in the susceptibility of HER2-low/non-overexpressing, or clinically speaking, HER2 negative, breast cancer to HER2-targeted therapies.

HER2-low/non-overexpressing tumors can be defined as IHC 1+/2+ with ISH scores of less than 1.8 (HER2/CEP17 ratio) or less than 6 (HER2 copy number) [316]. HER2 levels are found to be higher in IHC 1+/2+ tumors *versus* IHC 0 tumors and normal or autologous breast tissue levels [322-323]. Greater than 50% of tumors can be defined in this way across multiple breast cancer subtypes including luminal A/B and basal with the exclusion of HER2 positive tumors [324-326]. This is a large proportion of all breast tumors which includes "triple negative" breast cancers (TNBCs). There is currently a recognized unmet clinical need in TNBC and the presence of low HER2 levels in the molecular subtypes associated with TNBC (basal-like/luminal) along with increased EGFR levels [327-329], makes HER2 a potential target in this breast cancer subtype through mechanisms outlined below, even in the absence of the genetic and phenotypic alterations associated with HER2-targeted therapy response.

Functional inhibition of HER2 and/or multiple members of the HER family through the previously described monoclonal antibody therapies (trastuzumab and pertuzumab) and TKIs (laptinib, neratinib, afatinib, dacomitinib) may inhibit growth of HER2-low breast cancer cells and should not be discounted as a putative mechanism of action in HER2-low tumors. Furthermore, the presence of a well-defined clinical target at low but significantly elevated levels on malignantly transformed cells could be exploited by monoclonal antibody therapies, ADCs and immunotherapies.

Antibody Dependent Cell-Mediated Cytotoxicity

Along with disrupting HER2 signaling pathways, trastuzumab induces ADCC in HER2 positive tumor cells through immune effector cells, including CD56 positive NK cells [330]. The contribution of the immune response to the efficacy of this therapy has not been fully resolved. As outlined above, *in vivo* mouse studies suggest that engagement of the host immune response is essential for therapy efficacy [70]. In a pilot pre-surgical study, strong CD56 positive NK cell tumor infiltration was associated with improved patient response to trastuzumab in HER2 positive breast cancer patients [60]. It has also been shown that high levels of tumor infiltrating lymphocytes (TILs) were significantly associated with higher rates of pathologic complete remission in response to neo-adjuvant trastuzumab in HER2-positive patients and the addition of an immunomodulatory therapy to trastuzumab increased tumor regression in a mouse model [331]. Increased TILs have also been associated with patient response to the HER2 targeted monoclonal antibody therapies. Pertuzumab, like trastuzumab, also induces a strong ADCC response but it targets a distinct region of the HER2 protein, and has the potential to augment trastuzumab activity [157]. Its mechanism of action, inhibiting dimerization of HER2 with EGFR and HER3, may also prove efficacious in HER2-low tumors dependent on alternate HER signaling pathways [136]. Pre-clinical and clinical evidence is building for a significant role for the immune-mediated response to monoclonal antibody therapies in HER2-positive disease. HER2-low breast cancer cells contain enough HER2 protein to bind trastuzumab and initiate ADCC mediated by immune cells *in vitro* [323, 332] and may also be susceptible to these immune-mediated effects. Differences in circulating immune cell composition and cytokine profiles have been reported between HER2-positive and HER2-negative patient populations [333]. However, peripheral blood mononuclear cells (PBMCs) from breast cancer patients have shown impaired NK activity compared to PBMCs from healthy individuals and a competent ADCC response alone is not the only pre-requisite for a strong immune response, which is also dependent on multiple factors including tumor immune evasion strategies, microenvironment, and immune cell infiltration [334, 335].

Adaptive Immunity

There is evidence for the role of the adaptive immune response to anti-HER2 therapy. Using immunocompetent wild-type (WT) BALB/c mice inoculated with a syngeneic HER2 breast cancer cell line, Park *et al.*, demonstrated that the efficacy of a mouse anti-HER2 antibody was significantly reduced in Rag1-knockout mice, lacking adaptive immunity [336]. The anti-HER2 antibody retained some effect in the Rag1-knockout mice, which the authors attributed to the direct effects of the antibody. The same study found that depletion of CD8 positive T cells in WT BALB/c mice reduced response to the anti-HER2 therapy. WT BALB/c mice with no detectable tumor growth 30 days following anti-HER2 treatment were also resistant to tumor re-challenge, evidence of immune memory. Additional results suggesting anti-HER2 antibody response was related to HMGB-1 (high-mobility group box 1) activated

MyD88-dependent toll-like receptor (TLR) signaling in combination with a second study that established the role of NK cells and type 1 interferons (IFNs) [337], led Mortenson and Fu to propose that activation of NK cell-mediated ADCC by the anti-HER2 antibody, promotes HMGB-1 release, stimulates MyD88 dependent TLRs, and thereby causes the release of type-1 IFNs to prime the adaptive immune system [334]. This scenario suggests that the initiation of an adaptive immune response to monoclonal antibody therapies is possible in HER2-low tumors in the right circumstances.

Interestingly, the HER2 E75 vaccine, developed to prevent disease reoccurrence in high risk patients, showed most clinical efficacy in the subset of patients with lymph node-positive (DFS, 90.2% *versus* 79.1%, p = 0.13), HER2 IHC 1+/2+ (DFS, 94.0% *versus* 79.4%, p = 0.04), or grade 1/2 (DFS, 98.4% *versus* 86.0%, p = 0.01) tumors [338].

Cancer Stem Cells (CSCs)

Wicha and colleagues have proposed that the efficacy of HER2 blockade in patients without HER gene amplification might be understood through the cancer stem cell hypothesis. The model is based on the existence of a small subset of tumor stem cells that drive tumorigenesis in many human cancers, including breast cancer [339]. The dependency of these breast cancer stem cell populations on HER2 has been demonstrated in pre-clinical HER2 positive models and has most recently provided evidence for the targeting of a HER2-dependent stem cell population in ER positive HER2 negative breast cancer, as the basis for the efficacy of trastuzumab in the NSABP-B31 and N9831 adjuvant clinical trials [340-344].

Tyrosine Kinase Inhibitors (TKIs)

Lapatinib has been shown to increase the levels of HER2 on the surface of HER2 positive MCF7-HER2 breast cancer cells by stabilizing HER2 in an inactive conformation [343]. The increased levels of HER2 have translated to increased levels of trastuzumab-mediated ADCC in pre-clinical HER2-expressing breast cancer and oesophageal cell line models [343, 344]. However, lapatinib in combination with capecitabine has shown no benefit in HER2-negative patients

[345] and it is unlikely that a lapatinib/trastuzumab combination will be attempted in HER2-low patients without a proven benefit for trastuzumab in that setting. Neratinib and afatinib may have efficacy in HER2-low cancers due to their ability to irreversibly inhibit multiple HER family members [272, 289, 290].

T-DM1

The trastuzumab-emtansine ADC T-DM1 has a tolerable safety profile and has shown efficacy in HER2-positive breast cancer patients [177, 188]. T-DM1 retains ADCC and HER2 cell signaling inhibition capabilities in combination with the presence of a highly toxic chemotherapeutic agent suggesting that it may have greater potential than trastuzumab when targeting HER2 low breast tumors directly [178, 179]. Chemotherapeutic agents have been shown to alter the immune response [346], and it remains to be seen if the addition of emtansine has any effect on the immune response to trastuzumab.

HER2 TARGETED THERAPIES IN NON-BREAST TUMOURS

Amplification or overexpression of HER2 has also been reported in a range of non-breast solid tumors, including 4-20% of gastro-esophageal, 7-16% of pancreatic, 3-15% of bladder, 2-8% of lung, 6-11% of endometrial and 2-18% of ovarian cancers [347-356]. HER2 overexpression and/or gene amplification has been associated with poor prognosis in esophageal, pancreatic, bladder, lung, endometrial and ovarian cancer [357-365]. However, a study of 924 gastric cancer patients reported that HER2 overexpression did not correlate with patient outcome [366].

Trastuzumab has shown activity in preclinical models of HER2 positive pancreatic, ovarian, endometrial and gastric cancer [61, 367-371]. Three trials evaluated trastuzumab in HER2 positive gastric or gastro-esophageal junction cancer patients. A phase II study of first line treatment with trastuzumab and cisplatin was conducted in patients with advanced gastric cancer. Based on 17 assessable patients, preliminary data reported a 35% ORR (1CR and 5 PR) and 3% SD with an acceptable toxicity profile [372].

A phase III open label trial (ToGA) was designed to assess whether trastuzumab added to cisplatin and 5-fluorouracil or capecitabine improved efficacy compared to chemotherapy alone in patients with HER2 positive locally advanced or metastatic gastric cancer. Trastuzumab was administered in combination with chemotherapy for six cycles and continued until disease progression. Of 3,807 patients screened 810 (21.3%) were HER2 positive. Trastuzumab improved OS (13.8 *versus* 11.1 months) (HR 0.74; $p < 0.0046$). The addition of trastuzumab also improved PFS (HR 0.71; $p < 0.0002$) and ORR (CR or PR) (odds ratio 1.70; $p < 0.0017$) [373]. Based on these results trastuzumab combined with cisplatin and capecitabine or 5-fluorouracil is approved, for the treatment of patients with previously untreated HER2 positive advanced gastric cancer or gastro-esophageal junction adenocarcinoma [374]. Two phase III trials are currently evaluating (i) pertuzumab in combination with trastuzumab and (ii) T-DM1 in patients with HER2 positive advanced gastric cancer.

Lapatinib has also shown preclinical activity in preclinical studies of pancreatic cancer, lung cancer, bladder cancer, endometrial cancer and gastro-esophageal cancer [375-381]. A phase II study of lapatinib in NSCLC reported that lapatinib monotherapy did not induce a significant number of tumor regressions [382]. A phase II study of lapatinib as second-line treatment for patients with locally advanced or metastatic transitional cell carcinoma did not meet its primary endpoint of ORRs (CR or PR, defined by RECIST) greater than 10% [383]. However, HER2 and/or EGFR status were not used to select patients for either of these studies. Wulfing *et al.* reported improved OS in a subset of patients with tumors which overexpressed EGFR and/or HER2 [383].

A phase II clinical trial of lapatinib as monotherapy in patients with either EGFR and/or HER2 positive, previously treated, advanced adenocarcinoma of the esophagus or gastroesophageal junction achieved no CRs or PRs, and 2 SDs in 21 evaluable patients [384]. Lapatinib also demonstrated modest single agent activity as first line treatment in a phase II trial in patients with advanced gastric cancer [385]. However, patients were not selected based on EGFR and/or HER2 status. Lapatinib is currently being tested in combination with chemotherapy in gastric cancer and a phase II study of first line lapatinib and capecitabine was recently reported, with promising efficacy [386].

A phase II trial of lapatinib monotherapy was conducted in patients with treatment-refractory HER2 amplified gastro-esophageal, bladder, ovarian, or uterine tumors [387]. However, the study closed early due to low response rate in addition to slow screening and enrollment. After 12 weeks of lapatinib treatment, 1 (3%) patient had a CR, 9 (28%) had SD, and 20 (63%) had progressive disease.

The irreversible TKIs, neratinib, afatinib and dacomitinib are being tested in NSCLC, due to their activity against EGFR, which is mutated in 10-30% of NSCLC [388-390]. Afatinib and dacomitinib are both currently in phase III trials in NSCLC cancer, while neratinib is in phase II studies.

In summary, the limited efficacy observed in non-breast tumors suggest that although the HER2-amplification is present outside of breast cancer, it is not the dominant driver in these tumors that it is in HER2 positive breast cancer.

CONCLUSION AND FUTURE CHALLENGES

Trastuzumab has become the cornerstone of targeted therapy for HER2 positive breast since its FDA approval in 1998. It is a very successful drug prolonging OS in HER2 positive metastatic breast cancer patients. For patients with early stage breast cancer, trastuzumab treatment has dramatically improved prognosis. In a recent clinical trial report, the invasive DFS for HER2 positive breast cancer patients who received adjuvant trastuzumab and chemotherapy, with approximately 3 years median follow-up, was 92% [391]. For patients with metastatic HER2 positive breast cancer, trastuzumab with chemotherapy produces durable CRs in approximately 9.5% of the population. Studies on long-term remissions following lapatinib treatment are not yet available. As impressive as these improvements are, there is still a need to develop additional treatment options for patients with metastatic HER2 positive breast cancer.

Based on the recent results of the ALTTO trial [250], the future of TKIs for HER2 positive breast cancer remains unclear. With the approval of pertuzumab in combination with trastuzumab as first-line therapy for metastatic disease and T-DM1 for trastuzumab refractory disease, one of the key questions now is will lapatinib or the newer irreversible TKIs offer significant improvement compared to, or in addition to, the dual antibody approach or T-DM1. Further preclinical studies comparing combinations of the TKIs with trastuzumab or T-DM1 and/or pertuzumab will help to inform future combination clinical trials. These studies could also have important health economic implications as the cost of dual antibody treatment may be prohibitive for a lot of healthcare systems.

Although mechanisms of resistance to trastuzumab and lapatinib have been extensively studied, we do not, as yet, have clinically validated biomarkers to better select the patients, within the HER2 positive subtype, who are most likely to benefit from therapy. The identification of these biomarkers is of paramount importance to improve patient outcomes and also from the health economics perspective.

In addition to HER2 targeted monoclonal antibodies and TKIs, gene therapy approaches involving anti-sense oligonucleotides, small interfering RNAs and microRNAs [392-402], as well as vaccine approaches [for review see ref 403] are also being investigated for HER2 positive breast cancer.

Another approach to improve response to HER2 targeted therapies is to combine HER2 targeting with therapies that target downstream signaling pathways, in particular the PI3K/AKT/mTOR pathway. Data from ongoing clinical trials will determine if targeting these pathways along with HER2 will lead to clinical benefit.

In summary, the development of HER2 targeted therapeutics has been one of the major success stories in the era of targeted therapies for cancer, and it is anticipated that the next generation of HER2 targeted agents, either alone or in combination will lead to further improvements in outcome for patients with HER2 positive breast cancer.

ACKNOWLEDGEMENTS

The authors acknowledge the financial support of Science Foundation Ireland (08/SRC/B1410), the Irish Research Council, and the Cancer Clinical Research Trust/the Caroline Foundation.

CONFLICT OF INTEREST

JC has received research funding and speaker's fees from Roche and GSK. DC/NOD have received research funding from Roche. AC/NOD/JC have received research funding from Boehringer Ingelheim. NOD has received research funding from GSK. BB received a speaker's honorarium from Roche.

REFERENCES

[1] Slamon DJ, Clark GM, Wong SG, Levin WJ, Ullrich A, McGuire WL. Human breast cancer: correlation of relapse and survival with amplification of the HER-2/neu oncogene. Science. 1987; 235: 177-82.

[2] Pal SK, Pegram M. HER2 targeted therapy in breast cancer...beyond Herceptin. Rev Endocr Metab Disord. 2007; 8: 269-77.

[3] Cho HS, Mason K, Ramyar KX, Stanley AM, Gabelli SB, Denney DW, Jr., *et al*. Structure of the extracellular region of HER2 alone and in complex with the Herceptin Fab. Nature. 2003; 421: 756-60.

[4] Daly JM, Jannot CB, Beerli RR, Graus-Porta D, Maurer FG, Hynes NE. Neu differentiation factor induces ErbB2 down-regulation and apoptosis of ErbB2-overexpressing breast tumor cells. Cancer Res. 1997; 57: 3804-11.

[5] Tzahar E, Waterman H, Chen X, Levkowitz G, Karunagaran D, Lavi S, *et al*. A hierarchical network of interreceptor interactions determines signal transduction by Neu differentiation factor/neuregulin and epidermal growth factor. Mol Cell Biol. 1996; 16: 5276-87.

[6] Yarden Y. The EGFR family and its ligands in human cancer. signalling mechanisms and therapeutic opportunities. Eur J Cancer. 2001; 37 Suppl 4: S3-8.

[7] Zhang Q, Park E, Kani K, Landgraf R. Functional isolation of activated and unilaterally phosphorylated heterodimers of ERBB2 and ERBB3 as scaffolds in ligand-dependent signaling. Proc Natl Acad Sci U S A. 2012; 109: 13237-42.

[8] Sliwkowski MX. Pari passu dimers of dimers. Proc Natl Acad Sci U S A. 2012;109:13140-1.

[9] Ozcelik C, Erdmann B, Pilz B, Wettschureck N, Britsch S, Hubner N, *et al*. Conditional mutation of the ErbB2 (HER2) receptor in cardiomyocytes leads to dilated cardiomyopathy. Proc Natl Acad Sci U S A. 2002; 99: 8880-5.

[10] Finkle D, Quan ZR, Asghari V, Kloss J, Ghaboosi N, Mai E, *et al*. HER2-targeted therapy reduces incidence and progression of midlife mammary tumors in female murine mammary tumor virus huHER2-transgenic mice. Clin Cancer Res. 2004; 10: 2499-511.

[11] Meyer D, Birchmeier C. Multiple essential functions of neuregulin in development. Nature. 1995; 378: 386-90.

[12] Morris JK, Lin W, Hauser C, Marchuk Y, Getman D, Lee KF. Rescue of the cardiac defect in ErbB2 mutant mice reveals essential roles of ErbB2 in peripheral nervous system development. Neuron. 1999; 23: 273-83.

[13] Gassmann M, Lemke G. Neuregulins and neuregulin receptors in neural development. Current opinion in neurobiology. 1997; 7: 87-92.

[14] Lee KF, Simon H, Chen H, Bates B, Hung MC, Hauser C. Requirement for neuregulin receptor erbB2 in neural and cardiac development. Nature. 1995; 378: 394-8.

[15] Andrechek ER, White D, Muller WJ. Targeted disruption of ErbB2/Neu in the mammary epithelium results in impaired ductal outgrowth. Oncogene. 2005; 24: 932-7.

[16] Press MF, Cordon-Cardo C, Slamon DJ. Expression of the HER-2/neu proto-oncogene in normal human adult and fetal tissues. Oncogene. 1990; 5: 953-62.

[17] Bast RC, Jr., Pusztai L, Kerns BJ, MacDonald JA, Jordan P, Daly L, *et al.* Coexpression of the HER-2 gene product, p185HER-2, and epidermal growth factor receptor, p170EGF-R, on epithelial ovarian cancers and normal tissues. Hybridoma. 1998; 17: 313-21.

[18] Danova M, Giordano M, Torelli F, Franchini G, Cappellano F, Riccardi A, *et al.* HER-2/neu oncogene expression and DNA ploidy in normal human kidney and renal cell carcinoma. Eur J Histochem. 1992; 36: 279-88.

[19] Garratt AN, Ozcelik C, Birchmeier C. ErbB2 pathways in heart and neural diseases. Trends Cardiovasc Med. 2003; 13: 80-6.

[20] Negro A, Brar BK, Lee KF. Essential roles of Her2/erbB2 in cardiac development and function. Recent Prog Horm Res. 2004; 59: 1-12.

[21] Pugatsch T, Abedat S, Lotan C, Beeri R. Anti-erbB2 treatment induces cardiotoxicity by interfering with cell survival pathways. Breast Cancer Res. 2006; 8: R35.

[22] Padhy LC, Shih C, Cowing D, Finkelstein R, Weinberg RA. Identification of a phosphoprotein specifically induced by the transforming DNA of rat neuroblastomas. Cell. 1982; 28: 865-71.

[23] Chazin VR, Kaleko M, Miller AD, Slamon DJ. Transformation mediated by the human HER-2 gene independent of the epidermal growth factor receptor. Oncogene. 1992; 7: 1859-66.

[24] Di Fiore PP, Pierce JH, Kraus MH, Segatto O, King CR, Aaronson SA. erbB-2 is a potent oncogene when overexpressed in NIH/3T3 cells. Science. 1987; 237: 178-82.

[25] Hudziak RM, Schlessinger J, Ullrich A. Increased expression of the putative growth factor receptor p185HER2 causes transformation and tumorigenesis of NIH 3T3 cells. Proc Natl Acad Sci U S A. 1987; 84: 7159-63.

[26] Muthuswamy SK, Li D, Lelievre S, Bissell MJ, Brugge JS. ErbB2, but not ErbB1, reinitiates proliferation and induces luminal repopulation in epithelial acini. Nat Cell Biol. 2001; 3: 785-92.

[27] Benz CC, Scott GK, Sarup JC, Johnson RM, Tripathy D, Coronado E, *et al.* Estrogen-dependent, tamoxifen-resistant tumorigenic growth of MCF-7 cells transfected with HER2/neu. Breast Cancer Res Treat. 1992; 24: 85-95.

[28] Woods Ignatoski KM, Livant DL, Markwart S, Grewal NK, Ethier SP. The role of phosphatidylinositol 3'-kinase and its downstream signals in erbB-2-mediated transformation. Mol Cancer Res. 2003; 1: 551-60.

[29] Woods Ignatoski KM, Grewal NK, Markwart S, Livant DL, Ethier SP. p38MAPK induces cell surface alpha4 integrin downregulation to facilitate erbB-2-mediated invasion. Neoplasia. 2003; 5: 128-34.

[30] Yen L, You XL, Al Moustafa AE, Batist G, Hynes NE, Mader S, *et al.* Heregulin selectively upregulates vascular endothelial growth factor secretion in cancer cells and stimulates angiogenesis. Oncogene. 2000; 19: 3460-9.

[31] Menard S, Tagliabue E, Campiglio M, Pupa SM. Role of HER2 gene overexpression in breast carcinoma. J Cell Physiol. 2000; 182: 150-62.

[32] Ross JS, Fletcher JA, Bloom KJ, Linette GP, Stec J, Symmans WF, *et al.* Targeted therapy in breast cancer: the HER-2/neu gene and protein. Mol Cell Proteomics. 2004; 3: 379-98.

[33] Konecny G, Untch M, Arboleda J, Wilson C, Kahlert S, Boettcher B, *et al.* Her-2/neu and urokinase-type plasminogen activator and its inhibitor in breast cancer. Clin Cancer Res. 2001; 7: 2448-57.

[34] Ferretti G, Felici A, Papaldo P, Fabi A, Cognetti F. HER2/neu role in breast cancer: from a prognostic foe to a predictive friend. Curr Opin Obstet Gynecol. 2007; 19: 56-62.

[35] Wolff AC, Hammond ME, Hicks DG, Dowsett M, McShane LM, Allison KH, *et al.* Recommendations for human epidermal growth factor receptor 2 testing in breast cancer: American Society of Clinical Oncology/College of American Pathologists clinical practice guideline update. J Clin Oncol. 2013; 31: 3997-4013.

[36] Molina MA, Saez R, Ramsey EE, Garcia-Barchino MJ, Rojo F, Evans AJ, *et al.* NH(2)-terminal truncated HER-2 protein but not full-length receptor is associated with nodal metastasis in human breast cancer. Clin Cancer Res. 2002; 8: 347-53.

[37] Xia W, Liu LH, Ho P, Spector NL. Truncated ErbB2 receptor (p95ErbB2) is regulated by heregulin through heterodimer formation with ErbB3 yet remains sensitive to the dual EGFR/ErbB2 kinase inhibitor GW572016. Oncogene. 2004; 23: 646-53.

[38] Liu PC, Liu X, Li Y, Covington M, Wynn R, Huber R, *et al.* Identification of ADAM10 as a major source of HER2 ectodomain sheddase activity in HER2 overexpressing breast cancer cells. Cancer Biol Ther. 2006; 5: 657-64.

[39] Scaltriti M, Rojo F, Ocana A, Anido J, Guzman M, Cortes J, *et al.* Expression of p95HER2, a truncated form of the HER2 receptor, and response to anti-HER2 therapies in breast cancer. J Natl Cancer Inst. 2007; 99: 628-38.

[40] Carney WP, Neumann R, Lipton A, Leitzel K, Ali S, Price CP. Potential clinical utility of serum HER-2/neu oncoprotein concentrations in patients with breast cancer. Clin Chem. 2003; 49: 1579-98.

[41] Ludovini V, Gori S, Colozza M, Pistola L, Rulli E, Floriani I, *et al.* Evaluation of serum HER2 extracellular domain in early breast cancer patients: correlation with clinicopathological parameters and survival. Ann Oncol. 2008; 19: 883-90.

[42] Saez R, Molina MA, Ramsey EE, Rojo F, Keenan EJ, Albanell J, *et al.* p95HER-2 predicts worse outcome in patients with HER-2-positive breast cancer. Clin Cancer Res. 2006; 12: 424-31.

[43] Hudziak RM, Lewis GD, Winget M, Fendly BM, Shepard HM, Ullrich A. p185HER2 monoclonal antibody has antiproliferative effects *in vitro* and sensitizes human breast tumor cells to tumor necrosis factor. Mol Cell Biol. 1989; 9: 1165-72.

[44] Fendly BM, Winget M, Hudziak RM, Lipari MT, Napier MA, Ullrich A. Characterization of murine monoclonal antibodies reactive to either the human epidermal growth factor receptor or HER2/neu gene product. Cancer Res. 1990; 50: 1550-8.

[45] Harries M, Smith I. The development and clinical use of trastuzumab (Herceptin). Endocr Relat Cancer. 2002; 9: 75-85.

[46] Sarup JC, Johnson RM, King KL, Fendly BM, Lipari MT, Napier MA, *et al.* Characterization of an anti-p185HER2 monoclonal antibody that stimulates receptor function and inhibits tumor cell growth. Growth Regul. 1991; 1: 72-82.

[47] Baselga J, Mendelsohn J. Receptor blockade with monoclonal antibodies as anti-cancer therapy. Pharmacol Ther. 1994; 64: 127-54.

[48] Miller RA, Oseroff AR, Stratte PT, Levy R. Monoclonal antibody therapeutic trials in seven patients with T-cell lymphoma. Blood. 1983; 62: 988-95.

[49] Carter P, Presta L, Gorman CM, Ridgway JB, Henner D, Wong WL, *et al*. Humanization of an anti-p185HER2 antibody for human cancer therapy. Proc Natl Acad Sci U S A. 1992; 89: 4285-9.

[50] Roche. Herceptin Product Information.

[51] Hudis CA. Trastuzumab--mechanism of action and use in clinical practice. N Engl J Med. 2007; 357: 39-51.

[52] Slamon DJ, Leyland-Jones B, Shak S, Fuchs H, Paton V, Bajamonde A, *et al*. Use of chemotherapy plus a monoclonal antibody against HER2 for metastatic breast cancer that overexpresses HER2. N Engl J Med. 2001; 344: 783-92.

[53] Romond EH, Perez EA, Bryant J, Suman VJ, Geyer CE, Jr., Davidson NE, *et al*. Trastuzumab plus adjuvant chemotherapy for operable HER2-positive breast cancer. N Engl J Med. 2005; 353: 1673-84.

[54] Sliwkowski MX, Lofgren JA, Lewis GD, Hotaling TE, Fendly BM, Fox JA. Nonclinical studies addressing the mechanism of action of trastuzumab (Herceptin). Semin Oncol. 1999; 26: 60-70.

[55] Pegram M, Hsu S, Lewis G, Pietras R, Beryt M, Sliwkowski M, *et al*. Inhibitory effects of combinations of HER-2/neu antibody and chemotherapeutic agents used for treatment of human breast cancers. Oncogene. 1999; 18: 2241-51.

[56] Delord JP, Allal C, Canal M, Mery E, Rochaix P, Hennebelle I, *et al*. Selective inhibition of HER2 inhibits AKT signal transduction and prolongs disease-free survival in a micrometastasis model of ovarian carcinoma. Ann Oncol. 2005; 16: 1889-97.

[57] Nagata Y, Lan K-H, Zhou X, Tan M, Esteva FJ, Sahin AA, *et al*. PTEN activation contributes to tumor inhibition by trastuzumab, and loss of PTEN predicts trastuzumab resistance in patients. Cancer cell. 2004; 6: 117-27.

[58] Yakes FM, Chinratanalab W, Ritter CA, King W, Seelig S, Arteaga CL. Herceptin-induced inhibition of phosphatidylinositol-3 kinase and AKT Is required for antibody-mediated effects on p27, cyclin D1, and antitumor action. Cancer Res. 2002; 62: 4132-41.

[59] Liang K, Lu Y, Jin W, Ang KK, Milas L, Fan Z. Sensitization of breast cancer cells to radiation by trastuzumab. Mol Cancer Ther. 2003; 2: 1113-20.

[60] Junttila TT, Akita RW, Parsons K, Fields C, Lewis Phillips GD, Friedman LS, *et al*. Ligand-independent HER2/HER3/PI3K complex is disrupted by trastuzumab and is effectively inhibited by the PI3K inhibitor GDC-0941. Cancer Cell. 2009; 15: 429-40.

[61] Molina MA, Codony-Servat J, Albanell J, Rojo F, Arribas J, Baselga J. Trastuzumab (herceptin), a humanized anti-Her2 receptor monoclonal antibody, inhibits basal and activated Her2 ectodomain cleavage in breast cancer cells. Cancer Res. 2001; 61: 4744-9.

[62] Varchetta S, Gibelli N, Oliviero B, Nardini E, Gennari R, Gatti G, *et al*. Elements related to heterogeneity of antibody-dependent cell cytotoxicity in patients under trastuzumab therapy for primary operable breast cancer overexpressing Her2. Cancer Res. 2007; 67: 11991-9.

[63] De Santes K, Slamon D, Anderson SK, Shepard M, Fendly B, Maneval D, *et al*. Radiolabeled antibody targeting of the HER-2/neu oncoprotein. Cancer Res. 1992; 52: 1916-23.

[64] Cuello M, Ettenberg SA, Clark AS, Keane MM, Posner RH, Nau MM, *et al*. Down-regulation of the erbB-2 receptor by trastuzumab (herceptin) enhances tumor necrosis

factor-related apoptosis-inducing ligand-mediated apoptosis in breast and ovarian cancer cell lines that overexpress erbB-2. Cancer Res. 2001; 61: 4892-900.

[65] Klapper LN, Waterman H, Sela M, Yarden Y. Tumour-inhibitory antibodies to HER-2/ErbB-2 may act by recruiting c-Cbl and enhancing ubiquitination of HER-2. Cancer Res. 2000; 60: 3384-8.

[66] Austin CD, De Maziere AM, Pisacane PI, van Dijk SM, Eigenbrot C, Sliwkowski MX, *et al*. Endocytosis and sorting of ErbB2 and the site of action of cancer therapeutics trastuzumab and geldanamycin. Mol Biol Cell. 2004; 15: 5268-82.

[67] Gennari R, Menard S, Fagnoni F, Ponchio L, Scelsi M, Tagliabue E, *et al*. Pilot study of the mechanism of action of preoperative trastuzumab in patients with primary operable breast tumors overexpressing HER2. Clin Cancer Res. 2004; 10: 5650-5.

[68] Fornier MN, Seidman AD, Schwartz MK, Ghani F, Thiel R, Norton L, *et al*. Serum HER2 extracellular domain in metastatic breast cancer patients treated with weekly trastuzumab and paclitaxel: association with HER2 status by immunohistochemistry and fluorescence *in situ* hybridization and with response rate. Ann Oncol. 2005; 16: 234-9.

[69] Kostler WJ, Schwab B, Singer CF, Neumann R, Rucklinger E, Brodowicz T, *et al*. Monitoring of serum Her-2/neu predicts response and progression-free survival to trastuzumab-based treatment in patients with metastatic breast cancer. Clin Cancer Res. 2004; 10: 1618-24.

[70] Clynes RA, Towers TL, Presta LG, Ravetch JV. Inhibitory Fc receptors modulate *in vivo* cytoxicity against tumor targets. Nat Med. 2000; 6: 443-6.

[71] Arnould L, Gelly M, Penault-Llorca F, Benoit L, Bonnetain F, Migeon C, *et al*. Trastuzumab-based treatment of HER2-positive breast cancer: an antibody-dependent cellular cytotoxicity mechanism? Br J Cancer. 2006; 94: 259-67.

[72] Beano A, Signorino E, Evangelista A, Brusa D, Mistrangelo M, Polimeni MA, *et al*. Correlation between NK function and response to trastuzumab in metastatic breast cancer patients. J Transl Med. 2008; 6: 25.

[73] Izumi Y, Xu L, di Tomaso E, Fukumura D, Jain RK. Tumour biology: herceptin acts as an anti-angiogenic cocktail. Nature. 2002; 416: 279-80.

[74] Epstein M AR, Tchekmedyian N, *et al*. HER2-overexpressing human breast cancer xenografts exhibit increased angiogenic potential mediated by vascular endothelial growth factor (VEGF) Breast Cancer Res Treat. 2002; 76.

[75] Klos KS, Zhou X, Lee S, Zhang L, Yang W, Nagata Y, *et al*. Combined trastuzumab and paclitaxel treatment better inhibits ErbB-2-mediated angiogenesis in breast carcinoma through a more effective inhibition of AKT than either treatment alone. Cancer. 2003; 98: 1377-85.

[76] Wen XF, Yang G, Mao W, Thornton A, Liu J, Bast RC, Jr., *et al*. HER2 signaling modulates the equilibrium between pro- and antiangiogenic factors *via* distinct pathways: implications for HER2-targeted antibody therapy. Oncogene. 2006; 25: 6986-96.

[77] Shak S. Overview of the trastuzumab (Herceptin) anti-HER2 monoclonal antibody clinical program in HER2-overexpressing metastatic breast cancer. Herceptin Multinational Investigator Study Group. Semin Oncol. 1999; 26: 71-7.

[78] Baselga J, Tripathy D, Mendelsohn J, Baughman S, Benz CC, Dantis L, *et al*. Phase II study of weekly intravenous recombinant humanized anti-p185HER2 monoclonal antibody in patients with HER2/neu-overexpressing metastatic breast cancer. J Clin Oncol. 1996; 14: 737-44.

[79] Pegram MD, Lipton A, Hayes DF, Weber BL, Baselga JM, Tripathy D, *et al.* Phase II study of receptor-enhanced chemosensitivity using recombinant humanized anti-p185HER2/neu monoclonal antibody plus cisplatin in patients with HER2/neu-overexpressing metastatic breast cancer refractory to chemotherapy treatment. J Clin Oncol. 1998; 16: 2659-71.

[80] Cobleigh MA, Vogel CL, Tripathy D, Robert NJ, Scholl S, Fehrenbacher L, *et al.* Multinational study of the efficacy and safety of humanized anti-HER2 monoclonal antibody in women who have HER2-overexpressing metastatic breast cancer that has progressed after chemotherapy for metastatic disease. J Clin Oncol. 1999; 17: 2639-48.

[81] Tokuda Y, Watanabe T, Omuro Y, Ando M, Katsumata N, Okumura A, *et al.* Dose escalation and pharmacokinetic study of a humanized anti-HER2 monoclonal antibody in patients with HER2/neu-overexpressing metastatic breast cancer. Br J Cancer. 1999; 81: 1419-25.

[82] Baselga J, Carbonell X, Castaneda-Soto NJ, Clemens M, Green M, Harvey V, *et al.* Phase II study of efficacy, safety, and pharmacokinetics of trastuzumab monotherapy administered on a 3-weekly schedule. J Clin Oncol. 2005; 23: 2162-71.

[83] Leyland-Jones B, Gelmon K, Ayoub JP, Arnold A, Verma S, Dias R, *et al.* Pharmacokinetics, safety, and efficacy of trastuzumab administered every three weeks in combination with paclitaxel. J Clin Oncol. 2003; 21: 3965-71.

[84] Sawyer DB, Zuppinger C, Miller TA, Eppenberger HM, Suter TM. Modulation of anthracycline-induced myofibrillar disarray in rat ventricular myocytes by neuregulin-1beta and anti-erbB2: potential mechanism for trastuzumab-induced cardiotoxicity. Circulation. 2002; 105: 1551-4.

[85] Perez EA, Romond EH, Suman VJ, Jeong JH, Davidson NE, Geyer CE Jr, *et al.* Four-year follow-up of trastuzumab plus adjuvant chemotherapy for operable human epidermal growth factor receptor 2-positive breast cancer: joint analysis of data from NCCTG N9831 and NSABP B-31. J Clin Oncol. 2011; 29: 3366-73.

[86] Smith I, Procter M, Gelber RD, Guillaume S, Feyereislova A, Dowsett M, *et al.* 2-year follow-up of trastuzumab after adjuvant chemotherapy in HER2-positive breast cancer: a randomised controlled trial. Lancet. 2007; 369: 29-36.

[87] Goldhirsch A, Gelber RD, Piccart-Gebhart MJ, de Azambuja E, Procter M, Suter TM, *et al.* 2 years *versus* 1 year of adjuvant trastuzumab for HER2-positive breast cancer (HERA): an open-label, randomised controlled trial. Lancet. 2013; 382: 1021-8.

[88] Joensuu H, Bono P, Kataja V, Alanko T, Kokko R, Asola R, *et al.* Fluorouracil, Epirubicin, and Cyclophosphamide With Either Docetaxel or Vinorelbine, With or Without Trastuzumab, As Adjuvant Treatments of Breast Cancer: Final Results of the FinHer Trial. Journal of Clinical Oncology. 2009; 27: 5685-92.

[89] Au HJ, Eiermann W, Robert NJ, Pienkowski T, Crown J, Martin M, *et al.* Health-related quality of life with adjuvant docetaxel- and trastuzumab-based regimens in patients with node-positive and high-risk node-negative, HER2-positive early breast cancer: results from the BCIRG 006 Study. Oncologist. 2013; 18: 812-8.

[90] Slamon D, Eiermann W, Robert N, Pienkowski T, Martin M, Press M, *et al.* Adjuvant trastuzumab in HER2-positive breast cancer. N Engl J Med. 2011; 365: 1273-83.

[91] Viani GA, Afonso SL, Stefano EJ, De Fendi LI, Soares FV. Adjuvant trastuzumab in the treatment of her-2-positive early breast cancer: a meta-analysis of published randomized trials. BMC Cancer. 2007; 7: 153.

[92] Gianni L, Eiermann W, Semiglazov V, Manikhas A, Lluch A, Tjulandin S, *et al.* Neoadjuvant chemotherapy with trastuzumab followed by adjuvant trastuzumab *versus* neoadjuvant chemotherapy alone, in patients with HER2-positive locally advanced breast cancer (the NOAH trial): a randomised controlled superiority trial with a parallel HER2-negative cohort. Lancet. 2010; 375: 377-84.

[93] Untch M, Fasching PA, Konecny GE, Hasmüller S, Lebeau A, Kreienberg R, *et al.* Pathologic Complete Response After Neoadjuvant Chemotherapy Plus Trastuzumab Predicts Favorable Survival in Human Epidermal Growth Factor Receptor 2–Overexpressing Breast Cancer: Results From the TECHNO Trial of the AGO and GBG Study Groups. J Clin Oncol. 2011; 29: 3352-7.

[94] Untch M, Rezai M, Loibl S, Fasching PA, Huober J, Tesch H, *et al.* Neoadjuvant treatment with trastuzumab in HER2-positive breast cancer: results from the GeparQuattro study. J Clin Oncol. 2010; 28: 2024-31.

[95] Leveque D, Wisniewski S, Jehl F. Pharmacokinetics of therapeutic monoclonal antibodies used in oncology. Anticancer Res. 2005; 25: 2327-43.

[96] Pestalozzi BC, Brignoli S. Trastuzumab in CSF. J Clin Oncol. 2000;18:2349-51.

[97] Duchnowska R, Szczylik C. Central nervous system metastases in breast cancer patients administered trastuzumab. Cancer Treat Rev. 2005; 31: 312-8.

[98] Platini C, Long J, Walter S. Meningeal carcinomatosis from breast cancer treated with intrathecal trastuzumab. Lancet Oncol. 2006; 7: 778-80.

[99] Ismael G, Hegg R, Muehlbauer S, Heinzmann D, Lum B, Kim S-B, *et al.* Subcutaneous *versus* intravenous administration of (neo)adjuvant trastuzumab in patients with HER2-positive, clinical stage I-III breast cancer (HannaH study): a phase 3, open-label, multicentre, randomised trial. Lancet Oncol. 2012; 13: 869-78.

[100] Gullo G, Zuradelli M, Sclafani F, Santoro A, Crown J. Durable complete response following chemotherapy and trastuzumab for metastatic HER2-positive breast cancer. Ann Oncol. 2012; 23: 2204-5.

[101] Nahta R, Esteva FJ. HER-2-targeted therapy: lessons learned and future directions. Clin Cancer Res. 2003; 9: 5078-84.

[102] Nahta R, Esteva FJ. Trastuzumab: triumphs and tribulations. Oncogene.26:3637-43.

[103] Browne BC, O'Brien N, Duffy MJ, Crown J, O'Donovan N. HER-2 signaling and inhibition in breast cancer. Curr Cancer Drug Targets. 2009; 9: 419-38.

[104] Li J, Yen C, Liaw D, Podsypanina K, Bose S, Wang SI, *et al.* PTEN, a Putative Protein Tyrosine Phosphatase Gene Mutated in Human Brain, Breast, and Prostate Cancer. Science. 1997; 275: 1943-7.

[105] Mutter GL, Lin MC, Fitzgerald JT, Kum JB, Baak JP, Lees JA, *et al.* Altered PTEN expression as a diagnostic marker for the earliest endometrial precancers. J Natl Cancer Inst. 2000; 92: 924-30.

[106] Li D-M, Sun H. PTEN/MMAC1/TEP1 suppresses the tumorigenicity and induces G1 cell cycle arrest in human glioblastoma cells. Proc Natl Acad Sci USA. 1998; 95: 15406-11.

[107] Berns K, Horlings HM, Hennessy BT, Madiredjo M, Hijmans EM, Beelen K, *et al.* A functional genetic approach identifies the PI3K pathway as a major determinant of trastuzumab resistance in breast cancer. Cancer Cell. 2007; 12: 395-402.

[108] O'Brien NA, Browne BC, Chow L, Wang Y, Ginther C, Arboleda J, *et al.* Activated Phosphoinositide 3-Kinase/AKT Signaling Confers Resistance to Trastuzumab but not Lapatinib. Mol Can Ther. 2010; 9: 1489-502.

[109] Chandarlapaty S, Sakr RA, Giri D, Patil S, Heguy A, Morrow M, *et al.* Frequent Mutational Activation of the PI3K-AKT Pathway in Trastuzumab-Resistant Breast Cancer. Clin Can Res. 2012; 18: 6784-91.

[110] Perez EA, Dueck AC, McCullough AE, Chen B, Geiger XJ, Jenkins RB, *et al.* Impact of PTEN Protein Expression on Benefit From Adjuvant Trastuzumab in Early-Stage Human Epidermal Growth Factor Receptor 2–Positive Breast Cancer in the North Central Cancer Treatment Group N9831 Trial. J Clin Oncol. 2013; 31: 2115-22.

[111] Valabrega G, Montemurro F, Aglietta M. Trastuzumab: mechanism of action, resistance and future perspectives in HER2-overexpressing breast cancer. Ann Oncol. 2007;18:977-84.

[112] Lu Y, Zi X, Zhao Y, Mascarenhas D, Pollak M. Insulin-Like Growth Factor-I Receptor Signaling and Resistance to Trastuzumab (Herceptin). J Natl Can Inst. 2001; 93: 1852-7.

[113] Browne BC, Crown J, Venkatesan N, Duffy MJ, Clynes M, Slamon D, *et al.* Inhibition of IGF1R activity enhances response to trastuzumab in HER-2-positive breast cancer cells. Ann Oncol. 2011; 22: 68-73.

[114] Browne BC, Eustace AJ, Kennedy S, O'Brien NA, Pedersen K, McDermott MS, *et al.* Evaluation of IGF1R and phosphorylated IGF1R as targets in HER2-positive breast cancer cell lines and tumors. Breast Cancer Res Treat. 2012; 136: 717-27.

[115] Reinholz MM, Dueck AC, Chen B, Geiger X, McCullough AE, Jenkins RB, *et al.* Effect of IGF1R protein expression on benefit to adjuvant trastuzumab in early-stage HER2+ breast cancer in NCCTG N9831 trial. J Clin Oncol 2011; 29: Abstr 10503.

[116] Shattuck DL, Miller JK, Carraway KL, 3rd, Sweeney C. Met receptor contributes to trastuzumab resistance of Her2-overexpressing breast cancer cells. Cancer Res. 2008; 68: 1471-7.

[117] Dua R, Zhang J, Nhonthachit P, Penuel E, Petropoulos C, Parry G. EGFR over-expression and activation in high HER2, ER negative breast cancer cell line induces trastuzumab resistance. Breast Cancer Res Treat. 2010; 122: 685-97.

[118] Ritter CA, Perez-Torres M, Rinehart C, Guix M, Dugger T, Engelman JA, *et al.* Human breast cancer cells selected for resistance to trastuzumab *in vivo* overexpress epidermal growth factor receptor and ErbB ligands and remain dependent on the ErbB receptor network. Clin Cancer Res. 2007; 13: 4909-19.

[119] Gijsen M, King P, Perera T, Parker PJ, Harris AL, Larijani B, *et al.* HER2 Phosphorylation Is Maintained by a PKB Negative Feedback Loop in Response to Anti-HER2 Herceptin in Breast Cancer. PLoS Biol. 2010; 8: e1000563.

[120] Ali SM, Carney WP, Esteva FJ, Fornier M, Harris L, Kostler WJ, *et al.* Serum HER-2/neu and relative resistance to trastuzumab-based therapy in patients with metastatic breast cancer. Cancer. 2008; 113: 1294-301.

[121] Anido J, Scaltriti M, Bech Serra JJ, Santiago Josefat B, Todo FR, Baselga J, *et al.* Biosynthesis of tumorigenic HER2 C-terminal fragments by alternative initiation of translation. Embo J. 2006; 25: 3234-44.

[122] Scaltriti M, Rojo F, OcaÃ±a A, Anido J, Guzman M, Cortes J, *et al.* Expression of p95HER2, a Truncated Form of the HER2 Receptor, and Response to Anti-HER2 Therapies in Breast Cancer. J Natl Can Inst. 2007; 99: 628-38.

[123] Sperinde J, Jin X, Banerjee J, Penuel E, Saha A, Diedrich G, *et al.* Quantitation of p95HER2 in paraffin sections by using a p95-specific antibody and correlation with

outcome in a cohort of trastuzumab-treated breast cancer patients. Clin Cancer Res. 2010; 16: 4226-35.

[124] O'Brien NA, Browne BC, Chow L, Wang Y, Ginther C, Arboleda J, *et al.* Activated phosphoinositide 3-kinase/AKT signaling confers resistance to trastuzumab but not lapatinib. Mol Cancer Ther. 2010; 9: 1489-502.

[125] Price-Schiavi SA, Jepson S, Li P, Arango M, Rudland PS, Yee L, *et al.* Rat Muc4 (sialomucin complex) reduces binding of anti-ErbB2 antibodies to tumor cell surfaces, a potential mechanism for herceptin resistance. Int J Cancer. 2002; 99: 783-91.

[126] Nagy P, FriedlÃ¤nder E, Tanner M, Kapanen AI, Carraway KL, Isola J, *et al.* Decreased Accessibility and Lack of Activation of ErbB2 in JIMT-1, a Herceptin-Resistant, MUC4-Expressing Breast Cancer Cell Line. Cancer Res. 2005; 65: 473-82.

[127] Chen AC, Migliaccio I, Rimawi M, Lopez-Tarruella S, Creighton CJ, Massarweh S, *et al.* Upregulation of mucin4 in ER-positive/HER2-overexpressing breast cancer xenografts with acquired resistance to endocrine and HER2-targeted therapies. Breast Cancer Res Treat. 2012; 134: 583-93.

[128] Citri A, Kochupurakkal BS, Yarden Y. The achilles heel of ErbB-2/HER2: regulation by the Hsp90 chaperone machine and potential for pharmacological intervention. Cell Cycle. 2004; 3: 51-60.

[129] Chandarlapaty S, Scaltriti M, Angelini P, Ye Q, Guzman M, Hudis CA, *et al.* Inhibitors of HSP90 block p95-HER2 signaling in Trastuzumab-resistant tumors and suppress their growth. Oncogene. 2010; 29: 325-34.

[130] ViewPoints: Amgen looks to leapfrog rivals in Herceptin biosimilar race with Phase III trial in early stage breast cancer patients In: Desk V, editor. First Word Pharma2013.

[131] Im Y-H, Odarchenko P, Grecea D, Komov D, Valentynovych Anatoliy C, Gupta S, *et al.* Double-blind, randomized, parallel group, phase III study to demonstrate equivalent efficacy and comparable safety of CT-P6 and trastuzumab, both in combination with paclitaxel, in patients with metastatic breast cancer (MBC) as first-line treatment. J Clin Oncol. 2013; 31(suppl; abstr 629).

[132] Yin D, Barker KB, Li R, Meng X, Reich SD, Ricart AD, *et al.* A phase I pharmacokinetics trial comparing PF-05280014 (a potential biosimilar) and trastuzumab in healthy volunteers (REFLECTIONS B327-01). J Clin Oncol. 2013; 31(suppl; abstr 612).

[133] Chustecka Z. Biosimilar Trastuzumab (Hertraz) Approved in India. Medscape Medical News 2013.

[134] Mylan. Mylan-Biocon Receive First Indian Biosimilar Regulatory Approval for Herceptin®. 2013.

[135] Adams CW, Allison DE, Flagella K, Presta L, Clarke J, Dybdal N, *et al.* Humanization of a recombinant monoclonal antibody to produce a therapeutic HER dimerization inhibitor, pertuzumab. Cancer Immunol Immunother. 2006; 55: 717-27.

[136] Franklin MC, Carey KD, Vajdos FF, Leahy DJ, de Vos AM, Sliwkowski MX. Insights into ErbB signaling from the structure of the ErbB2-pertuzumab complex. Cancer Cell. 2004; 5: 317-28.

[137] Agus DB, Akita RW, Fox WD, Lewis GD, Higgins B, Pisacane PI, *et al.* Targeting ligand-activated ErbB2 signaling inhibits breast and prostate tumor growth. Cancer Cell. 2002; 2: 127-37.

[138] Lemmon MA, Bu Z, Ladbury JE, Zhou M, Pinchasi D, Lax I, *et al.* Two EGF molecules contribute additively to stabilization of the EGFR dimer. EMBO J 1997; 16: 281-94.

[139] Moriki T, Maruyama H, Maruyama IN. Activation of preformed EGF receptor dimers by ligand-induced rotation of the transmembrane domain. J Mol Biol. 2001; 311: 1011-26.

[140] Sako Y, Minoghchi S, Yanagida T. Single-molecule imaging of EGFR signalling on the surface of living cells. Nature Cell Biol. 2000; 2: 168-72.

[141] Garrett TP, McKern NM, Lou M, Elleman TC, Adams TE, Lovrecz GO, *et al.* The crystal structure of a truncated ErbB2 ectodomain reveals an active conformation, poised to interact with other ErbB receptors. Mol Cell. 2003; 11: 495-505.

[142] Klapper LN, Glathe S, Vaisman N, Hynes NE, Andrews GC, Sela M, *et al.* The ErbB-2/HER2 oncoprotein of human carcinomas may function solely as a shared coreceptor for multiple stroma-derived growth factors. Proc Natl Acad Sci U S A. 1999; 96: 4995-5000.

[143] Graus-Porta D, Beerli RR, Daly JM, Hynes NE. ErbB-2, the preferred heterodimerization partner of all ErbB receptors, is a mediator of lateral signaling. EMBO J. 1997; 16: 1647-55.

[144] Citri A, Yarden Y. EGF-ERBB signalling: towards the systems level. Nature Reviews Mol Cell Biol. 2006; 7: 505-16.

[145] Lee-Hoeflich ST, Crocker L, Yao E, Pham T, Munroe X, Hoeflich KP, *et al.* A central role for HER3 in HER2-amplified breast cancer: implications for targeted therapy. Cancer Res. 2008; 68: 5878-87.

[146] Kani K, Warren CM, Kaddis CS, Loo JA, Landgraf R. Oligomers of ERBB3 have two distinct interfaces that differ in their sensitivity to disruption by heregulin. J Biol Chem. 2005; 280: 8238-47.

[147] Lane HA, Motoyama AB, Beuvink I, Hynes NE. Modulation of p27/Cdk2 complex formation through 4D5-mediated inhibition of HER2 receptor signaling. Ann Oncol. 2001; 12 Suppl 1: S21-2.

[148] Le XF, Claret FX, Lammayot A, Tian L, Deshpande D, LaPushin R, *et al.* The role of cyclin-dependent kinase inhibitor p27Kip1 in anti-HER2 antibody-induced G1 cell cycle arrest and tumor growth inhibition. J Biol Chem. 2003; 278: 23441-50.

[149] Sims AH, Zweemer AJ, Nagumo Y, Faratian D, Muir M, Dodds M, *et al.* Defining the molecular response to trastuzumab, pertuzumab and combination therapy in ovarian cancer. Br J Can. 2012; 106: 1779-89.

[150] Clynes RA, Towers TL, Presta LG, Ravetch JV. Inhibitory Fc receptors modulate *in vivo* cytotoxicity against tumor targets. Nature Med. 2000; 6: 443-6.

[151] Alimandi M, Romano A, Curia MC, Muraro R, Fedi P, Aaronson SA, *et al.* Cooperative signaling of ErbB3 and ErbB2 in neoplastic transformation and human mammary carcinomas. Oncogene. 1995; 10: 1813-21.

[152] Wallasch C, Weiss FU, Niederfellner G, Jallal B, Issing W, Ullrich A. Heregulin-dependent regulation of HER2/neu oncogenic signaling by heterodimerization with HER3. Embo J. 1995; 14: 4267-75.

[153] Nagumo Y, Faratian D, Mullen P, Harrison DJ, Hasmann M, Langdon SP. Modulation of HER3 is a marker of dynamic cell signaling in ovarian cancer: implications for pertuzumab sensitivity. Mol Cancer Res. 2009; 7: 1563-71.

[154] Nahta R, Hung MC, Esteva FJ. The HER-2-targeting antibodies trastuzumab and pertuzumab synergistically inhibit the survival of breast cancer cells. Cancer Res. 2004; 64: 2343-6.

[155] Brockhoff G, Heckel B, Schmidt-Bruecken E, Plander M, Hofstaedter F, Vollmann A, *et al.* Differential impact of Cetuximab, Pertuzumab and Trastuzumab on BT474 and SK-BR-3 breast cancer cell proliferation. Cell Prolif. 2007; 40: 488-507.
[156] Arpino G, Gutierrez C, Weiss H, Rimawi M, Massarweh S, Bharwani L, *et al.* Treatment of human epidermal growth factor receptor 2-overexpressing breast cancer xenografts with multiagent HER-targeted therapy. J Natl Cancer Inst. 2007; 99: 694-705.
[157] Scheuer W, Friess T, Burtscher H, Bossenmaier B, Endl J, Hasmann M. Strongly enhanced antitumor activity of trastuzumab and pertuzumab combination treatment on HER2-positive human xenograft tumor models. Cancer Res. 2009; 69: 9330-6.
[158] Phillips GD, Fields CT, Li G, Dowbenko D, Schaefer G, Miller K, *et al.* Dual targeting of HER2-positive cancer with trastuzumab emtansine and pertuzumab: critical role for neuregulin blockade in antitumor response to combination therapy. Clin Cancer Res. 2014; 20: 456-68.
[159] Vogel CL, Cobleigh MA, Tripathy D, Gutheil JC, Harris LN, Fehrenbacher L, *et al.* Efficacy and safety of trastuzumab as a single agent in first-line treatment of HER2-overexpressing metastatic breast cancer. J Clin Oncol. 2002; 20: 719-26.
[160] Baselga J, Cortes J, Kim SB, Im SA, Hegg R, Im YH, *et al.* Pertuzumab plus trastuzumab plus docetaxel for metastatic breast cancer. N Engl J Med. 2012; 366: 109-19.
[161] Agus DB, Gordon MS, Taylor C, Natale RB, Karlan B, Mendelson DS, *et al.* Phase I clinical study of pertuzumab, a novel HER dimerization inhibitor, in patients with advanced cancer. J Clin Oncol. 2005; 23: 2534-43.
[162] Agus DB, Sweeney CJ, Morris MJ, Mendelson DS, McNeel DG, Ahmann FR, *et al.* Efficacy and safety of single-agent pertuzumab (rhuMAb 2C4), a human epidermal growth factor receptor dimerization inhibitor, in castration-resistant prostate cancer after progression from taxane-based therapy. J Clin Oncol. 2007; 25: 675-81.
[163] Herbst RS, Davies AM, Natale RB, Dang TP, Schiller JH, Garland LL, *et al.* Efficacy and safety of single-agent pertuzumab, a human epidermal receptor dimerization inhibitor, in patients with non small cell lung cancer. Clin Cancer Res. 2007; 13: 6175-81.
[164] Gordon MS, Matei D, Aghajanian C, Matulonis UA, Brewer M, Fleming GF, *et al.* Clinical activity of pertuzumab (rhuMAb 2C4), a HER dimerization inhibitor, in advanced ovarian cancer: potential predictive relationship with tumor HER2 activation status. J Clin Oncol. 2006; 24: 4324-32.
[165] Gianni L, Llado A, Bianchi G, Cortes J, Kellokumpu-Lehtinen PL, Cameron DA, *et al.* Open-label, phase II, multicenter, randomized study of the efficacy and safety of two dose levels of Pertuzumab, a human epidermal growth factor receptor 2 dimerization inhibitor, in patients with human epidermal growth factor receptor 2-negative metastatic breast cancer. J Clin Oncol. 2010; 28: 1131-7.
[166] Baselga J, Gelmon KA, Verma S, Wardley A, Conte P, Miles D, *et al.* Phase II trial of pertuzumab and trastuzumab in patients with human epidermal growth factor receptor 2-positive metastatic breast cancer that progressed during prior trastuzumab therapy. J Clin Oncol. 2010; 28: 1138-44.
[167] Gianni L, Pienkowski T, Im YH, Roman L, Tseng LM, Liu MC, *et al.* Efficacy and safety of neoadjuvant pertuzumab and trastuzumab in women with locally advanced, inflammatory, or early HER2-positive breast cancer (NeoSphere): a randomised multicentre, open-label, phase 2 trial. Lancet Oncol. 2012; 13: 25-32.

[168] Attard G, Kitzen J, Blagden SP, Fong PC, Pronk LC, Zhi J, *et al.* A phase Ib study of pertuzumab, a recombinant humanised antibody to HER2, and docetaxel in patients with advanced solid tumors. Br J Cancer. 2007; 97: 1338-43.

[169] Hurvitz SA, Hu Y, O'Brien N, Finn RS. Current approaches and future directions in the treatment of HER2-positive breast cancer. Cancer Treat Rev. 2013; 39: 219-29.

[170] Swain SM, Kim SB, Cortes J, Ro J, Semiglazov V, Campone M, *et al.* Pertuzumab, trastuzumab, and docetaxel for HER2-positive metastatic breast cancer (CLEOPATRA study): overall survival results from a randomised, double-blind, placebo-controlled, phase 3 study. Lancet Oncol. 2013; 14: 461-71.

[171] Schneeweiss A, Chia S, Hickish T, Harvey V, Eniu A, Hegg R, *et al.* Pertuzumab plus trastuzumab in combination with standard neoadjuvant anthracycline-containing and anthracycline-free chemotherapy regimens in patients with HER2-positive early breast cancer: a randomized phase II cardiac safety study (TRYPHAENA). Ann Oncol. 2013; 24: 2278-84.

[172] Minckwitz G von JB, I Bradbury, Azambuja E de, MJ Scullion, G Ross, KS Saini, and M Piccart-Gebhart Adjuvant Pertuzumab and Herceptin IN IniTial TherapY of Breast Cancer: APHINITY (BIG 4–11/BO25126/TOC4939g). Cancer Res. 2011; 71: Abstract nr OT1-02-4.

[173] Ellis PA, Barrios CH, Im Y, Patre M, Branle F, Perez EA. MARIANNE: A phase III, randomized study of trastuzumab-DM1 (T-DM1) with or without pertuzumab (P) compared with trastuzumab (H) plus taxane for first-line treatment of HER2-positive, progressive, or recurrent locally advanced or metastatic breast cancer (MBC). J Clin Oncol. 2011; 29 (suppl; abstr TPS102).

[174] Issell BF, Crooke ST. Maytansine. Cancer Treat Rev. 1978;5:199-207.

[175] Chari RV, Martell BA, Gross JL, Cook SB, Shah SA, Blattler WA, *et al.* Immunoconjugates containing novel maytansinoids: promising anticancer drugs. Cancer Res. 1992; 52: 127-31.

[176] Lewis Phillips GD, Li G, Dugger DL, Crocker LM, Parsons KL, Mai E, *et al.* Targeting HER2-positive breast cancer with trastuzumab-DM1, an antibody-cytotoxic drug conjugate. Cancer Res. 2008; 68: 9280-90.

[177] Krop IE, Beeram M, Modi S, Jones SF, Holden SN, Yu W, *et al.* Phase I study of trastuzumab-DM1, an HER2 antibody-drug conjugate, given every 3 weeks to patients with HER2-positive metastatic breast cancer. J Clin Oncol. 2010; 28: 2698-704.

[178] Barok M, Tanner M, Koninki K, Isola J. Trastuzumab-DM1 causes tumor growth inhibition by mitotic catastrophe in trastuzumab-resistant breast cancer cells *in vivo*. Breast Cancer Res. 2011; 13: R46.

[179] Junttila TT, Li G, Parsons K, Phillips GL, Sliwkowski MX. Trastuzumab-DM1 (T-DM1) retains all the mechanisms of action of trastuzumab and efficiently inhibits growth of lapatinib insensitive breast cancer. Breast Cancer Res Treat. 2011; 128: 347-56.

[180] Jumbe NL, Xin Y, Leipold DD, Crocker L, Dugger D, Mai E, *et al.* Modeling the efficacy of trastuzumab-DM1, an antibody drug conjugate, in mice. J Pharmacokinet Pharmacodyn. 2010; 37: 221-42.

[181] Poon KA, Flagella K, Beyer J, Tibbitts J, Kaur S, Saad O, *et al.* Preclinical safety profile of trastuzumab emtansine (T-DM1): mechanism of action of its cytotoxic component retained with improved tolerability. Toxicology and applied pharmacology. 2013; 273: 298-313.

[182] Lu D, Burris HA, 3rd, Wang B, Dees EC, Cortes J, Joshi A, *et al.* Drug interaction potential of trastuzumab emtansine (T-DM1) combined with pertuzumab in patients with HER2-positive metastatic breast cancer. Curr Drug Metab. 2012; 13: 911-22.

[183] Thon JN, Devine MT, Jurak Begonja A, Tibbitts J, Italiano JE, Jr. High-content live-cell imaging assay used to establish mechanism of trastuzumab emtansine (T-DM1)--mediated inhibition of platelet production. Blood. 2012; 120: 1975-84.

[184] Beeram M, Krop IE, Burris HA, Girish SR, Yu W, Lu MW, *et al.* A phase 1 study of weekly dosing of trastuzumab emtansine (T-DM1) in patients with advanced human epidermal growth factor 2-positive breast cancer. Cancer. 2012; 118: 5733-40.

[185] Girish S, Gupta M, Wang B, Lu D, Krop IE, Vogel CL, *et al.* Clinical pharmacology of trastuzumab emtansine (T-DM1): an antibody-drug conjugate in development for the treatment of HER2-positive cancer. Cancer Chemother Pharmacol. 2012; 69: 1229-40.

[186] Burris HA, 3rd, Rugo HS, Vukelja SJ, Vogel CL, Borson RA, Limentani S, *et al.* Phase II study of the antibody drug conjugate trastuzumab-DM1 for the treatment of human epidermal growth factor receptor 2 (HER2)-positive breast cancer after prior HER2-directed therapy. J Clin Oncol. 2011; 29: 398-405.

[187] Krop IE, LoRusso P, Miller KD, Modi S, Yardley D, Rodriguez G, *et al.* A phase II study of trastuzumab emtansine in patients with human epidermal growth factor receptor 2-positive metastatic breast cancer who were previously treated with trastuzumab, lapatinib, an anthracycline, a taxane, and capecitabine. J Clin Oncol. 2012; 30: 3234-41.

[188] Hurvitz SA, Dirix L, Kocsis J, Bianchi GV, Lu J, Vinholes J, *et al.* Phase II randomized study of trastuzumab emtansine *versus* trastuzumab plus docetaxel in patients with human epidermal growth factor receptor 2-positive metastatic breast cancer. J Clin Oncol. 2013; 31: 1157-63.

[189] Verma S, Miles D, Gianni L, Krop IE, Welslau M, Baselga J, *et al.* Trastuzumab emtansine for HER2-positive advanced breast cancer. N Engl J Med. 2012; 367: 1783-91.

[190] Krop I, Lin N, Blackwell K, Guardino E, Huober J, Lu M, *et al.* Efficacy and safety of trastuzumab emtansine (T-DM1) *vs* lapatinib plus capecitabine (XL) in patients with human epidermal growth factor receptor 2 (HER2)-positive metastatic breast cancer (MBC) and central nervous system (CNS) metastases: Results from a retrospective exploratory analysis of EMILIA. San Antonio Breast Cancer Symposium. 2013; Abstract [P4-12-27].

[191] Krop IE, Suter TM, Dirix L, Romieu G, Zamagni C, Citron ML, *et al.* Cardiac safety of trastuzumab emtansine (T-DM1) following anthracycline-based chemotherapy as (neo)adjuvant therapy for human epidermal growth factor receptor 2-positive (HER2+) early-stage breast cancer (EBC): Final data from TDM4874g. San Antonio Breast Cancer Symposium. 2013; Abstract [P2-15-03].

[192] Lewis Phillips G, C. F, Crocker L, Parsons K, Tibbitts J, Holden S, *et al.* Potent anti-tumor activity of trastuzumab-DM1 antibody-drug conjugate in combination with cytotoxic chemotherapeutic agents, antibodies or small molecule kinase inhibitors. Proceedings AACR Annual Meeting. 2008; Abstract: #2133.

[193] Fields CT, Crocker LM, Sliwkowski MX, Lewis Phillips GD. Dual targeting of HER2: Enhanced antitumor efficacy of trastuzumab-DM1 combined with pertuzumab. Proceedings AACR Annual Meeting. 2010; Abstract:#5607.

[194] Modi S, Elias AD, LoRusso P, Samant M, Guardino E, Althaus B, *et al.* Results from a phase Ib study of trastuzumab emtansine (T-DM1), paclitaxel (T), and pertuzumab (P) in

patients with HER2-positive metastatic breast cancer (MBC) previously treated with trastuzumab. J Clin Oncol. 2012; 30: Abstr 528.

[195] Elias A, Modi S, Krop IE, Pegram M, Ipe D, Guardino EA, *et al.* Results from a phase 2a study of trastuzumab emtansine, paclitaxel, and pertuzumab in patients with HER2-positive metastatic breast cancer. San Antonio Breast Cancer Symposium. 2013; Abstract:[P4-12-09].

[196] Martin M, Dewar J, Albanell J, Limentani S, Chang J, Strasak A, *et al.* Neoadjuvant trastuzumab emtansine and docetaxel, with or without pertuzumab, in patients with HER2-positive early-stage breast cancer: Results from a phase 1b/2a study. San Antonio Breast Cancer Symposium. 2013; Abstract: [P4-12-07].

[197] Matsui H, Takeshita A, Naito K, Shinjo K, Shigeno K, Maekawa M, *et al.* Reduced effect of gemtuzumab ozogamicin (CMA-676) on P-glycoprotein and/or CD34-positive leukemia cells and its restoration by multidrug resistance modifiers. Leukemia. 2002; 16: 813-9.

[198] Naito K, Takeshita A, Shigeno K, Nakamura S, Fujisawa S, Shinjo K, *et al.* Calicheamicin-conjugated humanized anti-CD33 monoclonal antibody (gemtuzumab zogamicin, CMA-676) shows cytocidal effect on CD33-positive leukemia cell lines, but is inactive on P-glycoprotein-expressing sublines. Leukemia. 2000; 14: 1436-43.

[199] Wong S, Bumbaca D, Yue Q, Halladay J, Kenny JR, Salphati L, *et al.* Nonclinical disposition, metabolism, and *in vitro* drug-drug interaction assessment of DM1, a component of trastuzumab emtansine (T-DM1). Mol Cancer Ther. 2011; 10: Abstract A136.

[200] Kovtun YV, Audette CA, Mayo MF, Jones GE, Doherty H, Maloney EK, *et al.* Antibody-maytansinoid conjugates designed to bypass multidrug resistance. Cancer Res. 2010; 70: 2528-37.

[201] Larkin A, O'Driscoll L, Kennedy S, Purcell R, Moran E, Crown J, *et al.* Investigation of MRP-1 protein and MDR-1 P-glycoprotein expression in invasive breast cancer: a prognostic study. Int J Cancer. 2004; 112: 286-94.

[202] Rybarova S, Hodorova I, Hajdukova M, Schmidtova K, Mojzis J, Kajo K, *et al.* Expression of MDR proteins in breast cancer and its correlation with some clinical and pathological parameters. Neoplasma. 2006; 53: 128-35.

[203] Xia W, Mullin RJ, Keith BR, Liu LH, Ma H, Rusnak DW, *et al.* Anti-tumor activity of GW572016: a dual tyrosine kinase inhibitor blocks EGF activation of EGFR/erbB2 and downstream Erk1/2 and AKT pathways. Oncogene. 2002; 21: 6255-63.

[204] Rusnak DW, Lackey K, Affleck K, Wood ER, Alligood KJ, Rhodes N, *et al.* The effects of the novel, reversible epidermal growth factor receptor/ErbB-2 tyrosine kinase inhibitor, GW2016, on the growth of human normal and tumor-derived cell lines *in vitro* and *in vivo*. Mol Cancer Ther. 2001; 1: 85-94.

[205] Burris HA, 3rd, Hurwitz HI, Dees EC, Dowlati A, Blackwell KL, O'Neil B, *et al.* Phase I safety, pharmacokinetics, and clinical activity study of lapatinib (GW572016), a reversible dual inhibitor of epidermal growth factor receptor tyrosine kinases, in heavily pretreated patients with metastatic carcinomas. J Clin Oncol. 2005; 23: 5305-13.

[206] Konecny GE, Pegram MD, Venkatesan N, Finn R, Yang G, Rahmeh M, *et al.* Activity of the dual kinase inhibitor lapatinib (GW572016) against HER-2-overexpressing and trastuzumab-treated breast cancer cells. Cancer Res. 2006; 66: 1630-9.

[207] O'Donovan N, Byrne AT, O'Connor AE, McGee S, Gallagher WM, Crown J. Synergistic interaction between trastuzumab and EGFR/HER-2 tyrosine kinase inhibitors in HER-2 positive breast cancer cells. Invest New Drugs. 2011; 29: 752-9.

[208] Altieri DC. Survivin, cancer networks and pathway-directed drug discovery. Nat Rev Cancer. 2008; 8: 61-70.

[209] Xia W, Bisi J, Strum J, Liu L, Carrick K, Graham KM, *et al.* Regulation of survivin by ErbB2 signaling: therapeutic implications for ErbB2-overexpressing breast cancers. Cancer Res. 2006; 66: 1640-7.

[210] Tanizaki J, Okamoto I, Fumita S, Okamoto W, Nishio K, Nakagawa K. Roles of BIM induction and survivin downregulation in lapatinib-induced apoptosis in breast cancer cells with HER2 amplification. Oncogene. 2011; 30: 4097-106.

[211] Mitchell C, Yacoub A, Hossein H, Martin AP, Bareford MD, Eulitt P, *et al.* Inhibition of MCL-1 in breast cancer cells promotes cell death *in vitro* and *in vivo*. Cancer Biol Ther. 2010; 10: 903-17.

[212] Kondo Y, Kanzawa T, Sawaya R, Kondo S. The role of autophagy in cancer development and response to therapy. Nat Rev Cancer. 2005; 5: 726-34.

[213] Tang Y, Hamed HA, Cruickshanks N, Fisher PB, Grant S, Dent P. Obatoclax and lapatinib interact to induce toxic autophagy through NOXA. Mol Pharmacol. 2012; 81: 527-40.

[214] Zhu X, Wu L, Qiao H, Han T, Chen S, Liu X, *et al.* Autophagy stimulates apoptosis in HER2-overexpressing breast cancers treated by lapatinib. J Cell Biochem. 2013; 114: 2643-53.

[215] Perez EA, Koehler M, Byrne J, Preston AJ, Rappold E, Ewer MS. Cardiac safety of lapatinib: pooled analysis of 3689 patients enrolled in clinical trials. Mayo Clin Proc. 2008; 3: 679-86.

[216] Shell SA, Lyass L, Trusk PB, Pry KJ, Wappel RL, Bacus SS. Activation of AMPK is necessary for killing cancer cells and sparing cardiac cells. Cell Cycle. 2008; 7: 1769-75.

[217] Xu J, Ji J, Yan XH. Cross-talk between AMPK and mTOR in regulating energy balance. Crit Reviews Food Sci Nutr. 2012; 52: 373-81.

[218] Burstein HJ, Storniolo AM, Franco S, Forster J, Stein S, Rubin S, *et al.* A phase II study of lapatinib monotherapy in chemotherapy-refractory HER2-positive and HER2-negative advanced or metastatic breast cancer. Ann Oncol. 2008; 19: 1068-74.

[219] Toi M, Iwata H, Fujiwara Y, Ito Y, Nakamura S, Tokuda Y, *et al.* Lapatinib monotherapy in patients with relapsed, advanced, or metastatic breast cancer: efficacy, safety, and biomarker results from Japanese patients phase II studies. Br J Cancer. 2009; 101: 1676-82.

[220] Blackwell KL, Pegram MD, Tan-Chiu E, Schwartzberg LS, Arbushites MC, Maltzman JD, *et al.* Single-agent lapatinib for HER2-overexpressing advanced or metastatic breast cancer that progressed on first- or second-line trastuzumab-containing regimens. Ann Oncol. 2009; 20: 1026-31.

[221] Gomez HL, Doval DC, Chavez MA, Ang PC, Aziz Z, Nag S, *et al.* Efficacy and safety of lapatinib as first-line therapy for ErbB2-amplified locally advanced or metastatic breast cancer. J Clin Oncol. 2008; 26: 2999-3005.

[222] Shimma N, Umeda I, Arasaki M, Murasaki C, Masubuchi K, Kohchi Y, *et al.* The design and synthesis of a new tumor-selective fluoropyrimidine carbamate, capecitabine. Bioorg Med Chem. 2000; 8: 1697-706.

[223] Budman DR, Soong R, Calabro A, Tai J, Diasio R. Identification of potentially useful combinations of epidermal growth factor receptor tyrosine kinase antagonists with

conventional cytotoxic agents using median effect analysis. Anticancer Drugs. 2006; 17: 921-8.

[224] Chu QS, Schwartz G, de Bono J, Smith DA, Koch KM, Versola MJ, *et al.* Phase I and pharmacokinetic study of lapatinib in combination with capecitabine in patients with advanced solid malignancies. J Clin Oncol. 2007; 25: 3753-8.

[225] Geyer CE, Forster J, Lindquist D, Chan S, Romieu CG, Pienkowski T, *et al.* Lapatinib plus capecitabine for HER2-positive advanced breast cancer. N Engl J Med. 2006; 355: 2733-43.

[226] Cameron D, Casey M, Press M, Lindquist D, Pienkowski T, Romieu CG, *et al.* A phase III randomized comparison of lapatinib plus capecitabine *versus* capecitabine alone in women with advanced breast cancer that has progressed on trastuzumab: updated efficacy and biomarker analyses. Breast Cancer Res Treat. 2008; 112: 533-43.

[227] Cameron D, Casey M, Oliva C, Newstat B, Imwalle B, Geyer CE. Lapatinib plus capecitabine in women with HER-2-positive advanced breast cancer: final survival analysis of a phase III randomized trial. Oncologist. 2010; 15: 924-34.

[228] Crown JP, Burris HA, 3rd, Boyle F, Jones S, Koehler M, Newstat BO, *et al.* Pooled analysis of diarrhea events in patients with cancer treated with lapatinib. Breast Cancer Res Treat. 2008; 112: 317-25.

[229] Pestalozzi BC, Zahrieh D, Price KN, Holmberg SB, Lindtner J, Collins J, *et al.* Identifying breast cancer patients at risk for Central Nervous System (CNS) metastases in trials of the International Breast Cancer Study Group (IBCSG). Ann Oncol. 2006; 17: 935-44.

[230] Gril B, Palmieri D, Bronder JL, Herring JM, Vega-Valle E, Feigenbaum L, *et al.* Effect of lapatinib on the outgrowth of metastatic breast cancer cells to the brain. J Natl Cancer Inst. 2008; 100: 1092-103.

[231] Lin NU, Dieras V, Paul D, Lossignol D, Christodoulou C, Stemmler HJ, *et al.* Multicenter phase II study of lapatinib in patients with brain metastases from HER2-positive breast cancer. Clin Cancer Res. 2009; 15: 1452-9.

[232] Bachelot T, Romieu G, Campone M, Dieras V, Cropet C, Dalenc F, *et al.* Lapatinib plus capecitabine in patients with previously untreated brain metastases from HER2-positive metastatic breast cancer (LANDSCAPE): a single-group phase 2 study. Lancet Oncol. 2013; 14: 64-71.

[233] Morikawa A, Peereboom DM, Smith QR, Thorsheim H, Lockman PR, Simmons AJ, *et al.* Clinical evidence for drug penetration of capecitabine and lapatinib uptake in resected brain metastases from women with metastatic breast cancer. J Clin Oncol. 2013; 31: Abstr 514.

[234] Chu I, Blackwell K, Chen S, Slingerland J. The dual ErbB1/ErbB2 inhibitor, lapatinib (GW572016), cooperates with tamoxifen to inhibit both cell proliferation- and estrogen-dependent gene expression in antiestrogen-resistant breast cancer. Cancer Res. 2005; 65: 18-25.

[235] Chu QS, Cianfrocca ME, Goldstein LJ, Gale M, Murray N, Loftiss J, *et al.* A phase I and pharmacokinetic study of lapatinib in combination with letrozole in patients with advanced cancer. Clin Cancer Res. 2008; 14: 4484-90.

[236] Johnston S, Pippen J, Jr., Pivot X, Lichinitser M, Sadeghi S, Dieras V, *et al.* Lapatinib combined with letrozole *versus* letrozole and placebo as first-line therapy for postmenopausal hormone receptor-positive metastatic breast cancer. J Clin Oncol. 2009; 27: 5538-46.

[237] Schwartzberg LS, Franco SX, Florance A, O'Rourke L, Maltzman J, Johnston S. Lapatinib plus letrozole as first-line therapy for HER-2+ hormone receptor-positive metastatic breast cancer. Oncologist. 2010; 15: 122-9.

[238] Di Leo A, Gomez HL, Aziz Z, Zvirbule Z, Bines J, Arbushites MC, *et al.* Phase III, double-blind, randomized study comparing lapatinib plus paclitaxel with placebo plus paclitaxel as first-line treatment for metastatic breast cancer. J Clin Oncol. 2008; 26: 5544-52.

[239] Guan Z, Xu B, DeSilvio ML, Shen Z, Arpornwirat W, Tong Z, *et al.* Randomized trial of lapatinib *versus* placebo added to paclitaxel in the treatment of human epidermal growth factor receptor 2-overexpressing metastatic breast cancer. J Clin Oncol. 2013; 31: 1947-53.

[240] LoRusso PM, Jones SF, Koch KM, Arya N, Fleming RA, Loftiss J, *et al.* Phase I and pharmacokinetic study of lapatinib and docetaxel in patients with advanced cancer. J Clin Oncol. 2008; 26: 3051-6.

[241] Fumoleau P, Dalenc F, Mailliez A, Veyret C, Bonneterre J, Guillemet C, *et al.* Phase I dose escalation study of oral lapatinib in combination with docetaxel in patients with HER2-positive locally advanced or metastatic breast cancer (LAMBC): Initial safety and tolerability results. J Clin Oncol. 2013; 31: Abstr e11529.

[242] Blackwell KL, Burstein HJ, Storniolo AM, Rugo H, Sledge G, Koehler M, *et al.* Randomized study of Lapatinib alone or in combination with trastuzumab in women with ErbB2-positive, trastuzumab-refractory metastatic breast cancer. J Clin Oncol. 2010; 28: 1124-30.

[243] Blackwell KL, Burstein HJ, Storniolo AM, Rugo HS, Sledge G, AKTan G, *et al.* Overall survival benefit with lapatinib in combination with trastuzumab for patients with human epidermal growth factor receptor 2-positive metastatic breast cancer: final results from the EGF104900 Study. J Clin Oncol. 2012; 30: 2585-92.

[244] Crown J, Kennedy MJ, Tresca P, Marty M, Espie M, Burris HA, *et al.* Optimally tolerated dose of lapatinib in combination with docetaxel plus trastuzumab in first-line treatment of HER2-positive metastatic breast cancer. Ann Oncol. 2013; 24: 2005-11.

[245] Baselga J, Bradbury I, Eidtmann H, Di Cosimo S, de Azambuja E, Aura C, *et al.* Lapatinib with trastuzumab for HER2-positive early breast cancer (NeoALTTO): a randomised, open-label, multicentre, phase 3 trial. Lancet. 2012; 379: 633-40.

[246] Azim HA, Jr., Agbor-Tarh D, Bradbury I, Dinh P, Baselga J, Di Cosimo S, *et al.* Pattern of rash, diarrhea, and hepatic toxicities secondary to lapatinib and their association with age and response to neoadjuvant therapy: analysis from the NeoALTTO trial. J Clin Oncol. 2013; 31: 4504-11.

[247] Hurvitz SA, Miller JM, Dichmann R, Perez AT, Patel R, Zehngebot LM, *et al.* Final analysis of a phase II 3-arm randomized trial of neoadjuvant trastuzumab or lapatinib or the combination of trastuzumab and lapatinib, followed by six cycles of docetaxel and carboplatin with trastuzumab and/or lapatinib in patients with HER2+ breast cancer (TRIO-US B07). San Antonio Breast Cancer Symposium. 2013; Abstract: [S1-02].

[248] Crown J, Coate L, Keane M, Kennedy J, O'Reilly S, Kelly C, *et al.* Randomized phase II study of pre-operative docetaxel, carboplatin with trastuzumab (TCH) and/or/lapatinib (L) in HER-2 positive (H+) breast cancer patients (BC pts). ICORG 10-05. San Antonio Breast Cancer Symposium. 2013; Abstract: [P4-12-25].

[249] Gradishar WJ. Emerging approaches for treating HER2-positive metastatic breast cancer beyond trastuzumab. Ann Oncol. 2013; 24: 2492-500.

[250] Piccart-Gebhart MJ, Holmes AP, Baselga J, De Azambuja A, Dueck AC, Viale G, *et al.* First results from the phase III ALTTO trial (BIG 2-06; NCCTG [Alliance] N063D) comparing one year of anti-HER2 therapy with lapatinib alone, trastuzumab alone, their sequence, or their combination in the adjuvant treatment of HER2-positive early breast cancer. J Clin Oncol 32: 5s, 2014 (suppl; abstr LBA4)

[251] Xia W, Husain I, Liu L, Bacus S, Saini S, Spohn J, *et al.* Lapatinib antitumor activity is not dependent upon phosphatase and tensin homologue deleted on chromosome 10 in ErbB2-overexpressing breast cancers. Cancer Res. 2007; 67: 1170-5.

[252] Scaltriti M, Chandarlapaty S, Prudkin L, Aura C, Jimenez J, Angelini PD, *et al.* Clinical benefit of lapatinib-based therapy in patients with human epidermal growth factor receptor 2-positive breast tumors coexpressing the truncated p95HER2 receptor. Clin Cancer Res. 2010; 16: 2688-95.

[253] Nahta R, Yuan LX, Du Y, Esteva FJ. Lapatinib induces apoptosis in trastuzumab-resistant breast cancer cells: effects on insulin-like growth factor I signaling. Mol Cancer Ther. 2007; 6: 667-74.

[254] Wang YC, Morrison G, Gillihan R, Guo J, Ward RM, Fu X, *et al.* Different mechanisms for resistance to trastuzumab *versus* lapatinib in HER2-positive breast cancers--role of estrogen receptor and HER2 reactivation. Breast Cancer Res. 2011; 13: R121.

[255] Xia W, Bacus S, Hegde P, Husain I, Strum J, Liu L, *et al.* A model of acquired autoresistance to a potent ErbB2 tyrosine kinase inhibitor and a therapeutic strategy to prevent its onset in breast cancer. Proc Natl Acad Sci U S A. 2006; 103: 7795-800.

[256] Liu L, Greger J, Shi H, Liu Y, Greshock J, Annan R, *et al.* Novel mechanism of lapatinib resistance in HER2-positive breast tumor cells: activation of AXL. Cancer Res. 2009; 69: 6871-8.

[257] Hafizi S, Dahlback B. Signalling and functional diversity within the Axl subfamily of receptor tyrosine kinases. Cytokine Growth Factor Rev. 2006; 17: 295-304.

[258] Dubrez-Daloz L, Dupoux A, Cartier J. IAPs: more than just inhibitors of apoptosis proteins. Cell Cycle. 2008;7:1036-46.

[259] Zhang Y, Zhu J, Tang Y, Li F, Zhou H, Peng B, *et al.* X-linked inhibitor of apoptosis positive nuclear labeling: a new independent prognostic biomarker of breast invasive ductal carcinoma. Diagn Pathol. 2011; 6: 49.

[260] Aird KM, Ghanayem RB, Peplinski S, Lyerly HK, Devi GR. X-linked inhibitor of apoptosis protein inhibits apoptosis in inflammatory breast cancer cells with acquired resistance to an ErbB1/2 tyrosine kinase inhibitor. Mol Cancer Ther. 2010 ;9: 1432-42.

[261] Rexer BN, Ham AJ, Rinehart C, Hill S, Granja-Ingram Nde M, Gonzalez-Angulo AM, *et al.* Phosphoproteomic mass spectrometry profiling links Src family kinases to escape from HER2 tyrosine kinase inhibition. Oncogene. 2011; 30: 4163-74.

[262] De Luca A, D'Alessio A, Gallo M, Maiello MR, Bode AM, Normanno N. Src and CXCR4 are involved in the invasiveness of breast cancer cells with acquired resistance to lapatinib. Cell Cycle. 2014; 13: 148-56.

[263] Huang C, Park CC, Hilsenbeck SG, Ward R, Rimawi MF, Wang YC, *et al.* beta1 integrin mediates an alternative survival pathway in breast cancer cells resistant to lapatinib. Breast Cancer Res. 2011; 13: R84.

[264] Bailey ST, Miron PL, Choi YJ, Kochupurakkal B, Maulik G, Rodig SJ, *et al.* Nuclear factor kappa B activation-induced anti-apoptosis renders HER2 positive cells drug resistant and accelerates tumor growth. Mol Cancer Res. 2013.

[265] Xia W, Bacus S, Husain I, Liu L, Zhao S, Liu Z, *et al.* Resistance to ErbB2 tyrosine kinase inhibitors in breast cancer is mediated by calcium-dependent activation of RelA. Mol Cancer Ther. 2010; 9: 292-9.

[266] Brady SW, Zhang J, Seok D, Wang H, Yu D. Enhanced PI3K p110alpha signaling confers acquired lapatinib resistance that can be effectively reversed by a p110alpha-selective PI3K inhibitor. Mol Cancer Ther. 2014; 13: 60-70.

[267] Eichhorn PJ, Gili M, Scaltriti M, Serra V, Guzman M, Nijkamp W, *et al.* Phosphatidylinositol 3-kinase hyperactivation results in lapatinib resistance that is reversed by the mTOR/phosphatidylinositol 3-kinase inhibitor NVP-BEZ235. Cancer Res. 2008; 68: 9221-30.

[268] Bian L, Wang T, Zhang SH, Zhang HQ, Guo YF, Du G, *et al.* Ki-67 index as a prognostic factor of subsequent lapatinib-based therapy in HER2-positive metastatic breast cancer with resistance to trastuzumab. Cancer Biol Ther. 2014;15.

[269] Finn RS, Press MF, Dering J, O'Rourke L, Florance A, Ellis C, *et al.* Quantitative ER and PgR Assessment as Predictors of Benefit from Lapatinib in Postmenopausal Women with Hormone Receptor-Positive, HER2-Negative Metastatic Breast Cancer. Clin Cancer Res. 2014; 20: 736-43.

[270] O'Neill F, Madden SF, Aherne ST, Clynes M, Crown J, Doolan P, *et al.* Gene expression changes as markers of early lapatinib response in a panel of breast cancer cell lines. Mol Cancer. 2012; 11: 41.

[271] O'Neill F, Madden SF, Clynes M, Crown J, Doolan P, Aherne ST, *et al.* A gene expression profile indicative of early stage HER2 targeted therapy response. Mol Cancer. 2013; 12: 69.

[272] Wissner A, Mansour TS. The development of HKI-272 and related compounds for the treatment of cancer. Arch Pharm (Weinheim). 2008; 341: 465-77.

[273] Rabindran SK, Discafani CM, Rosfjord EC, Baxter M, Floyd MB, Golas J, *et al.* Antitumor activity of HKI-272, an orally active, irreversible inhibitor of the HER-2 tyrosine kinase. Cancer Res. 2004; 64: 3958-65.

[274] Sanchez-Martin M, Pandiella A. Differential action of small molecule HER kinase inhibitors on receptor heterodimerization: therapeutic implications. Int J Cancer. 2012; 131: 244-52.

[275] Seyhan AA, Varadarajan U, Choe S, Liu W, Ryan TE. A genome-wide RNAi screen identifies novel targets of neratinib resistance leading to identification of potential drug resistant genetic markers. Mol Biosyst. 2012; 8: 1553-70.

[276] Canonici A, Gijsen M, Mullooly M, Bennett R, Bouguern N, Pedersen K, *et al.* Neratinib overcomes trastuzumab resistance in HER2 amplified breast cancer. Oncotarget. 2013; 4: 1592-605.

[277] Sato Y, Yashiro M, Takakura N. Heregulin induces resistance to lapatinib-mediated growth inhibition of HER2-amplified cancer cells. Cancer Sci. 2013; 104: 1618-25.

[278] Xia W, Petricoin EF, 3rd, Zhao S, Liu L, Osada T, Cheng Q, *et al.* An heregulin-EGFR-HER3 autocrine signaling axis can mediate acquired lapatinib resistance in HER2+ breast cancer models. Breast Cancer Res. 2013; 15: R85.

[279] Wong KK, Fracasso PM, Bukowski RM, Lynch TJ, Munster PN, Shapiro GI, *et al.* A phase I study with neratinib (HKI-272), an irreversible pan ErbB receptor tyrosine kinase inhibitor, in patients with solid tumors. Clin Cancer Res. 2009; 15: 2552-8.

[280] Hug B, Abbas R, Leister C, Burns J, Sonnichsen D. A single-dose, crossover, placebo- and moxifloxacin-controlled study to assess the effects of neratinib (HKI-272) on cardiac repolarization in healthy adult subjects. Clin Cancer Res. 2010; 16: 4016-23.

[281] Abbas R, Hug BA, Leister C, Burns J, Sonnichsen D. Pharmacokinetics of oral neratinib during co-administration of ketoconazole in healthy subjects. Br J Clin Pharmacol. 2011; 71: 522-7.

[282] Sendur MA, Aksoy S, Altundag K. Cardiotoxicity of novel HER2-targeted therapies. Curr Med Res Opin. 2013; 29: 1015-24.

[283] Jankowitz RC, Abraham J, Tan AR, Limentani SA, Tierno MB, Adamson LM, *et al.* Safety and efficacy of neratinib in combination with weekly paclitaxel and trastuzumab in women with metastatic HER2positive breast cancer: an NSABP Foundation Research Program phase I study. Cancer Chemother Pharmacol. 2013; 72: 1205-12.

[284] Gandhi L, Bahleda R, Tolaney SM, Kwak EL, Cleary JM, Pandya SS, *et al.* Phase I study of neratinib in combination with temsirolimus in patients with human epidermal growth factor receptor 2-dependent and other solid tumors. J Clin Oncol. 2014; 32: 68-75.

[285] Burstein HJ, Sun Y, Dirix LY, Jiang Z, Paridaens R, Tan AR, *et al.* Neratinib, an irreversible ErbB receptor tyrosine kinase inhibitor, in patients with advanced ErbB2-positive breast cancer. J Clin Oncol. 2010; 28: 1301-7.

[286] Chow LW, Xu B, Gupta S, Freyman A, Zhao Y, Abbas R, *et al.* Combination neratinib (HKI-272) and paclitaxel therapy in patients with HER2-positive metastatic breast cancer. Br J Cancer. 2013; 108: 1985-93.

[287] Awada A, Dirix L, Manso Sanchez L, Xu B, Luu T, Dieras V, *et al.* Safety and efficacy of neratinib (HKI-272) plus vinorelbine in the treatment of patients with ErbB2-positive metastatic breast cancer pretreated with anti-HER2 therapy. Ann Oncol. 2013; 24: 109-16.

[288] Martin M, Bonneterre J, Geyer CE, Jr., Ito Y, Ro J, Lang I, *et al.* A phase two randomised trial of neratinib monotherapy *versus* lapatinib plus capecitabine combination therapy in patients with HER2+ advanced breast cancer. Eur J Cancer. 2013; 49: 3763-72.

[289] Solca F, Dahl G, Zoephel A, Bader G, Sanderson M, Klein C, *et al.* Target binding properties and cellular activity of afatinib (BIBW 2992), an irreversible ErbB family blocker. J Pharmacol Exp Ther. 2012; 343: 342-50.

[290] Li D, Ambrogio L, Shimamura T, Kubo S, Takahashi M, Chirieac LR, *et al.* BIBW2992, an irreversible EGFR/HER2 inhibitor highly effective in preclinical lung cancer models. Oncogene. 2008; 27: 4702-11.

[291] Canonici A, Pedersen K, Browne B, McDermott M, Walsh N, Crown J, *et al.* Effect of afatinib alone and in combination with trastuzumab in HER2-positive breast cancer cell lines. J Clin Oncol. 2013; 31: Abstr 632.

[292] Harbeck N, Solca F, Gauler TC. Preclinical and clinical development of afatinib: a focus on breast cancer and squamous cell carcinoma of the head and neck. Future Oncol. 2014; 10: 21-40.

[293] Geuna E, Montemurro F, Aglietta M, Valabrega G. Potential of afatinib in the treatment of patients with HER2-positive breast cancer. Breast Cancer (Dove Med Press). 2012; 4: 131-7.

[294] Eskens FA, Mom CH, Planting AS, Gietema JA, Amelsberg A, Huisman H, *et al.* A phase I dose escalation study of BIBW 2992, an irreversible dual inhibitor of epidermal growth factor receptor 1 (EGFR) and 2 (HER2) tyrosine kinase in a 2-week on, 2-week off schedule in patients with advanced solid tumors. Br J Cancer. 2008; 98: 80-5.

[295] Marshall J, Hwang J, Eskens FA, Burger H, Malik S, Uttenreuther-Fischer M, *et al.* A Phase I, open-label, dose escalation study of afatinib, in a 3-week-on/1-week-off schedule in patients with advanced solid tumors. Invest New Drugs. 2013; 31: 399-408.

[296] Gordon MS, Mendelson DS, Gross M, Uttenreuther-Fischer M, Ould-Kaci M, Zhao Y, *et al.* A Phase I, open-label, dose-escalation study of continuous once-daily oral treatment with afatinib in patients with advanced solid tumors. Invest New Drugs. 2013; 31: 409-16.

[297] Yap TA, Vidal L, Adam J, Stephens P, Spicer J, Shaw H, *et al.* Phase I trial of the irreversible EGFR and HER2 kinase inhibitor BIBW 2992 in patients with advanced solid tumors. J Clin Oncol. 2010; 28: 3965-72.

[298] Vermorken JB, Rottey S, Ehrnrooth E, Pelling K, Lahogue A, Wind S, *et al.* A phase Ib, open-label study to assess the safety of continuous oral treatment with afatinib in combination with two chemotherapy regimens: cisplatin plus paclitaxel and cisplatin plus 5-fluorouracil, in patients with advanced solid tumors. Ann Oncol. 2013; 24: 1392-400.

[299] Marshall J, Shapiro GI, Uttenreuther-Fischer M, Ould-Kaci M, Stopfer P, Gordon MS. Phase I dose-escalation study of afatinib, an ErbB family blocker, plus docetaxel in patients with advanced cancer. Future Oncol. 2013; 9: 271-81.

[300] Awada AH, Dumez H, Hendlisz A, Wolter P, Besse-Hammer T, Uttenreuther-Fischer M, *et al.* Phase I study of pulsatile 3-day administration of afatinib (BIBW 2992) in combination with docetaxel in advanced solid tumors. Invest New Drugs. 2013; 31: 734-41.

[301] Lin NU, Winer EP, Wheatley D, Carey LA, Houston S, Mendelson D, *et al.* A phase II study of afatinib (BIBW 2992), an irreversible ErbB family blocker, in patients with HER2-positive metastatic breast cancer progressing after trastuzumab. Breast Cancer Res Treat. 2012; 133: 1057-65.

[302] Rimawi MF, Aleixo SB, Alarcon Rozas A, Nunes Matos Neto J, Caleffi M, Vinholesal JJF, *et al.* A neoadjuvant, randomized, open-label phase II trial of afatinib (A) *versus* trastuzumab (T) *versus* lapatinib (L) in patients (pts) with locally advanced HER2-positive breast cancer (BC). J Clin Oncol. 2012; 30: Abstr 606.

[303] Swanton C, Cromer J, Group S. Open-label, Phase II trial of afatinib, with or without vinorelbine (V), for the treatment of HER2-overexpressing inflammatory breast cancer (IBC). J Clin Oncol. 2012; 30: Abstr TPS650.

[304] Fry DW, Bridges AJ, Denny WA, Doherty A, Greis KD, Hicks JL, *et al.* Specific, irreversible inactivation of the epidermal growth factor receptor and erbB2, by a new class of tyrosine kinase inhibitor. Proc Natl Acad Sci U S A. 1998; 95: 12022-7.

[305] Kalous O, Conklin D, Desai AJ, O'Brien NA, Ginther C, Anderson L, *et al.* Dacomitinib (PF-00299804), an irreversible Pan-HER inhibitor, inhibits proliferation of HER2-amplified breast cancer cell lines resistant to trastuzumab and lapatinib. Mol Cancer Ther. 2012; 11: 1978-87.

[306] Engelman JA, Zejnullahu K, Gale CM, Lifshits E, Gonzales AJ, Shimamura T, *et al.* PF00299804, an irreversible pan-ERBB inhibitor, is effective in lung cancer models with EGFR and ERBB2 mutations that are resistant to gefitinib. Cancer Res. 2007; 67: 11924-32.

[307] Janne PA, Boss DS, Camidge DR, Britten CD, Engelman JA, Garon EB, *et al.* Phase I dose-escalation study of the pan-HER inhibitor, PF299804, in patients with advanced malignant solid tumors. Clin Cancer Res. 2011; 17: 1131-9.

[308] Takahashi T, Boku N, Murakami H, Naito T, Tsuya A, Nakamura Y, *et al.* Phase I and pharmacokinetic study of dacomitinib (PF-00299804), an oral irreversible, small molecule

inhibitor of human epidermal growth factor receptor-1, -2, and -4 tyrosine kinases, in Japanese patients with advanced solid tumors. Invest New Drugs. 2012; 30: 2352-63.

[309] Ruiz-Garcia A, Giri N, Labadie RR, Ni G, Boutros T, Richie N, *et al.* A phase I open-label study to investigate the potential drug-drug interaction between single-dose dacomitinib and steady-state paroxetine in healthy volunteers. J Clin Pharmacol. 2013; [Epub ahead of print].

[310] Bello CL, Smith E, Ruiz-Garcia A, Ni G, Alvey C, Loi CM. A phase I, open-label, mass balance study of [(14)C] dacomitinib (PF-00299804) in healthy male volunteers. Cancer Chemother Pharmacol. 2013; 72: 379-85.

[311] Breslin S, Corcoran C, Rani S, Crown J, O'Driscoll L. Assessment of neratinib-resistance and cross-resistance in HER2-overexpressing breast cancer cells. J Clin Oncol. 2013; 31: Abstr e11520.

[312] Canonici A, Pedersen K, Walsh N, Crown J, O'Donovan N. Effect of neratinib (N) alone and in combination with trastuzumab (T) in HER2-positive breast cancer (BC) cell lines. J Clin Oncol. 2012; 30: Abstr 632.

[313] Kang XH, Wang LF, Cao F, Fan FT, Xu ZY. [Tumour microenvironment elicits primary resistance to afatinib through HGF secretion]. Zhonghua Zhong Liu Za Zhi. 2013; 35: 732-6.

[314] Cortot AB, Repellin CE, Shimamura T, Capelletti M, Zejnullahu K, Ercan D, *et al.* Resistance to irreversible EGF receptor tyrosine kinase inhibitors through a multistep mechanism involving the IGF1R pathway. Cancer Res. 2013; 73: 834-43.

[315] Rani S, Germano S, Madden SF, Corcoran C, Breslin S, O'Brien NA, *et al.* Neuromedin U: A potential predictive biomarker for HER2-targeted drugs. J Clin Oncol. 2012; 30: Abstr 617.

[316] Wolff AC, Hammond ME, Hicks DG, Dowsett M, McShane LM, Allison KH, *et al.* Recommendations for human epidermal growth factor receptor 2 testing in breast cancer: American Society of Clinical Oncology/College of American Pathologists clinical practice guideline update. J Clin Oncol. 2013; 31: 3997-4013.

[317] Rakha EA, Ellis IO. Breast cancer: updated guideline recommendations for HER2 testing. Nat Rev Clin Oncol. 2014; 11: 8-9.

[318] Perez EA, Romond EH, Suman VJ, Jeong JH, Davidson NE, Geyer CE, Jr., *et al.* Four-year follow-up of trastuzumab plus adjuvant chemotherapy for operable human epidermal growth factor receptor 2-positive breast cancer: joint analysis of data from NCCTG N9831 and NSABP B-31. J Clin Oncol. 2011; 29: 3366-73.

[319] Paik S, Kim C, Wolmark N. HER2 status and benefit from adjuvant trastuzumab in breast cancer. N Engl J Med. 2008; 358: 1409-11.

[320] Perez EA, Reinholz MM, Hillman DW, Tenner KS, Schroeder MJ, Davidson NE, *et al.* HER2 and chromosome 17 effect on patient outcome in the N9831 adjuvant trastuzumab trial. J Clin Oncol. 2010; 28: 4307-15.

[321] Pogue-Geile KL, Kim C, Jeong JH, Tanaka N, Bandos H, Gavin PG, *et al.* Predicting degree of benefit from adjuvant trastuzumab in NSABP trial B-31. J Natl Cancer Inst. 2013; 105: 1782-8.

[322] Olsen DA, Ostergaard B, Bokmand S, Wamberg PA, Jakobsen EH, Brandslund I. HER-2 protein concentrations in breast cancer cells increase before immunohistochemical and fluorescence *in situ* hybridization analysis turn positive. Clin Chem Lab Med. 2007; 45: 177-82.

[323] Collins DM, O'Donovan N, McGowan PM, O'Sullivan F, Duffy MJ, Crown J. Trastuzumab induces antibody-dependent cell-mediated cytotoxicity (ADCC) in HER-2-non-amplified breast cancer cell lines. Ann Oncol. 2012; 23: 1788-95.

[324] Yanagawa M, Ikemot K, Kawauchi S, Furuya T, Yamamoto S, Oka M, *et al.* Luminal A and luminal B (HER2 negative) subtypes of breast cancer consist of a mixture of tumors with different genotype. BMC Res Notes.5: 376.

[325] Schnitt SJ. Classification and prognosis of invasive breast cancer: from morphology to molecular taxonomy. Mod Pathol. 2010; 23 Suppl 2: S60-4.

[326] Yanagawa M, Ikemot K, Kawauchi S, Furuya T, Yamamoto S, Oka M, *et al.* Luminal A and luminal B (HER2 negative) subtypes of breast cancer consist of a mixture of tumors with different genotype. BMC Res Notes. 2012; 5: 376.

[327] Corkery B, Crown J, Clynes M, O'Donovan N. Epidermal growth factor receptor as a potential therapeutic target in triple-negative breast cancer. Ann Oncol. 2009; 20: 862-7.

[328] Nogi H, Kobayashi T, Suzuki M, Tabei I, Kawase K, Toriumi Y, *et al.* EGFR as paradoxical predictor of chemosensitivity and outcome among triple-negative breast cancer. Oncol Rep. 2009; 21: 413-7.

[329] Rakha EA, Elsheikh SE, Aleskandarany MA, Habashi HO, Green AR, Powe DG, *et al.* Triple-negative breast cancer: distinguishing between basal and nonbasal subtypes. Clin Cancer Res. 2009; 15: 2302-10.

[330] Juranic ZD, Neskovic-Konstantinovic Z, Stanojkovic TP, Zizak Z, Srdic T, Stanojevic-Bakic N, *et al.* The antitumor immune response in HER-2 positive, metastatic breast cancer patients. J Transl Med. 2005; 3: 13.

[331] Loi S, Michiels S, Salgado R, Sirtaine N, Jose V, Fumagalli D, *et al.* Tumour infiltrating lymphocytes (TILs) indicate trastuzumab benefit in early-stage HER2-positive breast cancer (HER2+ BC). San Antonio Breast Cancer Symposium. 2013; Abstract: [S1-05].

[332] Carson WE, Parihar R, Lindemann MJ, Personeni N, Dierksheide J, Meropol NJ, *et al.* Interleukin-2 enhances the natural killer cell response to Herceptin-coated Her2/neu-positive breast cancer cells. Eur J Immunol. 2001; 31: 3016-25.

[333] Muraro E, Martorelli D, Turchet E, Miolo G, Scalone S, Comaro E, *et al.* A different immunologic profile characterizes patients with HER-2-overexpressing and HER-2-negative locally advanced breast cancer: implications for immune-based therapies. Breast Cancer Res. 2011; 13: R117.

[334] Mortenson ED, Fu YX. Adaptive Immune Responses and HER2/neu Positive Breast Cancer. Curr Pathobiol Rep. 2013; 1: 37-42.

[335] Whiteside TL, Vujanovic NL, Herberman RB. Natural killer cells and tumor therapy. Curr Top Microbiol Immunol. 1998; 230: 221-44.

[336] Park S, Jiang Z, Mortenson ED, Deng L, Radkevich-Brown O, Yang X, *et al.* The therapeutic effect of anti-HER2/neu antibody depends on both innate and adaptive immunity. Cancer Cell. 2010; 18: 160-70.

[337] Stagg J, Loi S, Divisekera U, Ngiow SF, Duret H, Yagita H, *et al.* Anti-ErbB-2 mAb therapy requires type I and II interferons and synergizes with anti-PD-1 or anti-CD137 mAb therapy. Proc Natl Acad Sci U S A. 2011; 108: 7142-7.

[338] Mittendorf EA, Clifton GT, Holmes JP, Clive KS, Patil R, Benavides LC, *et al.* Clinical trial results of the HER-2/neu (E75) vaccine to prevent breast cancer recurrence in high-risk patients: from US Military Cancer Institute Clinical Trials Group Study I-01 and I-02. Cancer. 2012; 118: 2594-602.

[339] Liu S, Wicha MS. Targeting breast cancer stem cells. J Clin Oncol. 2010;28:4006-12.

[340] Korkaya H, Wicha MS. HER-2, notch, and breast cancer stem cells: targeting an axis of evil. Clin Cancer Res. 2009; 15: 1845-7.

[341] Korkaya H, Paulson A, Iovino F, Wicha MS. HER2 regulates the mammary stem/progenitor cell population driving tumorigenesis and invasion. Oncogene. 2008; 27: 6120-30.

[342] Ithimakin S, Day KC, Malik F, Zen Q, Dawsey SJ, Bersano-Begey TF, *et al.* HER2 drives luminal breast cancer stem cells in the absence of HER2 amplification: implications for efficacy of adjuvant trastuzumab. Cancer Res. 2013; 73: 1635-46.

[343] Scaltriti M, Verma C, Guzman M, Jimenez J, Parra JL, Pedersen K, *et al.* Lapatinib, a HER2 tyrosine kinase inhibitor, induces stabilization and accumulation of HER2 and potentiates trastuzumab-dependent cell cytotoxicity. Oncogene. 2009; 28: 803-14.

[344] Mimura K, Kono K, Maruyama T, Watanabe M, Izawa S, Shiba S, *et al.* Lapatinib inhibits receptor phosphorylation and cell growth and enhances antibody-dependent cellular cytotoxicity of EGFR- and HER2-overexpressing esophageal cancer cell lines. Int J Cancer. 2011; 129: 2408-16.

[345] Press MF, Finn RS, Cameron D, Di Leo A, Geyer CE, Villalobos IE, *et al.* HER-2 gene amplification, HER-2 and epidermal growth factor receptor mRNA and protein expression, and lapatinib efficacy in women with metastatic breast cancer. Clin Cancer Res. 2008; 14: 7861-70.

[346] Weir GM, Liwski RS, Mansour M. Immune modulation by chemotherapy or immunotherapy to enhance cancer vaccines. Cancers. 2011; 3: 3114-42.

[347] Tapia C, Glatz K, Novotny H, Lugli A, Horcic M, Seemayer CA, *et al.* Close association between HER-2 amplification and overexpression in human tumors of non-breast origin. Mod Pathol. 2007; 20: 192-8.

[348] Yan B, Yau EX, Bte Omar SS, Ong CW, Pang B, Yeoh KG, *et al.* A study of HER2 gene amplification and protein expression in gastric cancer. J Clin Pathol. 2010; 63: 839-42.

[349] Thompson SK, Sullivan TR, Davies R, Ruszkiewicz AR. HER-2/neu Gene Amplification in Esophageal Adenocarcinoma and Its Influence on Survival. Ann Surg Oncol. 2011; 18: 2010-7.

[350] Tsiambas E, Karameris A, Dervenis C, Lazaris AC, Giannakou N, Gerontopoulos K, *et al.* HER2/neu expression and gene alterations in pancreatic ductal adenocarcinoma: a comparative immunohistochemistry and chromogenic *in situ* hybridization study based on tissue microarrays and computerized image analysis. JOP. 2006; 7: 283-94.

[351] Simonetti S, Russo R, Ciancia G, Altieri V, De Rosa G, Insabato L. Role of polysomy 17 in transitional cell carcinoma of the bladder: immunohistochemical study of HER2/neu expression and fish analysis of c-erbB-2 gene and chromosome 17. Int J Surg Pathol. 2009; 17: 198-205.

[352] Lae M, Couturier J, Oudard S, Radvanyi F, Beuzeboc P, Vieillefond A. Assessing HER2 gene amplification as a potential target for therapy in invasive urothelial bladder cancer with a standardized methodology: results in 1005 patients. Ann Oncol. 2010; 21: 815-9.

[353] Hirsch FR, Franklin WA, Veve R, Varella-Garcia M, Bunn PA, Jr. HER2/neu expression in malignant lung tumors. Semin Oncol. 2002; 29: 51-8.

[354] Fleming GF, Sill MW, Darcy KM, McMeekin DS, Thigpen JT, Adler LM, *et al.* Phase II trial of trastuzumab in women with advanced or recurrent, HER2-positive endometrial carcinoma: a Gynecologic Oncology Group study. Gynecol Oncol. 2010; 116: 15-20.

[355] McAlpine JN, Wiegand KC, Vang R, Ronnett BM, Adamiak A, Kobel M, *et al.* HER2 overexpression and amplification is present in a subset of ovarian mucinous carcinomas and can be targeted with trastuzumab therapy. BMC Cancer. 2009; 9: 433.

[356] Ramieri MT, Murari R, Botti C, Pica E, Zotti G, Alo PL. Detection of HER2 amplification using the SISH technique in breast, colon, prostate, lung and ovarian carcinoma. Anticancer Res. 2010; 30: 1287-92.

[357] Sato-Kuwabara Y, Neves JI, Fregnani JH, Sallum RA, Soares FA. Evaluation of gene amplification and protein expression of HER-2/neu in esophageal squamous cell carcinoma using Fluorescence *in situ* Hybridization (FISH) and immunohistochemistry. BMC Cancer. 2009; 9: 6.

[358] Komoto M, Nakata B, Amano R, Yamada N, Yashiro M, Ohira M, *et al.* HER2 overexpression correlates with survival after curative resection of pancreatic cancer. Cancer Sci. 2009; 100: 1243-7.

[359] Kruger S, Weitsch G, Buttner H, Matthiensen A, Bohmer T, Marquardt T, *et al.* HER2 overexpression in muscle-invasive urothelial carcinoma of the bladder: prognostic implications. Int J Cancer. 2002; 102: 514-8.

[360] Kolla SB, Seth A, Singh MK, Gupta NP, Hemal AK, Dogra PN, *et al.* Prognostic significance of Her2/neu overexpression in patients with muscle invasive urinary bladder cancer treated with radical cystectomy. Int Urol Nephrol. 2008; 40: 321-7.

[361] Liu L, Shao X, Gao W, Bai J, Wang R, Huang P, *et al.* The role of human epidermal growth factor receptor 2 as a prognostic factor in lung cancer: a meta-analysis of published data. J Thorac Oncol. 2010; 5: 1922-32.

[362] Santin AD, Bellone S, Van Stedum S, Bushen W, Palmieri M, Siegel ER, *et al.* Amplification of c-erbB2 oncogene: a major prognostic indicator in uterine serous papillary carcinoma. Cancer. 2005; 104: 1391-7.

[363] Slamon DJ, Godolphin W, Jones LA, Holt JA, Wong SG, Keith DE, *et al.* Studies of the HER-2/neu proto-oncogene in human breast and ovarian cancer. Science. 1989; 244: 707-12.

[364] Meden H, Marx D, Roegglen T, Schauer A, Kuhn W. Overexpression of the oncogene c-erbB-2 (HER2/neu) and response to chemotherapy in patients with ovarian cancer. Int J Gynecol Pathol. 1998; 17: 61-5.

[365] Serrano-Olvera A, Duenas-Gonzalez A, Gallardo-Rincon D, Candelaria M, De la Garza-Salazar J. Prognostic, predictive and therapeutic implications of HER2 in invasive epithelial ovarian cancer. Cancer Treat Rev. 2006; 32: 180-90.

[366] Grabsch H, Sivakumar S, Gray S, Gabbert HE, Muller W. HER2 expression in gastric cancer: Rare, heterogeneous and of no prognostic value - conclusions from 924 cases of two independent series. Cell Oncol. 2010; 32: 57-65.

[367] Pratesi G, Petrangolini G, Tortoreto M, Addis A, Zunino F, Calcaterra C, *et al.* Antitumor efficacy of trastuzumab in nude mice orthotopically xenografted with human pancreatic tumor cells expressing low levels of HER-2/neu. J Immunother. 2008; 31: 537-44.

[368] Kimura K, Sawada T, Komatsu M, Inoue M, Muguruma K, Nishihara T, *et al.* Antitumor effect of trastuzumab for pancreatic cancer with high HER-2 expression and enhancement of effect by combined therapy with gemcitabine. Clin Cancer Res. 2006; 12: 4925-32.

[369] Osipo C, Meeke K, Liu H, Cheng D, Lim S, Weichel A, *et al.* Trastuzumab therapy for tamoxifen-stimulated endometrial cancer. Cancer Res. 2005; 65: 8504-13.

[370] Matsui Y, Inomata M, Tojigamori M, Sonoda K, Shiraishi N, Kitano S. Suppression of tumor growth in human gastric cancer with HER2 overexpression by an anti-HER2 antibody in a murine model. Int J Oncol. 2005; 27: 681-5.

[371] Fujimoto-Ouchi K, Sekiguchi F, Yasuno H, Moriya Y, Mori K, Tanaka Y. Antitumor activity of trastuzumab in combination with chemotherapy in human gastric cancer xenograft models. Cancer Chemother Pharmacol. 2007; 59: 795-805.

[372] Cortés-Funes H, Rivera F, Alés I, Márquez A, Velasco A, Colomer R, *et al.* Phase II of trastuzumab and cisplatin in patients (pts) with advanced gastric cancer (AGC) with HER2/neu overexpression/amplification. J Clin Oncol. 2007; 25: Abstr 4613.

[373] Van Cutsem E, Kang Y, Chung H, Shen L, Sawaki A, Lordick F, *et al.* Efficacy results from teh ToGA trial: A phase III study of trastuzumab added to standard chemotherapy in firstline human epidermal growth factor receptor 2-positive advanced gastric cancer. J Clin Oncol. 2009; 27: LBA4509.

[374] De Vita F, Giuliani F, Silvestris N, Catalano G, Ciardiello F, Orditura M. Human epidermal growth factor receptor 2 (HER2) in gastric cancer: a new therapeutic target. Cancer Treat Rev. 2010; 36 Suppl 3: S11-5.

[375] Kimple RJ, Vaseva AV, Cox AD, Baerman KM, Calvo BF, Tepper JE, *et al.* Radiosensitization of epidermal growth factor receptor/HER2-positive pancreatic cancer is mediated by inhibition of AKT independent of ras mutational status. Clin Cancer Res. 2010; 16: 912-23.

[376] Komoto M, Nakata B, Nishii T, Kawajiri H, Shinto O, Amano R, *et al. In vitro* and *in vivo* evidence that a combination of lapatinib plus S-1 is a promising treatment for pancreatic cancer. Cancer Sci. 2010; 101: 468-73.

[377] Diaz R, Nguewa PA, Parrondo R, Perez-Stable C, Manrique I, Redrado M, *et al.* Antitumor and antiangiogenic effect of the dual EGFR and HER-2 tyrosine kinase inhibitor lapatinib in a lung cancer model. BMC Cancer. 2010; 10: 188.

[378] Kurtze I, Sonnemann J, Beck JF. KRAS-mutated non-small cell lung cancer cells are responsive to either co-treatment with erlotinib or gefitinib and histone deacetylase inhibitors or single treatment with lapatinib. Oncol Rep. 2011; 25: 1021-9.

[379] McHugh LA, Kriajevska M, Mellon JK, Griffiths TR. Combined treatment of bladder cancer cell lines with lapatinib and varying chemotherapy regimens--evidence of schedule-dependent synergy. Urology. 2007; 69: 390-4.

[380] Konecny GE, Venkatesan N, Yang G, Dering J, Ginther C, Finn R, *et al.* Activity of lapatinib a novel HER2 and EGFR dual kinase inhibitor in human endometrial cancer cells. Br J Cancer. 2008; 98: 1076-84.

[381] Kim JW, Kim HP, Im SA, Kang S, Hur HS, Yoon YK, *et al.* The growth inhibitory effect of lapatinib, a dual inhibitor of EGFR and HER2 tyrosine kinase, in gastric cancer cell lines. Cancer Lett. 2008; 272: 296-306.

[382] Ross HJ, Blumenschein GR, Jr., Aisner J, Damjanov N, Dowlati A, Garst J, *et al.* Randomized phase II multicenter trial of two schedules of lapatinib as first- or second-line monotherapy in patients with advanced or metastatic non-small cell lung cancer. Clin Cancer Res. 2010; 16: 1938-49.

[383] Wulfing C, Machiels JP, Richel DJ, Grimm MO, Treiber U, De Groot MR, *et al.* A single-arm, multicenter, open-label phase 2 study of lapatinib as the second-line treatment of patients with locally advanced or metastatic transitional cell carcinoma. Cancer. 2009; 115: 2881-90.

[384] Hecht JR, Urba SG, Koehler M, Ellis C, Gagnon R, Kemner A, *et al.* Lapatinib monotherapy in recurrent upper gastrointestinal malignancy: Phase II efficacy and biomarker analyses. ASCO Gastrointestinal Cancers Symposium. 2008: Abstr 43.

[385] Iqbal S, Goldman B, Lenz HJ, Fenoglio-Preiser CM, Blanke CD. S0413: A phase II SWOG study of GW572016 (lapatinib) as first line therapy in patients (pts) with advanced or metastatic gastric cancer. J Clin Oncol. 2007; 25: Abstr 4621.

[386] Pishvaian M, Sakaeva D, Hsieh RK, Rha SY, Caderillo-Ruiz G, Miller Jr. WH, *et al.* A global, multicenter phase II trial of lapatinib plus capecitabine in gastric cancer. J Clin Oncol. 2011; 29: Abstr 88.

[387] Galsky MD, Von Hoff DD, Neubauer M, Anderson T, Fleming M, Nagarwala Y, *et al.* Target-specific, histology-independent, randomized discontinuation study of lapatinib in patients with HER2-amplified solid tumors. Invest New Drugs. 2010; 30: 695-701.

[388] Kwak E. The role of irreversible HER family inhibition in the treatment of patients with non-small cell lung cancer. Oncologist. 2011; 16: 1498-507.

[389] Bowles DW, Weickhardt A, Jimeno A. Afatinib for the treatment of patients with EGFR-positive non-small cell lung cancer. Drugs Today (Barc). 2013; 49: 523-35.

[390] Majem M, Pallares C. An update on molecularly targeted therapies in second- and third-line treatment in non-small cell lung cancer: focus on EGFR inhibitors and anti-angiogenic agents. Clin Transl Oncol. 2013; 15: 343-57.

[391] Slamon DJ, Swain SM, Buyse M, Martin M, Geyer CE, Im Y-H, *et al.* Primary results from BETH, a phase 3 controlled study of adjuvant chemotherapy and trastuzumab ± bevacizumab in patients with HER2-positive, node-positive or high risk node-negative breast cancer. San Antonio Breast Cancer Symposium. 2013; Abstract: [S1-03].

[392] Piva R, Spandidos DA, Gambari R. From microRNA functions to microRNA therapeutics: novel targets and novel drugs in breast cancer research and treatment (Review). Int J Oncol. 2013; 43: 985-94.

[393] Fang C, Zhao Y, Guo B. MiR-199b-5p targets HER2 in breast cancer cells. J Cell Biochem. 2013; 114: 1457-63.

[394] Wu Y, Zhang Y, Wang M, Li Q, Qu Z, Shi V, *et al.* Downregulation of HER3 by a novel antisense oligonucleotide, EZN-3920, improves the antitumor activity of EGFR and HER2 tyrosine kinase inhibitors in animal models. Mol Cancer Ther. 2013; 12: 427-37.

[395] Chan DP, Deleavey GF, Owen SC, Damha MJ, Shoichet MS. Click conjugated polymeric immuno-nanoparticles for targeted siRNA and antisense oligonucleotide delivery. Biomaterials. 2013; 34: 8408-15.

[396] Zhang K, Hao L, Hurst SJ, Mirkin CA. Antibody-linked spherical nucleic acids for cellular targeting. J Am Chem Soc. 2012; 134: 16488-91.

[397] Liu X, Nakamura K, Cheng D, Peng C, Xiao N, Liu Y, Chen L, Rusckowski M, Hnatowich DJ. Her2/neu small interfering RNA delivered in culture by a streptavidin nanoparticle. Curr Drug Deliv. 2012; 9: 431-6.

[398] Sun J, Xu Y, Song S, Wu Z, Duan H. Antisense oligodeoxynucleotide targeting HER2 mRNA sensitized docetaxel in breast cancer treatment. Pharm Biol. 2011; 49: 1167-72.

[399] Lu H, Wang D, Kazane S, Javahishvili T, Tian F, Song F, *et al.* Site-specific antibody-polymer conjugates for siRNA delivery. J Am Chem Soc. 2013; 135: 13885-91.

[400] Nishimura Y, Mieda H, Ishii J, Ogino C, Fujiwara T, Kondo A. Targeting cancer cell-specific RNA interference by siRNA delivery using a complex carrier of affibody-displaying bio-nanocapsules and liposomes. J Nanobiotechnology. 2013; 11: 19.

[401] Wang Y, Liu P, Du J, Sun Y, Li F, Duan Y. Targeted siRNA delivery by anti-HER2 antibody-modified nanoparticles of mPEG-chitosan diblock copolymer. J Biomater Sci Polym Ed. 2013; 24: 1219-32.

[402] Kozłowska A, Mackiewicz J, Mackiewicz A. Therapeutic gene modified cell based cancer vaccines. Gene. 2013; 525: 200-7.

[403] Milani A, Sangiolo D, Montemurro F, Aglietta M, Valabrega G. Active immunotherapy in HER2 overexpressing breast cancer: current status and future perspectives. Ann Oncol. 2013; 24: 1740-8.

INDEX

A

Atta-ur-Rahman & M. Iqbal Choudhary (Eds)

B

C

D

E

F

G

H

I

K

L

N

O

P

R

S

T

V

W

X

Y

Made in United States
North Haven, CT
04 November 2026

21727471R00230